Effective SLP Interventions for Children with Cerebral Palsy

NDT/Traditional/Eclectic

Effective SLP Interventions for Children with Cerebral Palsy

NDT/Traditional/Eclectic

Fran Redstone, PhD, CCC-SLP, C/NDT

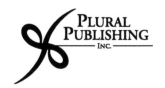

PLURAL
PUBLISHING
INC.

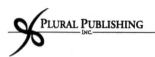
PLURAL PUBLISHING
INC.

5521 Ruffin Road
San Diego, CA 92123

e-mail: info@pluralpublishing.com
Website: http://www.pluralpublishing.com

Typeset in 11/13 Garamond by Flanagan's Publishing Services, Inc.
Printed in the United States of America by McNaughton & Gunn, Inc.
17 16 15   2 3 4 5

Library of Congress Cataloging-in-Publication Data

Redstone, Fran, author, editor of compilation.
  Effective SLP interventions for children with cerebral palsy : NDT/traditional/
eclectic / Fran Redstone.
       p. ; cm.
  Effective speech-language pathology interventions for children with cerebral
palsy
  Includes bibliographical references and index.
  ISBN-13: 978-1-59756-473-1 (alk. paper)
  ISBN-10: 1-59756-473-7 (alk. paper)
  I. Title. II. Title: Effective speech-language pathology interventions for chil-
dren with cerebral palsy.
  [DNLM: 1. Cerebral Palsy—rehabilitation. 2. Child. 3. Infant. 4. Speech-
Language Pathology—methods. WS 342]
  RJ496.C4
  618.92'836—dc23
                              2013047458

Contents

Preface

This book was written by clinicians who have spent their professional lives helping children with cerebral palsy. Most of these master clinicians have been trained and certified in neurodevelopmental treatment (NDT). The training provided by NDT subsumes all three disciplines that are typically involved in the treatment of children with cerebral palsy: speech, physical, and occupational therapy. All of the contributors to this book acknowledge the importance of motor control in the typical development of communication and its significance in the treatment of children with neuromotor disorders.

It is anticipated that the knowledge and expertise of these therapists will shorten the learning curve for new clinicians who are interested in working with this very special group of children. In addition, it is hoped that the dedication and enthusiasm of the contributors for their chosen field of expertise will engage the reader. It is this enjoyment that has been the impetus for their many years of practice. Although other professionals often experience burnout, these therapists have found fulfillment from the growth and progress they see in their young clients and their families.

The goal of this book is for all readers to become acquainted with the impact of a motor disorder on the development of communication. Perhaps some readers will become interested and will be motivated to work with these unique and very special youngsters.

Acknowledgments

I am grateful to all the contributors of this book who were so willing to give of their time and generously share their extensive knowledge. In addition, I'd like to offer special thanks to Robert Goldfarb who has helped me in this and many other endeavors. I must also express my appreciation to Joan Mohr who taught me a new approach to treating children with cerebral palsy and to Helen Mueller who pioneered so many specific speech and feeding techniques.

However, those who are closest to us are the ones who provide the most assistance and encouragement. Jon Folkman, my husband, has been a constant source of support and enjoyment for the last 36 years. In addition, he is computer savvy and a great editor! Also, the sheer pleasure of my son and his growing family has played a significant role in the production of this book.

Contributors

Cindy Geise Arroyo, DA, CCC-SLP
Associate Professor
Department of Communication Sciences and Disorders
Adelphi University
Garden City, New York
Chapter 10

Leslie Faye Davis, MS, CCC-SLP, NDT
Private Practice Consultant
Continuing Education Provider
Developmental Disabilities and Feeding-PreSpeech
North Woodmere, New York
Chapter 7

Majorie M. Palmer, MA, CCC-SLP, C/NDT
Neonatal/Pediatric Feeding Specialist
Founder/Director
NOMAS International
Former Clinical Instructor
University of California, San Francisco School of Medicine
Division of Gastroenterology, Hepatology, and Nutrition
Department of Pediatrics
San Francisco, California
Chapter 5

Fran Redstone, PhD, CCC-SLP, C/NDT
Associate Professor
Department of Communication Sciences and Disorders
Adelphi University
Garden City, New York
Chapters 1, 2, 4, 6, 7, 8, 9, and 12

Martine M. Smith, MSc, PhD
Associate Professor
Speech Language Pathology
Clinical Speech and Language Studies
Trinity College
Dublin, Leinster
Ireland
Chapter 11

Marilyn Seif Workinger, PhD, CCC-SLP
Emeritus Researcher
Marshfield Clinic Research Foundation
Marshfield, Wisconsin
Chapter 3

CHAPTER 1

The Development in Neurodevelopmental Treatment (NDT) for the SLP

Fran Redstone

The SLP and CP

Is it reasonable to expect a child with shallow breathing, open-mouth posture, and a tongue thrust, whose body is fixed in extension, to manipulate toys or interact with peers in a stimulating home or school environment? No, of course not, it is an exercise in frustration for the child and in futility for the child's unprepared speech-language pathologist (SLP). I know this because I've been there. Graduate training prepares educators and speech practitioners for dealing with the communication disorders of physically typical children, but this preparation seldom equips them to treat children with cerebral palsy who have sensorimotor impairments central to their speech/language/feeding disorder. These impairments affect respiration and feeding, as well as a child's interactions with the environment, family, and peers.

1

The goal of this text is to provide an understanding of how a sensorimotor impairment like cerebral palsy influences a child's speech/language/feeding, and to demonstrate how the SLP can use the knowledge of development and motor control to enhance speech and language development for the youngster with cerebral palsy. This information will be presented along with techniques that have been developed by highly skilled, experienced therapists. It is hoped that this book will facilitate the learning curve for the SLP treating children with neuromotor problems.

This book presents many areas of intervention that have been successfully addressed with Neurodevelopmental Treatment (NDT) principles including feeding, saliva control, sound production, interaction, augmentative and alternative communication (AAC), and literacy. NDT is one of the primary intervention approaches for children with cerebral palsy. It addresses the sensorimotor aspects of the disorder through the clinician guiding the child's motor output during functional activities. NDT was initially pioneered by Karl and Berta Bobath in the 1940s. But it has evolved significantly since that time because of the extensive clinical experience and increasingly sophisticated theoretical understanding of its practitioners.

The chapter authors will demonstrate how they use the knowledge and skills gained through NDT in functional activities and contexts. This has often led to the development of new approaches. The goal is to broaden the base of knowledge of SLPs who work with children with neuromotor deficits. However, it is also hoped that those who work primarily with children with cerebral palsy may consider taking continuing education courses to further this basic knowledge.

The information in this book should be integrated into the techniques generally cited as worthwhile for typically developing children. The approach whose principles are being presented is NDT. The present chapter deals with one aspect that is basic to this approach: the components of development and movement. This subsumes information about the coordination of the subsystems of the speech production system as well as the motor system. The second chapter describes the principles of motor learning and the theoretical bases for NDT. Other chapters illustrate the specific implications of cerebral palsy on function and how the principles of NDT enhance assessment and treatment. This book also includes techniques that have been developed by the authors over the years for addressing the needs of children with neuromotor problems. These techniques emphasize the importance of individualization for each and every child and the problem-solving nature of NDT.

The SLP must remember that children with cerebral palsy are not typically developing children. Cerebral palsy is a disorder of the central nervous system. It leads to neuromuscular impairments that interfere significantly with their development. This disorder is caused by a nonprogressive lesion in the immature brain that leads to motor functioning deficits (Bartlett & Palisano, 2000; Bax, 1964, 2001; Bennett, 1999) and has been described as a common developmental disability with motor impairment (Badawi et al., 2005; Treviranus & Roberts, 2003). Although the diagnosis of cerebral palsy is based on the movement characteristics and the distribution of muscle tone throughout the body (Bartlett & Palisano, 2000; Finnie, 2001; Langley & Thomas, 1991; Solomon & Charron, 1998), the International Workshop on the Definition and Classification of Cerebral Palsy has suggested that the traditional descriptions be used along with the functional consequences of the movement disorder, which include speech and feeding (Bax, Goldstein, Rosenbaum, Leviton, & Paneth, 2005).

Although I fervently hope that improved prenatal care and medical technology will put me out of business, I have found that most studies cite a relatively stable incidence of cerebral palsy of about 2 per 1,000 births (Andersen, Mjoen, & Vik, 2010). This figure is not diminishing probably due to the improved ability to save children in the NICU. Prematurity or low birth weight is the most prominent factor, leading to 40 to 50% of the cases of cerebral palsy. Half of the children who develop cerebral palsy have birth weights of 2,500 grams or less. The neural damage typically results from periventricular leukomalacia. Table 1–1 may facilitate triggering your memory from the last neurology course you took. The white matter (upper motor tracts) in the area around the ventricles of the developing fetus is quite vulnerable (Rais-Bahrami & Short, 2007). It might be worthwhile

Table 1–1. Neurology Terminology Pertinent to Cerebral Palsy

Terms	Definitions
Basal ganglia	Subcortical structures that are considered part of the extrapyramidal system. Consists of putamen, globus pallidus, and caudate nucleus.
Contralateral	On the opposite side.
Extrapyramidal tracts	Indirect system. Regulates reflexes, tone, and posture. Consists of several short pathways connecting many parts of the CNS.
Ipsilateral	On the same side.
Lower motor neuron system	Lies in the PNS. Consists of 12 cranial nerves and 31 spinal nerves. Originates in brainstem or spinal cord. Innervates muscle.
Periventricular leukomalacia (PVL)	Damage of the white matter near the lateral ventricles. More common in premature infants.
Pyramidal tracts	Direct motor system. Consists of corticospinal (for trunk and limbs) and corticobulbar tracts (for speech muscles).
Thalamus	Relay station for sensory information going to the cortex.
Tracts	Groups of axons within the CNS. Often referred to as pathways.
Upper motor neuron system	Part of the CNS that is responsible for skilled voluntary movement. Consists of pyramidal and extrapyramidal tracts.
White matter	Axons that are covered with myelin.

now to digress and discuss the neurology of cerebral palsy to emphasize the impact of damage or dysfunction within the central nervous system.

Basics of Cerebral Palsy

Children who are diagnosed with cerebral palsy all have damage to the central nervous system (Yeargin-Allsopp, Boyle, Van Naarden Braun, & Trevathan, 2008), specifically to the upper motor neuron (UMN) system. Figure 1–1 may facilitate visualizing the relationship between neural structures. The UMN system includes the pyramidal and extrapyramidal tracts and control circuits of the cerebellum and basal ganglia, which are described nicely by Halpern and Goldfarb (2013). The corticospinal and

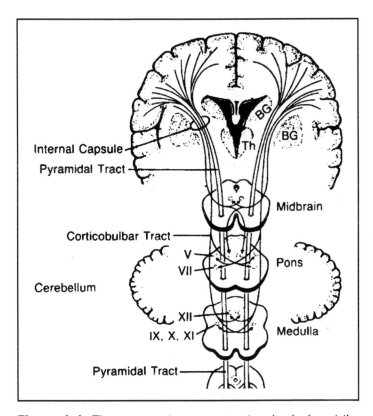

Figure 1–1. The upper motor neuron system beginning at the cortex. The corticobulbar tract and corticospinal tracts descend through the internal capsule and innervate lower motor neurons. Note subcortical, periventricular structures of the thalamus (Th) and the basal ganglia (BG) around the black area, which is the lateral ventricle. (Modified Figure 9–1. From *Treating disordered speech motor control, 2nd ed.* [*For Clinicians by Clinicians Series*] [p. 324], by D. Vogel and M. P. Cannito [Eds.], 2001, Austin, TX: Pro-Ed. Copyright 2001 by Pro-Ed, Inc. Adapted from *Clinical Management of Neurogenic Communicative Disorders* [pp. 1–96] by D. F. Johns [Ed.],1985, Austin, TX: Pro-Ed. Copyright 1985 Little, Brown. Reprinted with permission.)

corticobulbar tracts (white matter) of the pyramidal tract (direct pathway) are responsible for voluntary movement, and the extra-pyramidal system (indirect pathway) is an inhibiting influence that provides the background muscle tone and normal reflex patterns for coordinated movements. These pathways descend from the gray matter (neuronal cell bodies) in the cortex (Duffy, 2005) through the internal capsule to activate lower motor neurons in the spinal cord or brainstem. This is necessary for voluntary movements. We need to remember that most cranial nerves get information from both sides of the brain (bilateral innervation) and then transmit impulses to the muscles on the same side (ipsilateral). There is evidence that the nuclei of the hypoglossal nerves (CN XII) and the cervicofacial nerves are contralaterally innervated only (Seilel, King, & Drumright, 2005).

Other areas of the brain may not develop typically and may also lead to a diagnosis of cerebral palsy. These include sub-cortical areas such as the basal ganglia, the thalamus, and the pathways that connect these areas with each other and with the cortex that are likewise considered part of the extrapyramidal system. In addition, dysfunction of the cerebellum and its control circuits may also lead to the diagnosis of cerebral palsy. Cerebral palsy is an impairment of the central nervous system or upper motor neuron system. However, the pattern of damage within the UMN system in any specific child may be "idiosyncratic" (Bax, 2001) and the observation of a mixed clinical picture of central damage is not surprising because the pathways in the infant's brain are so proximate (Love & Webb, 2001). In fact, this also leads to the common associated problems we see in children with cerebral palsy. Further details of cerebral palsy and its associated problems are addressed in Chapter 3, "The ABCs of CP."

Speech Problems and Much More

Although children who are diagnosed with cerebral palsy do not necessarily have speech difficulties, too many do. Pelligrino (2007) reports that 30% of children with cerebral palsy have speech-language problems whereas Pennington, Goldbart, and Marshall (2005) note that 20% have *severe* communication problems. Andersen et al. (2010) found 35%. Bjornson et al.

(2003) note a range of 28 to 52%, and Sullivan et al. (2000) found that 78% of children diagnosed with cerebral palsy have speech disorders. This should not be surprising because speech is considered "the ultimate exemplar of complex, skilled motor behavior" (Smith, Goffman, & Stark, 1995, p. 87). However, the abnormal postures and muscle tone of cerebral palsy also affect mother–child interaction patterns (Hanzlik, 1990; Pennington & McConichie, 1999). It appears that parents of children with cerebral palsy are more directive, likely due to the lack of a quick response from the child with a motor impairment. In addition, feeding problems are noted to be as high as 90% (Arvedson & Brodsky, 2002; Calis et al., 2008; Sullivan et al., 2000).

Associated problems commonly occurring with cerebral palsy include cognition impairment (50–70%), language disturbance, learning disorder (Bishop, Brown, & Robson, 1990; Fennell & Dikel, 2001), seizures, and sensory impairments (Badawi et al., 2005). These problems may be primary, resulting from neurological damage in the same way as the onset of cerebral palsy. However, some language and cognitive deficits may be secondary to the motor impairment. This primary motor impairment influences the development of other systems such as speech, language, and cognition, because these are skills that typically develop through movement and manipulation of one's environment. Hanzlik (1990) relates parent behaviors such as excessive holding and physical guidance as causes for restricting exploration for cognitive growth. Additionally, Fennell and Dikel (2001) note that the cognitive and language skills of the child with athetoid cerebral palsy may be underestimated due to the severity of incoordination. This opinion is strongly supported by clinicians who have interacted with these children.

Speech-language pathologists (SLPs) often need to provide speech/language/feeding services to children with cerebral palsy. This may be in a hospital, clinic, special classroom, or a typical classroom. When we talk of serving children with cerebral palsy, we typically think of the child with severe impairments. However, as SLPs we should evaluate and monitor the speech/language skills of the child even with mild cerebral palsy and certainly with moderate cerebral palsy. Redstone (2004) found subtle but significant differences in the speech patterns and respiration of children with mild cerebral palsy. Mork (2001) studied the medical problems in a group of children with mild cerebral palsy and found specific problems including learning issues that, he asserts, deserve our attention. Again, graduate training prepares the SLP exceptionally well for dealing with the communication disorders of physically typical children, but this preparation, except for a course in augmentative and alternative communication (AAC), is quite limited with regard to children with cerebral palsy. Although AAC is important, it is not the only—or even the first—option that should be considered. Pennington and McConichie (1999) found that children with cerebral palsy were most likely to use natural forms of communication first, such as gross gesture and vocalization, when attempting interaction.

Intervention with this group of children is so difficult because cerebral palsy is such a heterogeneous group of developmental disorders. Therefore, there is no one answer, or one strategy, or one technique that will be appropriate for all these children. However, the one unifying concept is the motor impairment that affects movement and posture (Pelligrino, 2007), impacts neuromuscular coordination (Bobath, 1980; Langley & Thomas, 1991; Mecham, 2002), and causes activity limitations (Bax et al., 2005; Reddy, 2005) that affect all aspects of life (Hustad, Gorton, & Lee, 2010). This includes the development of interaction and communication, feeding and play skills, language and cognition.

The original static impairment changes the entire course of development (Boliek & Lohmeier, 1999; Campbell, 1991; Hodge & Wellman, 1999; Pinder & Olswang, 1995; Reddy, 2005). Unlike the adult with fully developed cognitive and linguistic systems who then has a stroke, the child with cerebral palsy is in the process of developing these functional systems (Bax, 2001; Caruso & Strand, 1999). Although the neural damage is nonprogressive, as the child's environment expands and the demands on the motor speech system increase, the clinical picture may change (McCauley & Strand, 1999).

The basis of early intervention (EI) is neural plasticity of the young brain, which is superior to that of the adult brain (Kragelob-Mann, 2005). The other important concept is the critical learning period, which is the first 2 years of life for oral skills related to feeding (Bahr, 2003). This is when learning is easiest.

The goal of EI is to diminish the effect of impairment. "Before the date of enactment of the Education for All Handicapped Children Act of 1975 (Public Law 94-142), the educational needs of millions of children with disabilities were not being fully met . . . " (U.S. Department of Education, 2012, section 601). However, as early as 1967 Bobath stressed the importance of early intervention for infants with cerebral palsy. Today, IDEA (2004) and EI have become part of our educational culture and the Bobath Approach has evolved into NDT.

Principles of Development

Young children are very variable and rarely develop in a linear fashion. Nonetheless, we typically evaluate a child based on developmental milestones that are presented sequentially. We learn about normal development because it enables us to better assess and treat. SLPs working with children with cerebral palsy need to know normal development in all areas, not just feeding and speech. This is due to the interrelationship of oral functioning with gross motor functioning. In a nutshell, the more we know about normal development, the better we will be at recognizing abnormal (Howle, 2002). However, the importance of a milestone lies in the essential competencies that enable the child to attain that milestone (Bly, 1983; Howle, 2002; Sheppard, 2008).

To fully understand several concepts of oral development that will be addressed in this section, a review of some general principles of development and control may be helpful. Development occurs from the head down; it is cephalocaudal. Children develop control of proximal structures prior to distal structures, and movements develop in straight planes prior to lateral ones. Dissociation, or separation of movement, is another requisite for precision of fine motor control. Dissociation is apparent when a child can extend an arm without the mouth also opening. Rotation is a type of dissociation in which there is movement around the body axis (Langley & Thomas, 1991), for example, when a child turns the body to reach a toy. Stability is the basis for the development of control with dissociation and rotation. The goal is for the child to have enough stability for controlled mobility within a function.

Development is more than just neural maturation (Alexander, Boehme, & Cupps, 1993; Bly, 1983). It is a "delicate balance between stability and mobility" (Morris, 1987, p. 79). Think of what happens to the infant in just 12 short months. The child adjusts to constant changes in neural maturation, skeletal growth, and environmental surroundings. According to Langley and Thomas (1991), the foundation of all movements depends on the development of postural control. When we look at a neonate, we see gravity-dependent, undifferentiated, reflex-controlled movements. Vocalizations are short, cries are undifferentiated, and feeding is reflex-dependent for safety. At 1 year of age, the infant has developed upright posture against gravity and is ambulating, eating table foods, and using single words for communication. Moreover, during this period the child has attained enough stability in an upright position to move one structure in an isolated fashion and to move distal structures. The child's stability and alignment allow for accomplishment of such functional tasks as feeding and speech, using many movement options (Figure 1–2).

Stability

Stability is a principle of motor development. The stability and alignment of the hips, trunk, shoulders, and head allow the graded, coordinated movements of the structures of the oral area for speech and feeding (Alexander et al., 1993; Jones-Owens, 1991; Pinder & Faherty, 1999). This postural stability also provides the foundation of arm movements for manipulation of objects and the child's ability to move within the environment to facilitate cognitive–linguistic development.

Initially, stability is attained through position in the young infant. For example, the 3-month-old uses positional flexion-abduction in prone in order to provide the necessary stability to raise the head in lieu of active postural control (Alexander et al., 1993). This is also the principle at work when we see a

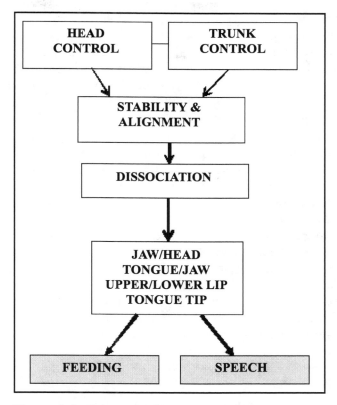

Figure 1–2. Schematic of the basis of feeding and speech control through stability/alignment and dissociation.

young infant use shoulder elevation during a transitional period for better head control.

Our proximal, or trunk muscles stabilize while we move other, more distal parts of our body. This has been referred to as dynamic stability (Bahr, 2001). Many of you will be thinking, "I don't need to know this. It is information for a physical therapist," but it is important for the SLP as well. The knowledge that control develops from proximal to distal tells us that the trunk is proximal to the head; the head is proximal to the jaw, and the jaw is proximal to the lips and tongue. This is the kind of information that we learn from normal development and can be used in treatment planning. Therefore, an SLP needs to know how to optimize trunk control for better oral control.

Dissociation

Dynamic stability is also a factor in the development of dissociated movements of oral structures. We think of the lips as a unit, but the lower lip moves at higher velocities than the upper lip (Seikel, King, & Drumright, 2005). I can move my tongue tip by using it in an isolated manner to make a /d/ or move my tongue without moving my larynx, and I chew using a rotary pattern. It also allows a child to use an index finger to activate an icon on an AAC device. Think of what you learned in your course on Anatomy and Physiology of the Speech Mechanism regarding the interaction of the extrinsic and intrinsic muscles of the tongue (Seikel et al., 2005). These two groups of muscles work together so that smooth, coordinated, graded movements of the tongue can be made for connected speech.

When we see rotation in the trunk, the shoulders and the pelvis will be in different planes because one side is flexing and the other is extending. This type of dissociated muscle usage in the thorax is necessary for the development of respiratory control for speech.

Straight Planes

Another principle of motor control and development important for the SLP to understand is that controlled movement occurs in straight planes first. This means that the tongue moves anterior/posterior before it lateralizes. It also means that when the young child is playing, reaching to the front will be easier than reaching to the side. These are all concepts SLPs should incorporate into assessment and treatment planning.

The more an SLP knows about the early development of feeding, speech, and language and the motor control basis for these skills, the more successful intervention will be. Using a general "developmental framework" is useful (Howle, 2002, p. 41), but not necessarily the specific milestones, because infants develop many movements at the same time (Howle, 2002). Kent (1999) suggests that development is often asynchronous due to the impact of interacting systems, but the knowledge of development is still a requisite for adequate assessment and treatment planning.

Development

A Starting Point: The Neonate

The apparent goal for the newborn's reflexes, position, and oral structures is safety. It has been stated that "nature has 'hardwired' the infant to meet its needs" (Seikel et al., 2005, p. 374). The small mandible and facial bones along with the sucking pads create a small intraoral space that allows for few options for tongue movement. The infant sucks using an anterior–posterior suckling movement with few degrees of freedom. High hyoid positioning in the neonate along with the physiological flexion provides greater safety during swallowing. This initial physiological flexion provides the stability for the jaw and proper positioning for tongue movement (Pinder & Faherty, 1999) for breast or bottle feeding. Flexion also allows the hands to be near the infant's mouth and provides oral stimulation, which is important for the development of normal oral sensitivity (Figure 1–3). Oral reflexes (suck/swallow, bite, root, gag) let the infant find food and ingest it safely prior to the development of adequate motor control. As the infant develops head control, these reflexes will be modified and/or disappear (Bahr, 2003; Pinder & Faherty, 1999).

If you have the opportunity to observe a newborn, note the oral posture. Invariably, it is a closed mouth posture. Neonates are nose breathers due to the physiological flexion and blockage of the small oral cavity by the tongue. This is strikingly different from the infants who are referred for therapy. The typical neonate is described as a belly breather with a respiratory rate that is fast and variable: 30 to 60 breaths per minute (Alexander et al., 1993). The fast rate is attributable to the lungs taking up the entire small thoracic space at birth (Seikel et al., 2005). Infant sounds are typically produced during random gross movements or cry. These sounds have nasal resonance due to the flexion and blockage of the small oral cavity by the tongue, and have been described as a "signal for attention" (Kamen, 1983, p. 234). In addition, the infant has a surprising ability to see and hear. An infant responds to faces and can differentiate voices at just a few weeks of age. As the child matures and develops control against gravity, there are changes in both structure and function.

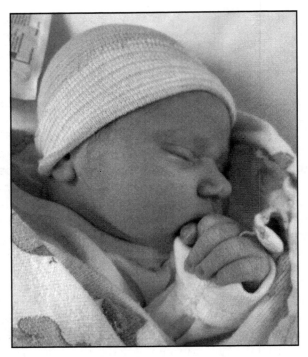

Figure 1–3. Neonatal flexion giving stability to the jaw and allowing for hand–mouth activity.

Three to 6 Months

The flexed, reflex-dominated neonate has been moving for the last 3 months under the influence of gravity. Extension has developed in the neck and upper back, and will continue down the back and over the hips. Active flexion, as opposed to the physiological flexion at birth, has developed into the upper thorax, and will continue into the abdomen. By 3 months we see cervical elongation with capital flexion. This is the beginning of the balance of extension and flexion (Redstone, 1991) and is reflected in the prone position when the 3-month-old maintains shoulder stability and props on forearms. The beginning of reaching with intent is seen, which enables the infant to learn about the immediate surrounding environment. Think of the implications of this in terms of content of language (Bloom & Lahey, 1978).

Interestingly, what the child reaches for is then brought to the mouth. The initial flexion led to oral stimulation, and now the ability to bring things to the mouth will increase the oral stimulation and continue the process of normalization of oral sensitivity (Figure 1–4).

By 6 months the infant has full head control due to the stability and alignment of head and trunk. This allows more dissociated oral movements, which are reflected in the functions of sound production and feeding. In addition, the child is learning by moving through the environment and is able to do this because of the increase in stability, dissociation, and a nice balance between extension and flexion. The child, even at this young age, has an enormous repertoire of movements, with many options for reaching a toy. This variety of movement options is what separates typical from atypical. This is seen in oral movements as well as gross motor movements. Good head control makes oral reflexes less necessary for safe feeding. The child has had quite a bit of oral stimulation from hand-to-mouth and object-to-mouth activities, and semisolids have been introduced. The child's oral structures have changed. Sucking pads

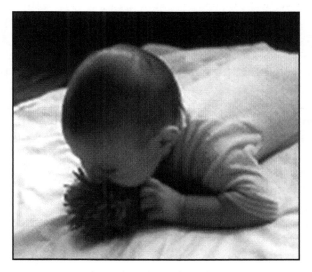

Figure 1–4. Reaching at 3 months of age leading to object-to-mouth activity. This further normalizes oral sensitivity.

are disappearing and there is greater pharyngeal space. Therefore, the tongue has more movement options. Although vowel sounds predominate in the sound repertoire of the infant's first 6 months, that is about to change.

Six to 9 Months

Extension has developed over the hips, along with antigravity flexion into the abdominal area (Bly, 1983). The child is crawling reciprocally on extended arms; is transitioning to sitting, kneeling, and sitting while playing or feeding; and might even pull up to stand. The child actively spoon feeds (Morris & Klein, 2000). In addition, some teeth may have emerged and, as a result, foods can be presented that have more texture and may allow for self-feeding. Trunk control is reflected in improved respiratory control for the long chains of babbling that are heard during this time.

This is a period of high babbling and the beginning of imitation. The variety and quantity of babbling has been used as a predictor of later language development (Bauman-Waengler, 2012; Mitchell & Kent, 1990). Open syllables predominate with many stop consonants. Although the movements for these sounds are easier because they entail total oral constriction (Green, Moore, Higashikawa, & Steeve, 2000), they require greater active control than past reflex-dominated movements, and are dependent on the newly developed head/trunk stability.

Think of the cognitive/linguistic development occurring at this period. Children are being stimulated by many new objects in the environment. Because they are propelling themselves through their surroundings, infants perceive stimulation from different viewpoints. Typically, a caregiver is labeling these new objects and experiences (Figure 1–5).

Ten Months to 1 Year

The infant has developed a significant amount of trunk stability by developing proximal musculature, with a sufficient balance of extension to hold him up against gravity in a stable bipedal

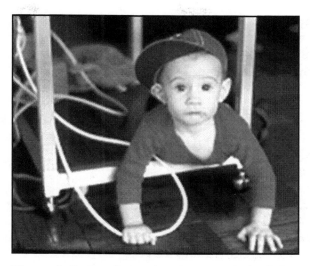

Figure 1–5. Crawling and environmental stimulation. Also, note trunk, elbow, and head extension with mouth closure indicating dissociation or independent movement of jaw from the rest of the body.

posture. This allows enough mobility and dissociation to shift weight, flex at the hip and knee, and begin to pull up to stand. Some children cruise around furniture and even take steps. However, equilibrium has not yet fully developed in the upright position. Children often look as if they are about to fall and attempt ambulation in a pattern using lateral flexion, although trunk rotation has been observed in crawling.

These same principles of stability, mobility, and dissociation are reflected orally when the infant safely eats table foods with tongue lateralization (Morris & Klein, 2000). The oral area is accommodating the child's attempts at self-feeding with utensils. The 1-year-old continues to babble, but now the vocalizations include greater variety of pitch and volume. This jargon babbling is used interactively as if to converse with a partner. The infant is also combining sounds to produce proto-words that are consistent sound combinations which are representative (Bauman-Waengler, 2012), and "real" words that are representative and whose form is consistent with the child's linguistic environment. However, the production of these words is quite variable

(Bauman-Waengler, 2012). Voiced nasals and stops still predominate, probably due to the ease of production noted earlier. Most researchers cite the high degree of individual differences in the development of sounds in children.

Most notable at this period is the interaction of the development of the gross motor system and the oral motor system. Because walking requires significant neural resources for the advanced levels of equilibrium, we may see a loss of oral control leading to drooling.

One to 2 Years

At this point the infant has attained all the basic motor components. Maturation, stimulation, experience, and practice are required to use these components functionally. Although some children take steps at 1 year, others don't begin until 15 months. The range of what is considered normal is large. This is true of speech development as well. Some children don't say their first words until 15 months, whereas others may begin just before 1 year. Although oral skills and respiratory control for speech continue to develop into adolescence, Bahr (2003) states that the critical period for oral skill development for feeding probably occurs within the first 2 to 3 years.

During this period, the feedforward system continues to develop motor programs so that the infant will become more efficient within functional tasks. This system is highly reliant on appropriate feedback, so that the child has a reference for what is correct. This depends on the responsiveness of people in the environment providing reinforcement for success, as well as an intact sensory system.

In terms of function, most children can walk, use stairs, and jump. Orally, they continue to normalize sensitivity by bringing things to their mouths and experience new tastes and textures of foods. They also self-feed using utensils, which adds a new dimension to oral control, due to competing neural resources. By 2 years of age, the child has developed dissociation of the lips, tongue, and jaw. In fact, the child now can drink from an open cup without biting the rim, because of internal jaw control (stability).

The biggest accomplishment is an increase in vocabulary (50-word stage) and the ability to put words together for communication. The child's intonation patterns vary with linguistic function (Bauman-Waengler, 2012). The most stable sounds are those that are functional and require the least coordination for production: nasals and stops.

Two+ Years

Refinement continues in all areas. For example, a preschooler's vocabulary triples, speech sound growth continues until at least 6 years of age, and respiratory control for speech may not be complete until adolescence. In the functional area of feeding, the 3-year-old is expected to be safe, efficient, and independent within a preschool classroom (Sheppard, 2008).

Theories regarding this development indicate that sound production may have an impact on vocabulary growth and this, in turn, is dependent on the stability of the trunk and head. In typical development, much depends on the early emergence and progress of motor skills. Children practice early behaviors that they learn during specific functions, and these then develop into true skills (Schmidt & Lee, 1999). Sheppard (2008) discusses this in relation to feeding skills, and notes that much depends on the timing of the introduction of various eating experiences. This, in turn, is dependent on the child's sensory and motor abilities and on cultural and parental preferences. See Pathways Foundation Developmental Chart in Figure 1–6.

Principles of Abnormal Development

To identify and understand abnormal development, one must first be familiar with what is normal. When we identify abnormal it is often because something is missing. All children desire to move. When children with cerebral palsy attempt to move without the necessary components, they learn to compensate in order to achieve the desired goal. These compensations are fairly predictable and are called "blocks" (Bly, 1983). Most blocks

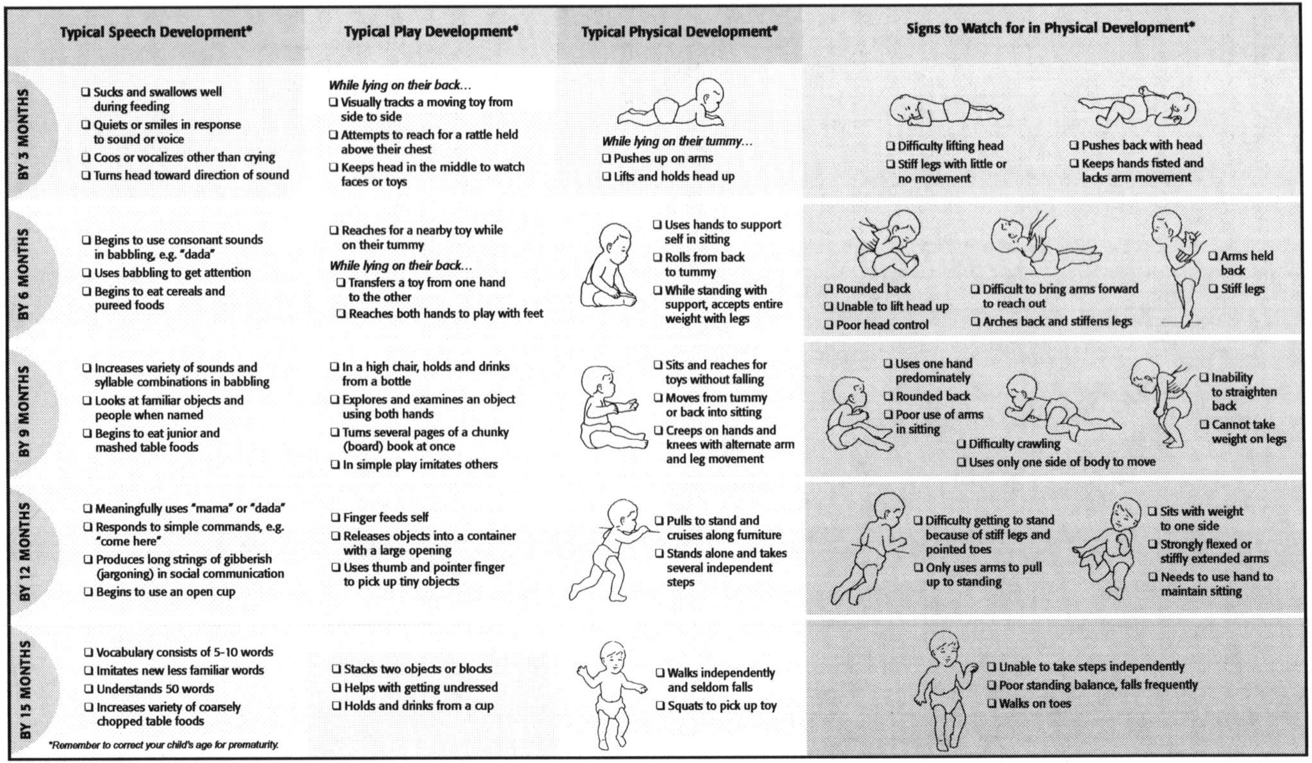

	Typical Speech Development*	Typical Play Development*	Typical Physical Development*	Signs to Watch for in Physical Development*
BY 3 MONTHS	☐ Sucks and swallows well during feeding ☐ Quiets or smiles in response to sound or voice ☐ Coos or vocalizes other than crying ☐ Turns head toward direction of sound	*While lying on their back...* ☐ Visually tracks a moving toy from side to side ☐ Attempts to reach for a rattle held above their chest ☐ Keeps head in the middle to watch faces or toys	☐ Pushes up on arms ☐ Lifts and holds head up	☐ Difficulty lifting head ☐ Stiff legs with little or no movement ☐ Pushes back with head ☐ Keeps hands fisted and lacks arm movement
BY 6 MONTHS	☐ Begins to use consonant sounds in babbling, e.g. "dada" ☐ Uses babbling to get attention ☐ Begins to eat cereals and pureed foods	☐ Reaches for a nearby toy while on their tummy *While lying on their back...* ☐ Transfers a toy from one hand to the other ☐ Reaches both hands to play with feet	☐ Uses hands to support self in sitting ☐ Rolls from back to tummy *While standing with support, accepts entire weight with legs*	☐ Rounded back ☐ Unable to lift head up ☐ Poor head control ☐ Difficult to bring arms forward to reach out ☐ Arches back and stiffens legs
BY 9 MONTHS	☐ Increases variety of sounds and syllable combinations in babbling ☐ Looks at familiar objects and people when named ☐ Begins to eat junior and mashed table foods	☐ In a high chair, holds and drinks from a bottle ☐ Explores and examines an object using both hands ☐ Turns several pages of a chunky (board) book at once ☐ In simple play imitates others	☐ Sits and reaches for toys without falling ☐ Moves from tummy or back into sitting ☐ Creeps on hands and knees with alternate arm and leg movement	☐ Uses one hand predominately ☐ Rounded back ☐ Poor use of arms in sitting ☐ Difficulty crawling ☐ Uses only one side of body to move ☐ Inability to straighten back ☐ Cannot take weight on legs
BY 12 MONTHS	☐ Meaningfully uses "mama" or "dada" ☐ Responds to simple commands, e.g. "come here" ☐ Produces long strings of gibberish (jargoning) in social communication ☐ Begins to use an open cup	☐ Finger feeds self ☐ Releases objects into a container with a large opening ☐ Uses thumb and pointer finger to pick up tiny objects	☐ Pulls to stand and cruises along furniture ☐ Stands alone and takes several independent steps	☐ Difficulty getting to stand because of stiff legs and pointed toes ☐ Only uses arms to pull up to standing ☐ Sits with weight to one side ☐ Strongly flexed or stiffly extended arms ☐ Needs to use hand to maintain sitting
BY 15 MONTHS	☐ Vocabulary consists of 5–10 words ☐ Imitates new less familiar words ☐ Understands 50 words ☐ Increases variety of coarsely chopped table foods	☐ Stacks two objects or blocks ☐ Helps with getting undressed ☐ Holds and drinks from a cup	☐ Walks independently and seldom falls ☐ Squats to pick up toy	☐ Unable to take steps independently ☐ Poor standing balance, falls frequently ☐ Walks on toes

*Remember to correct your child's age for prematurity.

Figure 1–6. Growth and developmental chart indicating sequences in gross motor, fine motor, and oral-motor areas in typical and atypical children. (From: Pathways *Assure Baby's Physical Development* brochure, Pathways.org, 800-955-2445. Reprinted with permission)

20

are based on abnormal extensor muscle activity, even in children with basic low tone. This imbalance of flexion and extension leads to lack of stability and compensations that are often described as "fixing." The child learns to move in this abnormal way, which gets reinforced through use. Kleim and Jones (2008) refer to this as "interference" (p. S233). These are movements that are easy to perform but are not efficient and impede learning. In general, we talk about neural plasticity in positive terms, whereas interference is negative.

The blocks that most directly compromise oral functioning are neck blocks leading to head hyperextension. These are due to lack of head control due to shortening of neck extensors and lack of developing neck flexion. Think of how important this is for safe swallows! Try this interactive experience.

> Throw your head back so you are in head hyperextension and then swallow. How does it feel? Does it make swallowing harder or easier?
>
> In the same position, attempt diadochokinesis. Now try it with normal head alignment. Which is faster?

Shoulder blocks lead to lack of weight bearing on forearms and interfere with reaching and manipulation skill development. This block impacts cognitive and language development, because the child is unable to fully explore the environment. The SLP should be aware that this block may also interfere with the ability to use a communication system. Pelvic blocks lead to poor abdominal muscle activity. This, in turn, affects respiratory control. The compensations that children employ vary with the child's experiences and motivation.

Development in Context

As stated previously, the knowledge of development is important, because it gives us an idea of what is required at each level. It helps the therapist prepare the child for the next level.

Head control at 6 months of age enables graded jaw, lip, and tongue movement that we see in feeding and sound production. Trunk control enables the respiratory musculature control that drives the speech production system. Head and trunk alignment allows for the integration of visual, auditory, and tactile stimuli for cognitive/linguistic development and appropriate interpersonal interaction. This knowledge will permit SLPs to provide better clinical services to their young clients. Bobath and Bobath (1984) state that the therapist must know what is needed immediately and what is necessary for future functionality.

However, as noted previously, the range of normal in the infant is particularly large. Determination of "normal" for a specific child often depends on the clinical judgment of the evaluator, along with input from the family. Rosenbaum (2007) says we need to "blend population-based data with our clinical experience and the perspectives of the people who know children best—their parents!" (p. 5).

There have been several factors that have led clinicians and some researchers to assert that developmental milestones have been changing (Hadders-Algra, 2007). One factor noted has been lack of prone positioning. Sudden infant death syndrome (SIDS) has been reduced dramatically with the recommendation that infants sleep in supine (American Academy of Pediatrics, 2000; Dewey, Fleming, Golding, & ALSPAC Study Team, 1998). However, motor milestones have been demonstrated to be slower in children who sleep in supine (Davis, Moon, Sachs, & Ottolini, 1998; Dewey et al., 1998; Jantz, Blosser, & Fruechting, 1997). Nonetheless, it is typical that by 18 months of age the discrepancy between prone and supine sleepers does not exist (Dewey et al., 1998). This developmental discrepancy has been studied for gross motor milestones, but nothing has been published regarding milestones in other areas such as feeding, speech, or language, although these are functional areas heavily dependent on gross motor development. Clinical observations of young children, and the identification of many children for early intervention speech services, often note delays without the presence of abnormal patterns. Obviously, this is an area that requires more research. In fact, Hadders-Algra (2007) invites us to explore this change in development rather than merely readjusting the norms.

Conclusions and Summary

The knowledge of the underlying neurological impairment of a child with cerebral palsy, along with the knowledge of the components and milestones of development, will enhance the clinical services the SLP provides. We learn what is expected and understand what is missing. Although both typical and atypical development are somewhat predictable, every child, typical or not, is different, and we, as SLPs, can never use a recipe approach. Below are some principles to remember when planning treatment for the child with cerebral palsy.

Ten Items for Improving Intervention

1. Cerebral palsy is a motor disorder resulting from CNS impairment.
2. Children with cerebral palsy are a heterogeneous group.
   a. Some have a motor disorder only. Do not assume other disorders.
   b. Some children have multiple challenges.
3. Feeding and speech are motor skills.
4. Motor development starts with head control.
5. The SLP needs to understand how motor development affects oral motor development.
   a. Head control is needed.
   b. Stability is required for dissociated movements of the oral area.
   c. Trunk control is needed for head control and respiration for speech.
6. There is a broad range of individual differences in typical development.
7. Children rarely work on one level at a time.
8. Abnormal development is predictable.
   a. Blocks are patterns that interfere with development.
   b. Most blocks include hyperextension.
9. A flexible developmental therapy approach is appropriate.

    a. Learning the components needed for each milestone aids treatment planning.

    b. Preparation for the future milestones is necessary.

10. Assessment of the oral area should be conducted with the knowledge that alignment and gross motor movements affect oral functioning.

Think Critically for Self-Study or Classroom Discussion

1. Identify two items from infant development that can be translated to intervention procedures for the child with cerebral palsy.
2. Why is midline orientation so important for oral development?
3. Why are infant vocalizations so nasal in the first few months?
4. Describe two movements that are indications of dissociation.
5. Why is a distal point such as the pelvis important to the SLP?

References

Alexander, R., Boehme, R., & Cupps, B. (1993). *Normal development of functional motor skills*. San Antonio, TX: Therapy Skill Builders.

Andersen, G., Mjoen, T. R., & Vik, T. (2010). Prevalence of speech problems and the use of augmentative and alternative communication in children with cerebral palsy: A registry-based study in Norway. *Perspectives on Augmentative and Alternative Communication, 19*, 12–20.

Arvedson, J. C., & Brodsky, I. (2002). *Pediatric swallowing and feeding: Assessment and management*. (2nd ed.). San Diego, CA: Singular.

Badawi, N., Felix, J. F., Kurinuzuk, J. J., Dixon, G., Watson, L., Keogh, J. M., . . . Stanley, F. J. (2005). Cerebral palsy following term newborn encephalopathy: A population-based study. *Developmental Medicine & Child Neurology, 47*, 293–298.

Bahr, D. C. (2001). *Oral motor assessment and treatment: Ages and stages.* Boston, MA: Allyn & Bacon.

Bahr, D. C. (2003). Typical versus atypical oral motor function in the pediatric population: Beyond the checklist. *Perspectives on Swallowing and Swallowing Disorders, 12,* 4–12.

Bartlett, D. J., & Palisano, R. J. (2000). A multivariate model of determinants of motor change for children with cerebral palsy. *Physical Therapy, 80,* 598–614.

Bauman-Waengler, J. (2012). *Articulation and phonological impairments: A clinical focus* (4th ed.). Boston, MA: Allyn & Bacon.

Bax, M. (1964). Terminology and classification of cerebral palsy. *Developmental Medicine & Child Neurology, 6,* 295–307.

Bax, M. (2001). Medical aspects of cerebral palsy. In N. R. Finnie (Ed.), *Handling the young child with cerebral palsy at home* (3rd ed., pp. 8–17). Boston, MA: Butterworth-Heinemann.

Bax, M., Goldstein, M., Rosenbaum, P., Leviton, A., & Paneth, N. (2005). Proposed definition and classification of cerebral palsy. *Developmental Medicine & Child Neurology, 47,* 571–576.

Bennett, F. C. (1999). Diagnosing cerebral palsy—the earlier the better. *Contemporary Pediatrics, 16,* 65–73.

Bishop, D. V. M., Brown, B. B., & Robson, J. (1990). The relationship between phoneme discrimination, speech perception, and language comprehension in cerebral-palsied individuals. *Journal of Speech and Hearing Research, 23,* 210–219.

Bjornson, K. F., McLaughlin, J. F., Loeser, J. D., Nowak-Cooperman, K. M., Russel, M., Bader, K. A., & Desmond, S. A. (2003). Oral motor, communication, and nutritional status of children during intrathecal baclofen therapy: A descriptive pilot study. *Archives of Physical Medicine and Rehabilitation, 84,* 500–506.

Bloom, L., & Lahey, M. (1978). *Language development and language disorders.* New York, NY: Wiley.

Bly, L. (1983). *The components of normal movement during the first year of life.* Oak Park, IL: Neurodevelopmental Treatment Association.

Bobath, B. (1967). The very early treatment of cerebral palsy. *Developmental Medicine & Child Neurology, 9,* 373–390.

Bobath, K. (1980). *A neurophysiological basis for the treatment of cerebral palsy.* London, UK: Lippincott.

Bobath, K., & Bobath, B. (1984). The neuro-developmental treatment. In D. Scrutton (Ed.), *Management of the motor disorders of children with cerebral palsy. Clinics in Developmental Medicine* (pp. 6–18). Philadelphia, PA: Lippincott.

Boliek, C. A., & Lohmeier, H. (1999). From the big bang to the brain. *Journal of Communication Disorders, 32,* 271–276.

Calis, E. A. C., Veugelers, R., Sheppard, J. J., Tobboel, D., Evenhuis, H. M., & Penning, C. (2008). Dysphagia in children with severe generalized cerebral palsy and intellectual disability. *Developmental Medicine & Child Neurology, 50,* 625–630.

Campbell, S. K. (1991). Central nervous system dysfunction in children. In S. K. Campbell (Ed.), *Pediatric neurologic physical therapy* (pp. 1–17). New York, NY: Churchill Livingston.

Caruso, A. J., & Strand, E. A. (1999). Motor speech disorders in children: Definitions, background, and a theoretical framework. In A. J. Caruso & E. A. Strand, (Eds.), *Clinical management of motor speech disorders in children* (pp. 1–28). New York, NY: Thieme.

Davis, B. E., Moon, R. Y., Sachs, H. C., & Ottolini, M. C. (1998). Effects of sleep position on infant motor development. *Pediatrics, 102,* 1135–1140.

Dewey, C., Fleming, P., Golding, J., & ALSPAC Study Team. (1998). Does supine sleeping position have any adverse effects on the child? II. Development in the first 18 months. *Pediatrics, 101,* 98. URL: http://www.pediatrics.org/cgi/content/full/101/1/e5

Fennell, E. B., & Dikel, T. N. (2001). Cognitive and neuropsychological functioning in children with cerebral palsy. *Journal of Child Neurology, 16,* 58–63.

Finnie, N. R. (2001). *Handling the young child with cerebral palsy* (3rd ed.). Oxford, UK: Butterworth-Heinemann.

Green, J. R., Moore, C. A, Higashikawa, M., & Steeve, R. W. (2000). The physiologic development of speech motor control: Lip and jaw coordination. *Journal of Speech, Language, and Hearing Research, 43,* 239–255.

Hadders-Algra, M. (2007). Atypical performance: How do we deal with that? *Developmental Medicine & Child Neurology, 49,* 403.

Halpern, H., & Goldfarb, R. (2013). *Language and motor speech disorders in adults* (3rd ed.). Burlington, MA: Jones & Bartlett Learning.

Hanzlik, J. R. (1990). Nonverbal interaction patterns of mothers and their infants with cerebral palsy. *Education and Training in Mental Retardation, 25,* 333–343.

Hodge, M. M., & Wellman, L. (1999). Management of children with dysarthria. In A. J. Caruso & E. A. Strand (Eds.), *Clinical management of motor speech disorders in children* (pp. 209–280). New York, NY: Thieme.

Howle, J. M. (2002). *Neurodevelopmental treatment approach: Theoretical foundations and principles of clinical practice.* Laguna Beach, CA: NDTA.

Hustad, K. C., Gorton, K., & Lee, J. (2010). Classification of speech and language profiles in 4-year-old children with cerebral palsy:

A prospective preliminary study. *Journal of Speech, Language, and Hearing Research, 53*, 1496–1513.

Jantz, J. W., Blosser, C. D., & Fruechting, L. A. (1997). A motor milestone change noted with a change in sleep position. *Archives of Pediatrics & Adolescent Medicine, 151*, 565–568.

Jones-Owens, L. (1991). Prespeech assessment and treatment. In M. B. Langley & L. J. Lombardino (Eds.), *Neurodevelopmental strategies for managing communication disorders in children with severe motor dysfunction* (pp. 49–80). Austin, TX: Pro-Ed.

Kamen, R. S. (1983). Speech and language development. In R. Alexander, R. Boehme, & B. Cupps, *Normal development of functional motor skills* (pp. 221–235). San Antonio, TX: Therapy Skill Builders.

Kent, R. D. (1999). Motor control: Neurophysiology and functional development. In A. J. Caruso & E. A. Strand (Eds.), *Clinical management of motor speech disorders in children* (pp. 29–72). New York, NY: Thieme.

Kragelob-Mann, I. (2005). Cerebral palsy: Towards developmental neuroscience. *Developmental Medicine & Child Neurology, 47*, 435.

Langley, M. B., & Thomas, C. (1991). Introduction to the neurodevelopmental approach. In M. B. Langley & L. J. Lombardino (Eds.), *Neurodevelopmental strategies for managing communication disorders in children with severe motor dysfunction* (pp. 1–28). Austin, TX: Pro-Ed.

Love, R. J., & Webb, W. G. (2001). *Neurology for the speech-language pathologist* (4th ed.). Boston, MA: Butterworth-Heinemann.

McCauley, R. J., & Strand, E. A. (1999). Treatment of children exhibiting phonological disorders with motor speech impairment. In A. J. Caruso & E. A. Strand (Eds.), *Clinical management of motor speech disorders in children* (pp. 187–208). New York, NY: Thieme.

Mecham, M. J. (2002). *Cerebral palsy* (3rd ed.). Austin, TX: Pro-Ed.

Mitchell, P. R., & Kent, R. D. (1990). Phonetic variation in multisyllable babbling. *Journal of Child Language, 17*, 247–265.

Mork, M. (2001). Medical problems and needs of follow-up in a group of children with mild cerebral palsy [Electronic version]. *Tidsskr Nor Laegeforen (Journal of the Norwegian Medical Association), 121*, 1566–1569. Retrieved August 18, 2012, from http://www.ncbi.nlm.nih.gov/pubmed/11446039?dopt=Abstract

Morris, S. E. (1987). Therapy for the child with cerebral palsy: Interacting frameworks. *Seminars in Speech and Language, 8*, 71–86.

Morris, S. E., & Klein, M. D. (2000). *Pre-feeding skills: A comprehensive resource for feeding development.* San Antonio, TX: Therapy Skill Builders.

Pelligrino, L. (2007). Cerebral palsy. In M. L. Batshaw, L. Pelligrino, & N. J. Roizen (Eds.), *Children with disabilities* (pp. 387–408). Baltimore, MD: Paul H. Brookes.

Pennington, L., Goldbart, J., & Marshall, J. (2005). Speech and language therapy to improve the communication skills of children with cerebral palsy. *Developmental Medicine & Child Neurology, 47*, 57–63.

Pennington, L., & McConachie, H. (1999). Mother-child interaction revisited: Communication with non-speaking physically disabled children. *International Journal of Language & Communication Disorders, 34*, 391–416.

Pinder, G. L., & Faherty, A. S. (1999). Issues in pediatric feeding and swallowing. In A. J. Caruso and E. A. Strand (Eds.), *Clinical management of motor speech disorders in children* (pp. 281–318). New York, NY: Thieme.

Pinder, G. L., & Olswang, L. B. (1995). Development of communicative intent in young children with cerebral palsy: A treatment efficacy study. *Infant-Toddler Intervention, 5*, 51–70.

Rais-Bahrami, K., & Short, B. L. (2007). Premature and small-for-dates infants. In M. L. Batshaw, L. Pelligrino, & N. J. Roizen (Eds.), *Children with disabilities* (pp. 107–124). Baltimore, MD: Paul H. Brookes.

Reddy, S. K. (2005). Commentary on definition and classification of cerebral palsy. *Developmental Medicine & Child Neurology, 47*, 508–509.

Redstone, F. (1991). Respiratory components of communication. In M. B. Langley & L. J. Lombardino (Eds.), *Neurodevelopmental strategies for managing communication disorders in children with severe motor dysfunction* (pp. 29–48). Austin, TX: Pro-Ed.

Redstone, F. (2004). The effects of seating position on the respiratory patterns of preschoolers with cerebral palsy. *International Journal of Rehabilitation Research, 27*, 283–288.

Rosenbaum, P. (2007). Certainty and uncertainty of determinants of long-term developmental outcome: Lessons from longitudinal studies. *Developmental Medicine & Child Neurology, 49*, s110, 5.

Seikel, J. A., King, D. W., & Drumwright, D. G. (2005). *Anatomy and physiology for speech, language, and hearing* (4th ed.). Clifton Park, NY: Delmar, Cengage.

Sheppard, J. J. (2008). Using motor learning approaches for treating swallowing and feeding disorders: A review. *Language, Speech, and Hearing Services in Schools, 39*, 227–236.

Smith, A., Goffman, L., & Stark, R. (1995). Speech motor control. *Seminars in Speech and Language, 16*, 87–98.

Solomon, N. P., & Charron, S. (1998). Speech breathing in able-bodied children and children with cerebral palsy: A review of the literature and implications for clinical intervention. *American Journal of Speech-Language Pathology, 7,* 61–78.

Sullivan, P. B., Lambert, B., Rose, M., Ford-Adams, M., Johnson, A., & Griffiths, P. (2000). Prevalence and severity of feeding and nutritional problems in children with neurological impairment: Oxford feeding study. *Developmental Medicine & Child Neurology, 42,* 674–680.

Treviranus, J., & Roberts, V. (2003). Supporting competent motor control of AAC systems. In J. C. Light, D. R. Beukelman, & J. Reichle (Eds.), *Communicative competence for individuals who use AAC: From research to effective practice* (pp. 199–240). Baltimore, MD: Paul H. Brookes.

U.S. Department of Education. (2012). IDEA 2004: Building the legacy. Amendments to IDEA. Section 601. http://www.ed.gov/part-c/statutes

Yeargin-Allsopp, M., Boyle, C., Braun, K. V. N., & Trevathan, E. (2008). The epidemiology of developmental disabilities. In P. J. Accardo (Ed.), *Capute & Accardo's neurodevelopmental disabilities in infancy and childhood* (pp. 61–104). Baltimore, MD: Paul H. Brookes.

CHAPTER 2

The ABCs of NDT

Fran Redstone

Introduction

Cerebral palsy has traditionally been defined as a neuromuscular deficit caused by a nonprogressive lesion in the immature brain that leads to impaired motor functioning (Bartlett & Palisano, 2000; Bax, 1964, 2001; Bennett, 1999). It is an aggregate of developmental disorders of movement and posture that result in varied clinical manifestations and activity limitations (Bax, Goldstein, Rosenbaum, Leviton, & Paneth, 2005; Reddy, 2005). It is described as the "most common developmental disability with associated motor impairment" (Treviranus & Roberts, 2003) that affects many areas of functioning. Carr (2005) points to the work of the International Workshop on the Definition and Classification of Cerebral Palsy and notes that the functional consequences of the movement disorder also incur oral-motor involvement (Bax et al., 2005). The specific underlying neurological deficits associated with cerebral palsy are addressed in the next chapter.

Suffice it to say, it is not unexpected that children with cerebral palsy may have communication disorders (Pennington, Goldbart, & Marshall, 2005) and associated problems such as cognition, language, and learning deficits (Bishop, Brown, & Robson, 1990), as well as seizures and sensory impairments (Badawi et al., 2005) that impact communication.

Although clinicians cannot cure the underlying neuronal damage, they can alleviate some of its effects on development through intervention. Neurodevelopmental treatment (NDT) is one such intervention that addresses the sensorimotor aspects of speech/swallowing and play/interaction directly, and communication indirectly. The purpose of this chapter is to review current theories of motor control and development and demonstrate the implications of these theories for the treatment of children with cerebral palsy through the framework of NDT. This book describes many areas of intervention that have been successfully addressed with NDT principles including feeding, saliva control, sound production, interaction, augmentative and alternative communication (AAC), and literacy. The chapter authors will demonstrate how they use the knowledge and skills gained through NDT in functional activities and contexts. This has often led to the development of new approaches to therapy. The goal of this book is to broaden the knowledge base of SLPs who work with children with neuromotor deficits. However, it is also hoped that those who work primarily with children with cerebral palsy may consider taking continuing education courses to further this basic knowledge.

Theories of Motor Control and Development and the Child with Cerebral Palsy

The child with cerebral palsy will develop differently than the child with a typical motor system (Boliek & Lohmeier, 1999) who has normal underlying neurological integrity. The motor impairment of cerebral palsy directly influences the effector muscles of the speech production subsystems (respiration, phonation, articulation, resonance) and swallowing mechanism as it does other motor systems.

A number of authors (ASHA, 2004; Ballard, 2001; Clark, 2005; Mann, 2002; Steele, 2006; Yorkston, 1996) note that the field of speech-language pathology lacks good evidence in many areas of intervention on which to base clinical decisions. Specifically, Pennington, Goldbart, and Marshall (2004) note that evidence is lacking to support speech and language treatment strategies for children with cerebral palsy. Therefore, Clark and Clark (2002) suggest that clinicians use their understanding of theoretical foundations as a basis for decisions regarding intervention. Clark (2005) and Steele (2006) also recommend the use of a "theory-driven approach" to patient care until such time as a body of empirical evidence for the practices used by speech language pathologists becomes available. It may be worthwhile to investigate the underlying theories behind many techniques used by SLPs including NDT. When clinicians work with children with cerebral palsy, Kamm, Thelen, and Jensen (1990) suggest that knowledge of movement science will aid them in providing a more holistic intervention.

In some ways, one might consider NDT a nonspeech neuromuscular approach that has been much maligned in recent speech literature. However, Clark and associates studied motor control using a nonspeech task because these researchers feel that motor principles are "common to both speech and nonspeech oral control" (Clark, Robin, McCullagh & Schmidt, 2001, p. 1017). In addition, Ballard (2001) notes that it is worthwhile for SLPs to explore the more extensive research base in the field of motor learning and control when presented with a client with speech motor control issues. This is the approach being used by Cerny, Panzarella, and Stathopoulos (1997) and Sapienza (2007) regarding strengthening of expiratory muscles for patients with neuromotor disorders. Because cerebral palsy is primarily a motor disorder (Bax, 2001; Bax et al., 2005; Nashner, Shumway-Cook, & Marin, 1983) that affects many areas of development, it is appropriate for SLPs to study theories of motor control and be familiar with NDT.

Bernstein's Dilemma

Current theories of motor control began when Bernstein (1967) suggested that the major obstacle in developing motor control is the great number of moving parts that need to be organized. Therefore, a person needs to simplify this process by reducing the elements or degrees-of-freedom (DOF) within a function so that each muscle does not need to be individually controlled.

Another factor that needs to be considered is the redundancy within our systems. This allows us to accomplish a movement in many different ways. This is referred to as motor equivalency (Sporns & Edelman, 1993). Bernstein notes that repetition is important but that we never repeat the same movement exactly. He believes that repetition leads to modification in order to attain a goal (Reed & Bril, 1996).

Various theories have developed to explain the process of simplification. Many authors suggest that this is accomplished using synergies. These are movement patterns that are often referred to as coordinated structures (Sporns & Edelman, 1993), functional units (Howle, 2002), or programs (Schmidt, 2003). Most researchers agree that the development of these synergies depends on the task at hand, the constraints of the body, and the environment (Mathiowetz & Haugen, 1994).

In support of these newer theories, we see that typical infants reduce the degrees-of-freedom by stabilizing parts of their body, in order to function within a new task. In the area of speech development, it has been hypothesized that the speech sounds that develop early (stops) are those whose total constriction controls the degrees-of-freedom (Green, Moore, Higashikawa, & Steeve, 2000). The concept of "fixing" describes the way in which a child with cerebral palsy may attempt to control the degrees-of-freedom (Howle, 2002). Bly (1983) states that the child with hypotonia lacks stability from which to move and learns to "hold himself artificially" (p. 42). This child may continue with the "rigid" movement because the nervous system may not allow the flexibility and variety of movement selection that is available to a physically typical child.

The constraints on the body of a child born with a neuro-motor deficit may be markedly different from that of a typical child. This includes the deficits stemming from the primary sensory and muscle tone issues as well as the associated problems mentioned previously.

Generalized Motor Program

Early hierarchical theories could not adequately explain how so many contractions are controlled at once (Schmidt & Lee,

2005). Bernstein hypothesized that programs are developed and selected based on the goal of the movement (Schmidt & Lee, 2005). This concept was then incorporated into Schmidt's Generalized Motor Program (GMP) (Schmidt, 1975), which states that we have memories of movements that are stored centrally and retrieved when we plan to move. This is commonly referred to as a closed-looped or feed-forward system. Although Bernstein used the term synergy, Schmidt uses schema. Schemas develop through experience and lead to motor learning. This theory states that a single program can be used for related movements to meet task demands (Mass et al., 2010). This allows for greater efficiency, storage, and speed of movements. This is important since speech is both fast and flexible. Schmidt (2003) notes that sensory information from feedback is slow. This is particularly important for SLPs because speech movements are fast.

Neuronal Group Selection Theory

The Neuronal Group Selection Theory (NGST) was conceived because researchers felt that programs too narrowly defined how movement arises. This theory emphasizes the importance of neural diversity, which allows a child to select a movement that matches the needs of a task (Sporns & Edelman, 1993). Selection of neuronal groups is based on the varied sensory information that results from a child's experiences. A functional synergy is developed that is a set of related movements to perform a task. The movements repeated during early experiences strengthen the synaptic connections (Hadders-Algra, 2000) used to produce the movements. Development occurs by sensing the adaptive value of movements to perform a task. This value is determined through sensory inputs. Hadders-Algra (2000) believes that the "role of sensory information in motor development is larger than previously presumed" (p. 570). This theory emphasizes sensory inputs for feedback, which allows for flexibility of movements, thus accounting for motor equivalence. This is important for the speech system because it involves both *fast* and *flexible* movements.

In support of this theory, Nashner et al. (1983) studied postural control in children with cerebral palsy and found that they had ineffective feedback systems. Neilson and O'Dwyer (1984) investigated athetoid movements using EMGs and discovered that their subject with athetoid cerebral palsy had poor motor feedback leading to the propagation of inappropriate movement. One may postulate that if feedback is enhanced, subsequent movements may be improved.

The central nervous system of a child with cerebral palsy incurred an injury early in development and lacks the typical neuronal diversity. This will impact both the movement patterns (Touwen, 1998) and sensory system of the affected child. In general, children with cerebral palsy have a paucity of movement patterns, whereas the typical child has many motor strategies available. This paucity then impacts further development of neuronal diversity because this child receives less sensory information.

Dynamic Systems Theory

The Dynamic Systems Theory (DST) (Thelen, 1991, 1995; Thelen & Smith, 2002; Kamm et al., 1990) describes infants as problem solvers who make adaptive choices based on the properties of their bodies and the task at hand. Interestingly, Thelen treats speech as another motor activity; moreover, she views language or symbolic thought in much the same way as she does walking, as emergent from activity. DST states that neural substrates for a task are not pre-established but are "softly organized" (Ruark & Moore, 1997, p. 1374). Thelen (1995) states that "developmental change is not planned but arises within a context . . . " (p. 82). This usually occurs through exploration in a supportive environment that allows the child to find solutions for specific tasks (Thelen, 1995). The child with cerebral palsy may need supports for this to occur.

According to the DST, each individual has many interacting systems. Movement patterns emerge through the self-organization of one's system with the environment (Mathiowetz & Haugen, 1994). Stable patterns emerge for a given task. Thelen (1991) labels this preferred, stable pattern an attractor. However, we are reminded that our system is *flexible,* and a task can be accomplished in many ways. This accounts for motor equivalence. Sensory information is used to evaluate the movement and to determine new demands of the environment. Change (development) occurs during "phase shifts" in which a new attractor is established (Thelen, 1991). Proponents of this theory (Kamm et al., 1990) describe development of a skill as *stability–phase shift–new movement*. Another way of saying this is that there is a stable pattern that is used and then a new variable is introduced, and a new set of movements are selected (Thelen, 1991). This theory does not state which of the many systems is most important. Personal systems, including centrally stored information, and environmental subsystems influence behavior. This is particularly important when discussing children with cerebral palsy, because we know that their personal characteristics vary from the typically developing child.

Discussion of Theories

While, in this author's clinical point of view, the brief summaries presented show general agreement, researchers involved in the development of these theories feel strongly about their differences. In fact DST has been referred to as "the so-called dynamical systems perspective" (Schmidt, 2003, p. 366), whereas others say that movement is possible without programs (Sporns & Edelman, 1993). The developers of these theories emphasize the differences between certain aspects of each theory. Bernstein and Schmidt highlight the closed-loop system and importance of programs. NGST focuses on feedback. DST appears to be a hybrid, emphasizing internal as well as external factors.

Although "camps" have formed and will not "be swayed by the arguments of the 'enemy'" (Schmidt, 2003, p. 368), it is acknowledged by the different "camps" that reducing the degrees-of-freedom is required and that information needs to be stored centrally for use in similar movements. They also agree that the environment plays a role in providing the purpose for performing the movement and the feedback of its success. In addition, the importance of sensory experiences is noted by all theorists, as is the significance of functional tasks.

Some of the differences may be semantic. Bernstein uses the term "synergy," whereas Schmidt's GMP states that what is stored centrally are "schemas." These are rules that have been developed with experience and practice. DST and NGST also use the term "synergy" to suggest that muscles are not controlled individually but "are organized into functional synergies that are constrained to act as a unit in a motor task" (Smith, McFarland, & Weber, 1986, p. 471). Variability and diversity are also used by several of the theorists. Thelen and Smith (2002) state that variability is "the essential ground for exploration and selection" (p. 342) of new behaviors. That is also the focus of NGST but, in this context, it relates to the importance of neural diversity to develop varied neural networks (Hadders-Algra, 2000).

For the SLP, it is important to note the areas of agreement: bodily constraints, sensory information, functional tasks, and varied experiences. For the SLP, this means that the child must have varied experiences with good feedback within functional tasks in order to develop the movement options to address the functions of swallowing, language learning, and communication.

Other Principles of Movement Science

Additionally, there are other principles of movement science supporting motor control and development that are quite important to the clinician working with children with motor disorders. These principles need to be incorporated into our sessions and stressed with caregivers. Most importantly, practice with repetition and intensity is required to impact the nervous system. We need to be sure that our sessions provide many opportunities for children to practice. We also need to instruct families how they can provide these opportunities in a natural environment during daily activities. This has been emphasized by many researchers (Kays & Robbins, 2007; Kleim & Jones, 2008; Yorkston, Beukelman, Strand, & Bell, 1999) and is the basis for early intervention.

Saliency is also extremely important: How meaningful is this experience to the child? And how enjoyable is it? This is closely related to active learning or the behavioral experiences (Kleim & Jones, 2008) we use in our session and is another principle that will impact skill development. Specificity is another concept that needs to be considered. It follows that if our desired outcome is improved swallowing, we need to practice swallowing. Remember, we need to provide many opportunities for the desired behavior—both within and outside of the therapy room.

Kamm et al. (1990) suggest that therapy should have the same goal as development: adaptability of movements. Specifically, the goals of intervention should be to improve stability, increase variability, and allow for greater exploration that will lead to change and development. It has been suggested that NDT enhances the probability for these goals to be achieved.

Neurodevelopmental Treatment—Principles

Neurodevelopmental treatment was developed in England by Berta Bobath in the 1940s and is often referred to as the "Bobath Approach." It is one of the most widely used therapeutic systems for children with cerebral palsy (Barry, 2001; Blauw-Hospers & Hadders-Algra, 2005; Campbell, 2002; Fetters & Kluzik, 1996; Howle, 2002; VanSant, 1991; Workinger, 2005). As initially conceived, NDT was static and passive, but it was appropriately based upon the prevailing motor control theories of the time that stressed reflex hierarchy and strict developmental sequence. This is no longer the case. NDT, like other interventions, has evolved (Mathiowetz & Haugen, 1994) by incorporating the observations and treatment techniques of experienced clinicians and integrating them with new motor-control theories (Howle, 2002). However, some authors inaccurately critique NDT as it was in 1960 (Kurtz, 2007; Mathiowetz & Haugen, 1994) completely unaware of the principles that have been developed and incorporated into mainstream NDT intervention during the last 50 years.

NDT is taught as a post-master's-degree 8-week certification course to the occupational therapist (OT), physical therapist (PT), and speech-language pathologist (SLP) treating children with cerebral palsy and other neuromotor disabilities. When a practitioner attains certification in NDT, this assumes competency and provides a certain degree of confidence to consumers. NDT has been described more as an "approach" than a prescribed set of intervention techniques (Palisano, 1991). It highlights the relationship between several processes of development, formerly viewed as discrete by practitioners working with children with cerebral palsy (VanSant, 1991). A basic tenet of NDT is an integrated approach to both treatment and development (Alexander, Boehme, & Cupps, 1993) that addresses skill acquisition in a holistic framework. NDT teaches clinicians to assess and analyze a child's movements in functional settings to determine what components may be missing or interfering with movement (Bly, 1983; Mohr, 1990). These components are then incorporated into an intervention plan. An NDT-trained SLP assesses and treats, if necessary, the scapula stability of a child who is not using his hands for the selection of symbols or manipulation of toys; or provides jaw stability if this interferes with lip and tongue movements for feeding and speech sound production; or enhances thoracic–abdominal control of a child not producing appropriate breath groups. The successful use of NDT, like other treatment protocols, depends greatly on the skill of the therapist.

The World Health Organization's International Classification of Function (ICF) gives professionals a framework to describe the effects of impairments on individuals (World Health Organization, 2001). For example, a child with cerebral palsy who has an impairment that includes abnormal muscle tone may also present functional disorders in swallowing, language, and sound production. NDT teaches (Howle, 2002) the World Health Organization's ICF emphasizing the importance of function, participation, and context. NDT speech pathologists address the motor impairment (abnormal muscle tone, lack of head control, jaw instability) while targeting discipline-specific objectives (lip closure, cause/effect, vocalization) through functional activities (e.g., eating, playing, speech) in an age-appropriate context.

Keesee (1976) reminds us that the goals of all the disciplines working with a young child with cerebral palsy often overlap since the initial concern is for "total body management" (p. 1360). NDT presents an integrated approach (Alexander et al., 1993) by addressing development and skill acquisition from a holistic framework. The principles and theoretical framework noted above are incorporated into NDT intervention. A unique aspect of NDT for the SLP is the facilitation of body alignment and postural control to attain stability in functional activities (Shumway-Cook & Woollacott, 2001) through therapeutic handling (Howle,

2002). For the SLP, postural control is the basis of oral/pharyngeal, respiratory/phonatory, and articulatory coordination for the functions of swallowing and communication (Howle, 2002). NDT could be another tool to attain these goals. An SLP could use NDT as the background for other traditional interventions. This is illustrated in Figure 2–1.

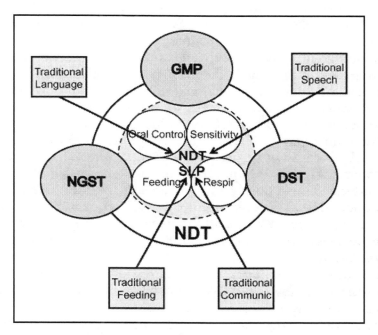

Figure 2–1. The gray circles represent the influence of the Dynamic Systems Theory (DST), Neuronal Group Selection Theory (NGST), and Generalized Motor Programs (GMP) on Neurodevelopmental Treatment (NDT) principles, which is represented as the outer circle. NDT speech interventions for feeding, respiration, oral control, and sensitivity are shown within the dashed circle, which is within the outer circle, demonstrating an NDT framework for these speech techniques. It also suggests that an NDT speech–language pathologist uses this background of NDT, along with other interventions that are shown as squares and that are utilized by SLPs to treat children with language, speech, and feeding disorders. (From "Neurodevelopmental Treatment in Speech-Language Pathology: Theory, Practice, and Research," *Communicative Disorders Review, 1,* 119–131. Plural Publishing, Inc., © 2007. Reprinted with permission.)

NDT Intervention

Therapeutic Handling

Kamm et al. (1990), proponents of DST, draw a parallel between the typically developing child and a therapist's young client. These authors state that treatment for a child with a disability should allow the youngster to seek more adaptive movements in a similar way to his typical counterpart. NDT strives to achieve this through facilitation of movement using therapeutic handling (Howle, 2002; Langley & Thomas, 1991). The ultimate goal of handling is to develop a functional skill. Facilitation is a handling strategy used in order to "make a posture or movement easier or more likely to occur" (Howle, 2002, p. 256). For example, the therapist may facilitate trunk rotation for improved muscle control for respiratory support, or jaw closure for chewing or sound production. Inhibition is another type of handling that restricts inefficient postures or movements (Howle, 2002). Originally, the Bobath approach emphasized "reflex-inhibiting postures," but quite early Bobath realized that passive positioning does not change movement or function (Howle, 2002). Today, NDT uses inhibitory handling to redirect an excessive or unintentional movement such as jaw extension during sound production or swallowing. It may be used to elongate a shortened muscle (hypertonus) to provide a greater range of movement, such as neck elongation for alignment of oral structures. Typically, inhibition and facilitation are used together through therapeutic handling.

Hands-to-midline is a goal often targeted by PT, OT, and SLP and it is an important motor milestone. It influences oral-motor and cognitive/linguistic development. It enables a child to learn about his or her environment, to play with toys, and to bring objects to his or her mouth. Kamm et al. (1990) describe the development of hands-to-midline, as *stability–phase shift–new movement.* A change in a subsystem (e.g., flexion) may lead to a change in stability (loss of ATNR), and a subsequent new movement pattern (hands-to-midline). It is through therapeutic handling that an NDT therapist helps a child develop stability and then the ability to cause a phase shift through experimentation.

Another example of this *stability–phase shift–new movement* that is associated with the goals of an SLP may be the development of chewing by introducing the child to new textures of food, which leads to oral exploration and the development of new oral movements (Alexander et al., 1993; Arvedson & Brodsky, 2002).

It may be argued that the therapist's handling during a functional task is causing changes in specific connections and may result in context-specific neuronal use. This, in turn, reduces the degrees-of-freedom. Touwen (1998) proposes that this adaptive variability is the essence of development. Selection of neuronal groups, paralleling NGST, is based on the varied sensory information that results from a child's experiences, which then strengthens the synaptic connections (Hadders-Algra, 2000). The motor system is being manipulated through the movement facilitated by the therapist. Sensory receptors send information back to the central nervous system leading to changes within the sensory system.

According to the DST a new behavior is learned through adapting to new demands. A skilled clinician introduces instability by providing new tasks or situations and enables children to discover the new "biomechanical dynamics of their actions" (Kamm et al., 1990, p. 774). The NGST proposes that therapists can change output of the child's motor system by influencing the input. NDT deals with these issues by having the clinician provide the support necessary for the child to be successful (Okimoto, Bundy, & Hanzlik, 2000; Pinder & Olswang, 1995) through therapeutic handling (facilitation and/or inhibition), use of equipment, or structured environment. NDT also emphasizes the importance of a child's participation in task-specific responses (Barry, 2001; Howle, 2002; Mohr, 1990) described by DST. The specific responses that occur within a context open further opportunities for a typical child's action and exploration (Thelen & Smith, 2002). However, children with cerebral palsy have a dearth of movement patterns and move stereotypically (Bly, 1991) when introduced to new stimuli. Generally, these children will not be able to make adaptive changes without help or facilitation. This becomes the duty of the clinician. Campbell (1997) describes the importance of a child's ability to explore and a therapist's responsibility to create programs that allow for this. Thelen and Smith (2002) state that a child's new experiences become part of the memory from which the youngster can generalize and subsequently utilize in similar situations. NDT strives to provide an environment in which variability can occur after stability has been established.

Again, it is through therapeutic handling techniques that the amount of stability and the number of degrees-of-freedom can be controlled. The handling is directed at developing the components of movement (postural alignment, weight bearing, weight shift, stability, and mobility) in functional activities. It is provided through key points of control, the areas where therapists place their hands to provide facilitation and inhibition during movement. These key points are typically proximal points such as the trunk, pelvis, or shoulders (Howle, 2002). Key points may also be on distal parts of the body such as the arms, legs, or even mandible, depending on the needs of the child and the movement being facilitated. These key points allow for greater freedom of movement by helping infants and children with neuromotor disorders to be actively involved in exploring their postural limits, just as typically developing children do. The provision of traditional techniques such as model/imitation, rate modification, breathing exercises, integral stimulation, or hand-over-hand activation that SLPs often use in a speech-language treatment session with physically typical children may not be as successful (Pennington, Goldbart, & Marshall, 2003; Pennington, Miller, Robson, & Sheen, 2010; Pennington, Smallman, & Farrier, 2006) when used with children with cerebral palsy, because these techniques are designed for the typical child's normal sensory system and its ability to respond motorically. However, if some preparation is provided using NDT handling, movement, and positioning, these traditional techniques are likely to be more effective.

NDT Feeding

Controversy Over the Relationship Between Feeding and Speech

There has been a fundamental disagreement between those who believe that speech is a skill adapted from earlier oral behaviors and those who feel that speech is independently developed. There are many proponents on both sides of this controversy. However, the connectivity between parts of the brain related to function has been studied and may shed light on these issues. Kays and Robbins (2007) suggest that neural networks within the brain indicate more shared regions between speech and feeding than previously thought. This is reiterated by Fox et al. (2006) discussing neural coupling of facial, oral, laryngeal, and respiratory muscles.

DST highlights the relationships among various systems in development. This would indicate a link between oral-skill and gross motor development (Thelen, 1995). This is further supported by the fact that feeding and speech share neural pathways, anatomical structures, and developmental patterns (Bahr, 2001, 2003; Culbertson & Tanner, 2012; Morris, 1985; Morris & Klein, 2000). However, some researchers highlight the distinctiveness of speech (Moore & Ruark, 1996; Ruark & Moore, 1997; Steeve & Moore, 2009; Steeve, Moore, Green, Reilly, & McMurtrey, 2008). These distinctive-speech advocates feel strongly that speech develops separately from other oral-motor skills, is unique, and does not emerge from early feeding behaviors. They seem to believe that the nervous system has separate and specific, pre-established substrates for both feeding and for speech. However, even they suggest there may be some common neural substrate that is present very early in development (Bahr, 2001). In addition, their emphasis on task specificity for the development of these skills is similar to that stressed by Thelen (1995).

Although these researchers feel that speech emerges separately from feeding, there is much common ground among theorists. For example, both the distinctive-speech advocates and DST theorists note that children *develop* task specific patterns based on function. Speech and feeding are two very different functions with completely different outcomes. Infants use the structures of the speech production system for feeding from birth in a reflex-bound mode, and subsequently use the same structures for feeding and speech in a voluntary manner with more dissociation and grading. However, the function of speech, according to NGST and DST, would appear to lead to different connections within the brain, subsuming a linguistic goal that is not part of the feeding process.

It seems that the controversy may be heightened once feeding is considered an oral-motor exercise or a nonspeech neuromuscular treatment. However, one hopes that no SLP with a master's degree would consider providing feeding therapy and expect to automatically improve articulation of /s/. On the other hand, it is inappropriate to deny the importance of this fundamental precursor of speech. Ultimately, imaging studies will teach us more about the neural connections for different functions and clarify the relationship between feeding and speech (Kays & Robbins, 2007).

NDT Feeding Intervention

Aside from the philosophical issues regarding a relationship between feeding and speech movements (Alexander, 1987; Lund, Appenteng, & Seguin, 1982; Moore & Ruark, 1996; Mueller, 1972; Mysak, 1980; Pinder & Faherty, 1999), the primary rationale for providing feeding/swallowing treatment for children with cerebral palsy stems from their frequent difficulties in this area (Reilly, Skuse, & Pobiete, 1996; Sullivan et al., 2000; Workinger, 2005). The prevalence of feeding disorders in this population has been reported to be as high as 80% (Rogers, Arvedson, Buck, Smart, & Msall, 1994), and these disorders have been associated with deficits in growth (Day et al., 2007).

In 1987 ASHA developed the first technical report dealing with feeding disorders and acknowledged that clinicians had been treating feeding disordered children with cerebral palsy for many years (ASHA, 2001). At that time, NDT was one of the few treatment programs to suggest specific feeding/swallowing techniques (Mueller, 1972, 2001). Many of these early principles and techniques are still in use today (Arvedson & Brodsky, 2002; Bahr, 2001; Hall, 2001; Redstone & West, 2004; West & Redstone, 2004; Wolf & Glass, 1992). Some of the protocols include positioning, mandibular stability through oral control, and normalization of oral sensitivity through an individualized, graded oral sensitivity program.

NDT hypothesizes that movements of the oral structures for feeding (and speech) require stability and alignment from the pelvis up. Providing this stability and alignment is the beginning of changing the environmental and bodily constraints for the child with cerebral palsy during a functional task. The more normal feeding movements resulting from improved alignment and stability are more efficient and lead to a successful, satiating task completion that supports all the theories presented previously.

Although most SLPs would agree that head control is necessary for the oral movements of a safe swallow (Arvedson & Brodsky, 2002; Larnert & Ekberg, 1995; Redstone & West, 2004; Seikel, King, & Drumright, 2000; West & Redstone, 2004), it needs to be emphasized that "trunk control is fundamental to head control" (Mohr, 1990, p. 1). Trunk control also depends on stability of the pelvis (Herman & Lange, 1999; Zemlin, 1998). Many children with cerebral palsy lack this stability, which may lead to poor development of jaw stability (Alexander et al., 1993; Hall, 2001; Redstone & West, 2004). In turn, lip and tongue movements depend on mandibular stability (Daniels, Brailey, & Foundas, 1999; Seikel et al., 2000; Tamura, Mizukami, Ayano, & Mukai, 2002).

NDT—Oral Control

Mandibular stability has been the target of much research (Green et al., 1997; Green et al., 2000). It has been found that the development of jaw stability precedes the development of the other articulators needed for speech such as the lips (Green, Moore, & Reilly, 2002; Green et al., 2000) and has been recognized as a prerequisite for both advanced feeding skills and speech (Arvedson & Brodsky, 2002; Bahr, 2001).

Dworkin et al. (2003) note that the jaw's function as the "prime mover" (p. 1018) for oral structures may put it at significant risk for breakdowns. These authors state that this structure is implicated in the "persistence of certain abnormal speech behaviors" (p. 1016) but is also central to the development of normal skills. Because of the importance of the mandible in both typical and atypical development, many intervention protocols targeting this structure have been established (Hayden & Square, 1984; Rosenfeld-Johnson, 1999), including NDT (Mueller, 1972; Redstone & West, 2004).

Jaw stability can be attained using the NDT technique of oral control (Mueller, 1972) which is therapeutic handling of the oral area. The clinician uses his or her hand to facilitate oral alignment and graded movements, and to inhibit inefficient movements and asymmetry. It is hypothesized that oral control does not force a movement but allows for greater possibilities of movement. According to DST, it allows for a change in the constraints of the child's environment, *a phase shift*, which then leads to the possibility of a new functional movement. NGST would state that the more normal input and successful completion of a functional task leads to strengthening of neural pathways. With the accumulation of many such experiences, a generalized motor program (GMP) will be developed and stored centrally for future use with similar tasks.

SLPs are well informed about prompting hierarchies for teaching language skills. Oral control can be considered a prompt. Like any prompt, therapeutic handling techniques such as oral control are faded as the client takes over actively. Oral control is used only after better head/trunk alignment and muscle tone have been attempted. In many instances, proximal stability can result in better functioning of a distal structure such as the mouth (Herman & Lange, 1999; West & Redstone, 2004), which would eliminate the need for oral control. Some reasons for using oral control stem from jaw instability as indicated by abnormal opening or asymmetry. This oral control will also facilitate improved tongue position and movement depending on the therapist's handling skills. And if administered correctly, oral control will help maintain head alignment, especially during periods of strong stimulation such as the approach of food or utensils.

Of course, oral control should be used Only When Needed (OWN)! Although a strategy such as upright positioning may be viewed as a general treatment principle for SLPs, oral control should be used more selectively. The clinician must know *exactly* why this technique is being used and carefully monitor its results. It is also important that oral control be used within a specific context such as eating or sound production (Sheppard, 2005). This technique has been addressed at length in previous publications (Mueller, 1972; Pinder & Faherty, 1999; Redstone & West, 2004) and is discussed further in Chapter 6.

NDT Intervention—Oral Sensitivity

NGST and DST both stress the importance of sensory input for the development of movement (Mathiowetz & Haugen, 1994; Sporns & Edelman, 1993). Miller (2002) highlights the importance of multiple sensory inputs on the functioning of the tongue during swallowing. Others recognize the importance of oral sensitivity for feeding (Dodrill et al., 2004) and chewing and swallowing (Engelen, van der Bilt, & Bosman, 2004). Miller (2002) describes the complex set of reflexes that are initiated through sensory input, modulating motor acts like speech and swallowing.

Children with cerebral palsy may have oral sensory problems that include hypo- or hypersensitivity (Arvedson & Brodsky, 2002; Workinger, 2005). These deficits may stem from primary neurological impairments, or they may result from secondary problems such as lack of flexion and midline orientation for hand-to-mouth behaviors (Pinder & Faherty, 1999). Improved sensory feedback will enhance future movements (Alexander, 1987; Bobath, 1980; Miller, 2002), and movements based on normal muscle tone can aid the further development of one's sensory system (Bahr, 2001; Ottenbacher, Bundy, & Short, 1983). Using NDT principles, speech clinicians improve sensitivity of the mouth through handling to attain more normal muscle tone, head flexion, and neck elongation (Alexander, 1987; Mueller, 1972). Subsequently, the clinician can focus on the attainment of midline orientation and the improvement of hands-to-mouth activities (Pinder & Faherty, 1999).

In addition, clinicians can develop an oral sensory program that will provide the child with graded input allowing more appropriate sensory processing (Arvedson & Brodsky, 2002; Mueller, 1972; Ottenbacher et al., 1983). Each program should be tailored to the needs of the child based on a careful oral assessment. This program may include oral tactile stimulation, graded input of new textures, and/or toothbrushing (Arvedson & Brodsky, 2002; Pinder & Faherty, 1999). The goal is to increase the possibility of a more normal, successful motor response through manipulation of the sensory environment (Alexander, 1987).

NDT Intervention—Respiration/Phonation

Boliek and Lohmeier (1999) discuss DST in relation to speech breathing and vocalization and demonstrate the relationship between these motor based systems and the linguistic system of the developing child. These authors note that as typical children develop better respiratory control, they can begin to use longer breath groups to reflect an increasing linguistic complexity. As greater control is achieved and longer breath groups are possible, the child with cerebral palsy may be able to more accurately demonstrate his language skills as well. Through therapeutic handling, NDT helps the child develop this control. Handling will include elongation of the trunk and provision of improved head/trunk alignment. Therapeutic handling can be incorporated into each treatment session as well as the child's daily routines at home and in the classroom. Through handling, movement, and positioning, children can develop more movement options and be successful in their attempts to vocalize. However, it is important to encourage many attempts to phonate functionally, at the appropriate level for each child, during each session.

The features of DOF, NGST, and DST that include task orientation, active participation, appropriate response, and sensory feedback are addressed using an NDT approach for improved phonation and speech sound production. Chapter 7 will discuss these topics more fully.

NDT—Language, Play, and Interaction

Anderson, Hinojosa, and Strauch (1987) discuss the use of NDT during the integration of play into an OT session. They note that play provides a rehearsal for later "real" experiences and allows for repetition and interaction. These aspects of play are also important to an SLP who may wish to prepare the child's trunk for phonation and the oral area for articulator movements during the activity. Many treatment protocols (Rosenfeld-Johnson, 1999; Hayden & Square, 1984) assert the importance of these components but acknowledge that motorically typical children already have normal tone and alignment. It is the child with movement and coordination problems who requires particular attention to these elements if the child is to benefit from the play experience.

Kamm et al. (1990) discuss DST as it relates to the field of physical therapy, but this theory may be equally useful for the SLP who works with a child with a compromised motor system. These authors state that a clinician can change a system by altering its constraints. For example, the clinician can change a task by having the child push instead of pull, thereby decreasing the probability of upper extremity flexion, shoulder elevation, and head hyperextension. Another change can involve the positioning of a child to better maintain normal muscle tone (Bergen & Colangelo, 1985; Nwaobi, Brubaker, Cusick, & Sussman, 1983).

These concerns are as applicable to an SLP as they are to a physical therapist, because head/neck extension and increased muscle tone will interfere with oral alignment, oral-motor movements, and will hinder midline orientation for hand-to-mouth activities and the manipulation of toys during play. Additionally, a slight change in the placement of materials from above eye level to below eye level during language stimulation can increase the possibility of a response through vocalization or gesture without an increase in muscle tone.

Conclusion

Although there is little documentation to support the assertion that most SLPs believe that the trunk and intervention for trunk stability is solely the purview of the PT, this appears to be the case, based on the author's 45 years of experience, personal communication with graduate students, and clinicians who treat children with cerebral palsy. Knowledge of normal and abnormal movement patterns may not be necessary for clinicians working with motorically typical children. However, clinicians who treat children with cerebral palsy and other neuromotor disorders must be aware of these patterns and how they influence coordinated swallowing and speech production. In addition, it is important to note that SLP goals and objectives for a child remain discipline specific: language reception and expression, speech sound production, interaction, and swallowing. This does not change with NDT training.

An advantage of a speech clinician knowing NDT is that most teams working with children with cerebral palsy include a physical and occupational therapist who have already been introduced to NDT during their professional academic coursework. In fact, NDT has been described as "synonymous with pediatric PT" (VanSant, 1991). However, as things now stand, the speech-language pathologist becomes aware of this intervention only through exposure to the other disciplines. Nonetheless, familiarity with NDT principles and techniques can only enhance the ability of PTs, OTs, and SLPs to work together successfully.

Another attribute of NDT that is difficult to quantify, but important to the SLP, is the entirely new perspective it provides for assessing children with cerebral palsy. SLPs are knowledgeable about the specific movements necessary for speech production and the coordination required between the several levels of the speech production system. However, the specifics regarding the relationship between a stable trunk and its implications for speech, especially for the child with cerebral palsy, are less widely disseminated.

It appears that NDT is supported by prevailing theories of motor control and development. Until controlled studies are conducted with large numbers of homogeneous participants, a treatment approach that is theory-driven, such as NDT, may be a useful tool.

---

10 Items to Improve Intervention

1. Do not be afraid to move the child to attain better head/trunk alignment.
2. Proper positioning will provide alignment and stability.
3. Facilitate efficient, graded movements in the oral area through positioning, handling, and oral control (OWN).
4. Offer enjoyable and meaningful experiences to the child that are novel and attainable.
5. Provide the child with success in functional tasks.
6. Provide many opportunities within the session for repetition and practice.
7. Know the rationale for all techniques used and use them only when needed (OWN).
8. Look for changes immediately with your handling—or change your technique.
9. Facilitate head/trunk alignment through appropriate positioning of stimuli (food and language) and avoid hyperextension of head.
10. Use NDT as the background for other traditional SLP interventions.

**Think Critically for Self-Study
or Classroom Discussion**

1. Compare and contrast the different theories presented in this chapter.
2. How do the theories support your work with children with cerebral palsy?
3. You and a PT are both addressing a child's head and trunk alignment. What is an SLP goal that might use this technique? What might the PT's goal be?
4. Which is an appropriate goal for an SLP?
   a. Joey will attain lip closure for cup drinking. (Yes, this is a functional SLP goal)
   b. Joey will attain head/trunk alignment? (No) Why?
5. How can you incorporate NDT principles into the following:
   a. A literacy session?
   b. A board game with a peer?
   c. The preschool classroom?

References

Alexander, R. (1987). Oral-motor treatment for infants and young children with cerebral palsy. *Seminars in Speech and Language, 8,* 87–100.

Alexander, R., Boehme, R., & Cupps, B. (1993). *Normal development of functional motor skills.* San Antonio, TX: Therapy Skill Builders.

American Speech-Language-Hearing Association. (2001). Roles of speech-language pathologists in swallowing and feeding disorders: Technical report. *ASHA 2002 Desk Reference, 3,* 181–199.

American Speech-Language-Hearing Association. (2004). *Evidence-based practice in communication disorders: An introduction* (Technical report). Retrieved from http//:www.asha.org/members/desk ref-journals/deskref/default

Anderson, J., Hinojosa, J., & Strauch, C. (1987). Integrating play in neurodevelopmental treatment. *The American Journal of Occupational Therapy, 41,* 421–426.

Arvedson, J. C., & Brodsky, I. (2002). *Pediatric swallowing and feeding: Assessment and management* (2nd ed.). San Diego, CA: Singular.

Badawi, N., Felix, J. P., Kurinozuk, J. J., Dixon, G., Watson, L., Keogh, J. M., & Stanley, F. J. (2005). Cerebral palsy following term newborn encephalopathy: A population-based study. *Developmental Medicine & Child Neurology, 47,* 293–298.

Bahr, D. C. (2001). *Oral motor assessment and treatment: Ages and stages.* Boston, MA: Allyn & Bacon.

Bahr, D. C. (2003). Typical versus atypical oral motor function in the pediatric population: Beyond the checklist. *Perspectives in Swallowing and Swallowing Disorders, 12,* 4–12.

Ballard, K. J. (2001). Principles of motor learning and treatment of AOS. *Neurophysiology and Neurogenic Speech and Language Disorders Newsletter, 11,* 13–18.

Barry, M. (2001). Evidence-based practice in pediatric physical therapy. *PT Magazine Continuing Education Series No. 22,* 38–51.

Bartlett, D. J., & Palisano, R. J. (2000). A multivariate model of determinants of motor change for children with cerebral palsy. *Physical Therapy, 80,* 598–614.

Bax, M. (1964). Terminology and classification of cerebral palsy. *Developmental Medicine & Child Neurology, 6,* 295–307.

Bax, M. (2001). Medical aspects of cerebral palsy. In N. R. Finnie, *Handling the young child with cerebral palsy at home* (3rd ed., pp. 8–17). Boston, MA: Butterworth-Heinemann.

Bax, M., Goldstein, M., Rosenbaum, P., Leviton, A., & Paneth, N. (2005). Proposed definition and classification of cerebral palsy. *Developmental Medicine & Child Neurology, 47,* 571–576.

Bennett, F. C. (1999). Diagnosing cerebral palsy—the earlier the better. *Contemporary Pediatrics, 16,* 65–73.

Bergen, A. F., & Colangelo, C. (1985). *Positioning the client with central nervous system deficits: The wheel chair and other adaptive equipment* (2nd ed.). Valhalla, NY: Valhalla Rehabilitation.

Bernstein, N. A. (1967). *The co-ordination and regulation of movements.* Oxford, UK: Pergamon Press.

Bishop, D. V. M., Brown, B. B., & Robson, J. (1990). The relationship between phoneme discrimination, speech perception, and language comprehension in cerebral-palsied individuals. *Journal of Speech and Hearing Research, 23,* 210–219.

Blauw-Hospers, C. H., & Hadders-Algra, M. (2005). A systematic review of the effects of early intervention on motor development. *Developmental Medicine & Child Neurology, 47,* 421–432.

Bly, L. (1983). *The components of normal movement during the first year of life.* Oak Park, IL: Neurodevelopmental Treatment Association.

Bly, L. (1991). A historical and current view of the basis of NDT. *Pediatric Physical Therapy, 3,* 131–136.

Bobath, K. (1980). *A neurophysiological basis for the treatment of cerebral palsy*. London, UK: Heinemann.

Boliek, C. A., & Lohmeier, H. (1999). From the big bang to the brain. *Journal of Communication Disorders, 32,* 271–276.

Campbell, S. K. (1997). Therapy programs for children that last a lifetime. *Physical & Occupational Therapy in Pediatrics, 17,* 1–15.

Campbell, S. K. (2002). Foreword. In J. M. Howle, *Neurodevelopmental treatment approach* (pp. xiii–xiv). Laguna Beach, CA: Neuro-Developmental Treatment Association.

Carr, L. (2005). Commentary on definition and classification of cerebral palsy. *Developmental Medicine & Child Neurology, 47,* 508.

Cerny, F. J., Panzarella, K. J., & Stathopoulos, E. (1997). Expiratory muscle conditioning in hypotonic children with low vocal intensity levels. *Journal of Medical Speech-Language Pathology, 5,* 141–152.

Clark, E. G., & Clark, E. A. (2002). Using evidence-based practice to guide decision making in AAC. *Perspectives on Augmentative and Alternative Communication, 11,* 6–9.

Clark, H. M. (2005). Therapeutic exercise in dysphagia management: Philosophies, practices, and challenges. *Perspectives on Swallowing and Swallowing Disorders (Dysphagia), 14,* 24–27.

Clark, H. M., Robin, D. A., McCullagh, G., & Schmidt, R. A. (2001). Motor control in children and adults during a non-speech oral task. *Journal of Speech, Language, and Hearing Research, 44,* 1015–1025.

Culbertson, W., & Tanner, D. C. (2012). Observations on speech and swallowing. In R. Goldfarb (Ed.), *Translational speech-language pathology and audiology* (pp. 233–238). San Diego, CA: Plural.

Daniels, S. K., Brailey, K., & Foundas, A. L. (1999). Lingual discoordination and dysphagia following acute stroke: Analyses of lesion localization. *Dysphagia, 14,* 85–92.

Day, S. M., Strauss, D. J., Vachon, P. J., Rosenbloom, L., Shavelle, R. M., & Wu, Y. W. (2007). Growth patterns in a population of children and adolescents with cerebral palsy. *Developmental Medicine & Child Neurology, 49,* 167–171.

Dodrill, P., McMahon, S., Ward, E., Weir, K., Donovan, T., & Riddle, B. (2004). Long-term oral sensitivity and feeding skills of low-risk preterm infants. *Early Human Development, 76,* 23–37.

Dworkin, J. P., Meleca, R. J., & Stachler, R. J. (2003). More on the role of the mandible in speech production: Clinical correlates of Green, Moore, and Reilly's (2002) findings. *Journal of Speech, Language, and Hearing Research, 46,* 1016–1021.

Engelen, L., Van der Bilt, A., & Bosman, F. (2004). Relationship between oral sensitivity and masticatory performance. *Journal of Dental Research, 83,* 388–392.

Fetters, L., & Kluzik, J. (1996). The effects of neurodevelopmental treatment versus practice on the reaching of children with spastic cerebral palsy. *Physical Therapy, 76,* 346–358.

Fox, C. M., Ramig, L. O., Ciucci, M. R., Sapir, S., McFarland, D. H., & Farley, B. G. (2006). The science and practice of LSVT/LOUD: Neural plasticity-principled approach to treating individuals with Parkinson disease and other neurological disorders. *Seminars in Speech and Language, 27,* 283–299.

Green, J. R., Moore, C. A., Higashikawa, M., & Steeve, R. W. (2000). The physiologic development of speech motor control: Lip and jaw coordination. *Journal of Speech, Language, and Hearing Research, 43,* 239–255.

Green, J. R., Moore, C. A., & Reilly, K. J. (2002). The sequential development of jaw and lip control for speech. *Journal of Speech, Language, and Hearing Research, 45,* 66–79.

Green, J. R., Moore, C. A., Ruark, J. L., Rodda, P. R., Morvee, W. T., & Vanwitzenburg, M. J. (1997). Development of chewing in children from 12 to 48 months: Longitudinal study of EMG patterns. *The Journal of Neurophysiology, 77,* 2704–2716.

Hadders-Algra, M. (2000). The neuronal group selection theory: A framework to explain variation in normal motor development. *Developmental Medicine & Child Neurology, 42,* 566–572.

Hall, K. D. (2001). *Pediatric dysphagia: Resource guide.* San Diego, CA: Singular, Thomson Learning.

Hayden, D. A., & Square, P. A. (1984). Motor speech treatment hierarchy: A systems approach. *Clinical Communication Disorders, 4,* 162–174.

Herman, J. H., & Lange, M. L. (1999). Seating and positioning to manage spasticity after brain injury. *NeuroRehabilitation, 12,* 105–117.

Howle, J. M. (2002). *Neurodevelopmental treatment approach: Theoretical foundations and principles of clinical practice.* Laguna Beach, CA: NDTA.

Kamm, K., Thelen, E., & Jensen, J. L. (1990). A dynamical systems approach to motor development. *Physical Therapy, 70,* 763–775.

Kays, S., & Robbins, J. (2007). Framing oral motor exercise in principles of neural plasticity. *Perspectives in Neurophysiology and Neurogenic Speech and Language Disorders, 17,* 11–17.

Keesee, P. D. (1976). Abnormal postural reflex activity and voice usage deviations in cerebral palsy. *Physical Therapy, 56,* 1358–1360.

Kurtz, L. A. (2007). Physical therapy and occupational therapy. In M. L. Batshaw, L. Pelligrino, & N. J. Roizen (Eds.), *Children with disabilities* (pp. 571–579). Baltimore, MD: Paul H. Brookes.

Langley, M. B., & Thomas, C. (1991). Introduction to the neurodevelopmental approach. In M. B. Langley & L. J. Lombardino (Eds.), *Neurodevelopmental strategies for managing communication dis-*

orders in children with severe motor dysfunction (pp.1–28). Austin, TX: Pro-Ed.

Larnert, G., & Ekberg, O. (1995). Positioning improves the oral and pharyngeal swallowing function in children with cerebral palsy. *Acta Pediatrica, 84*, 689–692.

Lund, J. P., Appenteng, K., & Seguin, J. J. (1982). Analogies and common features in the speech and masticatory control systems. In S. Grillner, B. Lundblom, & A. Persson (Eds.), *Speech motor control*. New York, NY: Pergamon Press.

Mann, G. C. (2002). How to distinguish between outcomes, effectiveness and efficacy studies in dysphagia research. *Perspectives on Swallowing and Swallowing Disorders (Dysphagia), 11*, 5–8.

Mass, E., Robin, D. A., Hula, S. N. A., Freedman, S. E., Wulf, G., Ballard, K. J., & Schmidth, R. A. (2010). Principles of motor learning in treatment of motor speech disorders. *American Journal of Speech-Language Pathology, 17*, 277–298.

Mathiowetz, V., & Haugen, J. B. (1994). Motor behavior research: Implications for therapeutic approaches to central nervous system dysfunction. *American Journal of Occupational Therapy, 48*, 733–745.

Miller, A. J. (2002). Oral and pharyngeal reflexes in the mammalian nervous system: Their diverse range in complexity and the pivotal role of the tongue. *Critical Review of Oral Biological Medicine, 13*, 409–425.

Mohr, J. D. (1990). Management of the trunk in adult hemiplegia: The Bobath concept. *Topics in Neurology, In-Touch Series, Lesson 1*, 1–11.

Moore, C. A., & Ruark, J. L. (1996). Does speech emerge from earlier appearing oral motor behaviors? *Journal of Speech and Hearing Research, 39*, 1034–1047.

Morris, S. E. (1985). Developmental implications for the management of feeding problems in neurologically impaired infants. *Seminars in Speech and Language, 6*, 293–315.

Morris, S. E., & Klein, M. D. (2000). *Pre-feeding skills: A comprehensive resource for feeding development*. San Antonio, TX: Therapy Skill Builders.

Mueller, H. (1972). Facilitating feeding and prespeech. In P. H. Pearson & C. E. Williams (Eds.), *Physical therapy services in the developmental disabilities* (pp. 283–310). Springfield, IL: Thomas.

Mueller, H. (2001). Feeding. In N. R. Finnie, *Handling the young child with cerebral palsy at home* (3rd ed., pp. 209–221). Boston, MA: Butterworth-Heinemann.

Mysak, E. D. (1980). *Neurospeech therapy for the cerebral palsied*. New York, NY: Teachers College Press.

Nashner, L. M., Shumway-Cook, A., & Marin, O. (1983). Stance posture control in select groups of children with cerebral palsy: Deficits in sensory organization and muscular coordination. *Experimental Brain Research, 49*, 393–409.

Neilson, P. D., & O'Dwyer, N. J. (1984). Reproducibility and variability of speech muscle activity in athetoid dysarthria of cerebral palsy. *Journal of Speech and Hearing Research, 27*, 502–517.

Nwaobi, O., Brubaker, C., Cusick, B., & Sussman, M. (1983). Electromyographic investigation of extensor activity in cerebral-palsied children in different seating positions. *Developmental Medicine & Child Neurology, 25*, 175–183.

Okimoto, A. M., Bundy, A., & Hanzlik, J. (2000). Playfulness in children with and without disability: Measurement and intervention. *The American Journal of Occupational Therapy, 54*, 73–82.

Ottenbacher, K., Bundy, A., & Short, M. A. (1983). The development and treatment of oral-motor dysfunction: A review of clinical research. *Physical & Occupational Therapy in Pediatrics, 3*, 1–13.

Palisano, R. J. (1991). Research on the effectiveness of neurodevelopmental treatment. *Pediatric Physical Therapy, 3*, 143–148.

Pennington, L., Goldbart, J., & Marshall, J. (2003). Speech and language therapy to improve the communication skills of children with cerebral palsy. *The Cochrane Database of Systematic Reviews, 3*, Art. No.: CD003466. doi:10.1002/14651858.CD003466

Pennington, L., Goldbart, J., & Marshall, J. (2005). Speech and language therapy to improve the communication skills of children with cerebral palsy. *Developmental Medicine & Child Neurology, 47*, 57–63.

Pennington, L., Miller, N., Robson, S., & Sheen, N. (2010). Intensive speech and language therapy for older children with cerebral palsy: A systems approach. *Developmental Medicine & Child Neurology, 52*, 337–344.

Pennington, L., Smallman, C., & Farrier, F. (2006). Intensive dysarthria therapy for older children with cerebral palsy: Findings from six cases. *Child Language Teaching and Therapy, 22*, 255–273.

Pinder, G. L., & Faherty, A. S. (1999). Issues in pediatric feeding and swallowing. In A. J. Caruso & E. A. Strand (Eds.), *Clinical management of motor speech disorders in children* (pp. 281–318). New York, NY: Thieme.

Pinder, G. L., & Olswang, L. B. (1995). Development of communicative intent in young children with cerebral palsy: A treatment efficacy study. *Infant-Toddler Intervention, 5*, 51–70.

Reddy, S. K. (2005). Commentary on definition and classification of cerebral palsy. *Developmental Medicine & Child Neurology, 47*, 508–509.

Redstone, F., & West, J. F. (2004). Postural control for feeding. *Pediatric Nursing, 30*, 97–100.

Reed, E. S., & Bril, B. (1996). Primacy of action in development. In N. A. Bernstein (author); M. L. Latash & M. T. Turvey (Eds.), *Dexterity and its development* (pp. 431–452). Mahwah, NJ: Lawrence Erlbaum Associates.

Reilly, S., Skuse, D., & Pobiete, X. (1996). Prevalence of feeding problems and oral motor dysfunction in children with cerebral palsy: A community survey. *Journal of Pediatrics, 129,* 877–882.

Rogers, B., Arvedson, J., Buck, G., Smart, P., & Msall, M. (1994). Characteristics of dysphagia in children with cerebral palsy. *Dysphagia, 9,* 60–73.

Rosenfeld-Johnson, S. (1999). *Oral-motor exercises for speech clarity.* Tucson, AZ: Innovative Therapists.

Sapienza, C. (2007). *Respiratory muscle strength training: Application and interpretation.* Presentation at the New York State Speech-Language-Hearing Association Convention. Buffalo, NY.

Schmidt, R. A. (1975). A schema theory of discrete motor skill learning. *Psychological Review, 82,* 225–260.

Schmidt, R. A., & Lee, T. D. (2005). *Motor control & learning: A behavioral emphasis* (4th ed.). Champaign, IL: Human Kinetics.

Seikel, J. A., King, D. W., & Drumwright, D. G. (2000). *Anatomy and physiology for speech, language, and hearing* (2nd ed.). San Diego, CA: Singular.

Sheppard, J. J. (2005). The role of sensorimotor therapy in the treatment of pediatric dysphagia. *Perspectives on Swallowing and Swallowing Disorders (Dysphagia), 14,* 6–10.

Shumway-Cook, A., & Woollacott, M. H. (2001). *Motor control. Theory and practical applications* (2nd ed.). Philadelphia, PA: Lippincott Williams & Wilkins.

Smith, A., McFarland, D. H., & Weber, C. M. (1986). Interactions between speech and finger movements: An exploration of the dynamic pattern perspective. *Journal of Speech and Hearing Research, 29,* 471–480.

Sporns, O., & Edelman, G. M. (1993). Solving Bernstein's problem: A proposal for the development of coordinated movement by selection. *Child Development, 64,* 960–981.

Steele, C. M. (2006). *Reflections on evidence-based-practice.* Retrieved April 8, 2006 from http://www.asha.org/about/membership-certification/divs/div13member/v13n4EBPSteele.htm

Steeve, R. W., & Moore, C. A. (2009). Mandibular motor control during the early development of speech and nonspeech behaviors. *Journal of Speech, Language, and Hearing Research, 52,* 1530–1554.

Steeve, R. W., Moore, C. A., Green, J. R., Reilly, K. J., & McMurtrey, J. R. (2008). Babbling, chewing, and sucking: Oromandibular coordination at 9 months. *Journal of Speech, Language, and Hearing Research, 51,* 1390–1404.

Sullivan, P. B., Lambert, B., Rose, M., Ford-Adams, M., Johnson, A., & Griffiths, P. (2000). The prevalence and severity of feeding and nutritional problems in children with neurological impairment: Oxford feeding study. *Developmental Medicine & Child Neurology, 42,* 674–680.

Tamura, F., Mizukami, M., Ayano, R., & Mukai, Y. (2002). Analysis of feeding function and jaw stability in bedridden elderly. *Dysphagia, 17,* 235–241.

Thelen, E. (1991). Motor aspects of emergent speech: A dynamic approach. In N. Krasnegor (Ed.), *Biobehavioral foundations of language acquisition* (pp. 339–362). Hillsdale, NJ: Erlbaum.

Thelen, E. (1995). Motor development: A new synthesis. *American Psychologist, 50,* 79–95.

Thelen, E., & Smith, L. (2002). *A dynamic systems approach to the development of cognition and action.* Cambridge, MA: MIT Press.

Touwen, B. C. L. (1998). The brain and development of function. *Developmental Review, 18,* 504–526.

Treviranus, J., & Roberts, V. (2003). Supporting competent motor control of AAC systems. In J. C. Light, D. R. Beukelman, & J. Reichle (Eds.), *Communicative competence for individuals who use AAC: From research to effective practice* (pp. 199–240). Baltimore, MD: Paul H. Brookes.

VanSant, A. F. (1991). Neurodevelopmental treatment and pediatric physical therapy: A commentary. *Pediatric Physical Therapy, 3,* 137–141.

West, J. F., & Redstone, F. (2004). Alignment during feeding and swallowing: Does it matter? A review. *Perceptual and Motor Skills, 98,* 349–358.

Wolf, L. S., & Glass, R. P. (1992). *Feeding and swallowing disorders in infancy: Assessment and management.* Tucson, AZ: Therapy Skill Builders.

Workinger, M. S. (2005). *Cerebral palsy resource guide for speech-language pathologists.* Clifton Park, NY: Thomson Delmar Learning.

World Health Organization. (2001). *International classification of functioning, disability and health.* Retrieved August 10, 2003, from http://www.who.int

Yorkston, K. M. (1996). Treatment efficacy: Dysarthria. *Journal of Speech, Language, and Hearing Research, 39,* S46–S57.

Yorkston, K. M., Beukelman, D. R., Strand, E. A., & Bell, K. R. (1999). *Management of motor speech disorders in children and adults* (2nd ed.). Austin, TX: Pro-Ed.

Zemlin, W. R. (1998). *Speech and hearing science: Anatomy and physiology* (3rd ed.). Boston, MA: Allyn & Bacon.

CHAPTER 3

ABCs of CP and Accompanying Motor Speech Disorders: An Overview

Marilyn S. Workinger

Introduction

There are approximately three-quarters of a million individuals in the United States with cerebral palsy (United Cerebral Palsy (UCP), 2013) with about 10,000 babies born each year who may develop the symptoms of cerebral palsy (Center for Disease Control and Prevention (CDCP), 2013). In order to provide the best possible services for these individuals, the speech-language pathologist (SLP) must have a basic understanding of the underlying disorder as well as the communication disorder itself. With limited time available for treatment and limited resources for accessing services, clinicians must be able to assess the communication disorder early and formulate an appropriate treatment program.

Definition of Cerebral Palsy

Although multiple definitions of cerebral palsy have appeared in the literature, each with a slightly different emphasis, collectively they are encompassed in a definition proposed at the International Workshop on Definition and Classification of Cerebral Palsy in 2004 stating: "Cerebral palsy describes a group of disorders of the development of movement and posture, causing activity limitation, that are attributed to non-progressive disturbances that occurred in the developing fetal or infant brain . . . " and may be accompanied by " . . . disturbances of sensation, cognition, communication, perception, and/or behavior, and/or by a seizure disorder" (Bax et al., 2005, p. 572).

Thus, the term "cerebral palsy" refers to a group of disorders. The lesion (damage to the brain) that causes cerebral palsy is nonprogressive and occurs early in brain development. The condition (symptoms caused by the damage to the brain) can change over time. The inability to develop normal movement patterns and postures is a result of the lesion, and individuals can demonstrate associated disorders, including disorders of sensation, communication, perception, cognition, and/or behavior. Seizure disorders are also common. The associated conditions present for any individual relate to the nature and extent of the lesion.

Classification of Cerebral Palsy

As with the definition of cerebral palsy, classification of the types of cerebral palsy has evolved over time. The terms used to define the types relate to muscle tone and movement characteristics. Howle (2002) defined muscle tone as " . . . the 'stiffness' or tension with which a muscle resists being lengthened" (p.128). She describes four classic types of cerebral palsy:

- Spastic: In this condition, muscles are stiff. Muscle tone is increased with velocity-dependent resistance to passive movement. Motor control is reduced. Movement synergies are abnormal and limited, and there is limited range of movement. Muscle activation and postural response is slow.

■ Dyskinetic: Movements appear uncontrolled and involuntary. Movements are abnormal in timing, direction, and spatial characteristics. Reversal of movement and/or latency of movement can be present. There is impaired postural stability. Athetosis, rigidity, and tremor are included in this category.

■ Hypotonic: In this condition, resting muscle tension is diminished. There is decreased ability to generate voluntary muscle force. Also seen are excessive joint flexibility and postural instability. This is often a transient condition with evolution to spasticity or athetosis.

■ Ataxic: Postural control is impaired and balance is disordered. There is imprecise control in timing of coordinated movement, and force is decreased during movement. This condition is frequently associated with hypotonia and tremor may be present.

The term "mixed" is often used to describe an individual who presents with more than one of the classic types of cerebral palsy. However, there may be changes to this system of classification including the elimination of the term "mixed" (Bax et al., 2005).

Typically, the motor disorder is also classified by degree and/or distribution. Monoplegia refers to involvement of a single extremity (rare). The term hemiplegia indicates involvement of the arm and leg on the same body side. Diplegia refers to involvement of all four limbs with greater involvement of the legs than the arms. Individuals who demonstrate quadriplegia or tetraplegia have involvement of all extremities with the arms and legs equally affected or the arms and upper body more severely involved than the legs. Triplegia refers to involvement of three extremities (rare), and paraplegia indicates involvement of only the legs (rare). Involvement of all four extremities with one body side more involved than the other could be described as double hemiplegia or quadriplegia with a superimposed hemiplegia.

Evaluation of the functional status of the individual using objective scales has been recommended. Scales most often used are the Gross Motor Function Classification System (GMFCS)

(Palisano et al., 1997) and the Manual Ability Classification System (MACS) (Eliasson et al., 2006). Recently, the Communication Function Classification System (CFCS) was developed for functional evaluation of communication skills (Hidecker et al., 2011). No formal scale for evaluation of speech and oromotor function is currently available.

Causes of Cerebral Palsy

The cause of cerebral palsy may be either congenital or acquired. Congenital causes are those occurring before or during birth and account for almost 90% of reported cases (United Cerebral Palsy, 2013). Acquired causes are those occurring after birth, before anatomical or physiological maturation of the brain is complete.

Among the most common risk factors for congenital cerebral palsy are low birth weight and premature birth. This is particularly true for infants weighing <1,500 grams and for infants born at, or before, 31 weeks gestation. Disruption of blood and oxygen supply to the brain, brain malformations, and infection in the mother are additional risk factors. Odding, Roebroeck, and Stam (2006) reported that multiple gestation pregnancies were a significant risk factor. The upper age limit for diagnosis of cerebral palsy remains controversial. The most frequent postnatal cerebral palsy causes are head injury, shaken baby syndrome, cerebrovascular events, and infection (such as meningitis) (CDC, 2013; UCP, 2013; Yeargin-Allsopp, Boyle, Braun, & Trevathan, 2008).

Menkes and Flores-Sarnat (2006) report that up to 10% of cases diagnosed as cerebral palsy may be due to chromosomal anomalies and continuous gene syndromes. Typically, these children have no clear etiology for their motor disorder, and often present with hypotonia or congenital anomalies. Kelley (2008) advises that children who are thought to have cerebral palsy may show metabolic disorders. These children can present as only having cerebral palsy for several years before regression or other symptoms emerge. Clinicians working with children diagnosed with cerebral palsy should be alert for signs of regression or other changes in medical status and report these to caregivers and/or medical providers.

Associated Conditions

In addition to the motor disorder, individuals diagnosed with cerebral palsy may demonstrate a broad array of associated conditions that can be present at birth or appear later in development. These associated conditions can have a profound effect on functional ability for communication and/or feeding and swallowing in either a child or adult and need to be considered in the treatment planning process.

Cognitive Deficits

Intellectual impairment is one of the most common associated disorders. Among children with cerebral palsy, prevalence of intellectual impairment varies from 20 to 70% (Beckung & Hagberg, 2002; Pelligrino, 2007; Sigurdardottir et al., 2008; Surveillance of Cerebral Palsy in Europe, 2002). However, scores over 85 have also been found (Sigurdardottir et al., 2008). Children with hemiplegia and diplegia exhibited higher scores than those with quadriplegia or dyskinesia, and children with spastic diplegia and quadriplegia performed more poorly on performance tasks than on verbal. Children who could not fully participate in standardized assessment because of motor involvement were assessed by alternate means, and 20% had developmental quotients greater than 85, underscoring the notion that motor involvement can mask the individual's true intellectual ability. When a child cannot participate in standardized testing we should not automatically assume low intellect.

Seizure Disorders

The prevalence of seizure disorders in children with cerebral palsy ranges from 27% to 50% (Kwong, Wong, & So, 1998; Nordmark, Hagglund, & Lagergren, 2001; Sigurdardottir et al., 2008). Children most likely to develop seizures include those with severe intellectual and/or motor involvement, brain malformation, infection, or gray matter injury (Pelligrino, 2007).

Visual Impairments

Visual impairments are common in individuals with cerebral palsy. A study of 164 patients revealed visual disturbance in 71% of participants (Schenk-Rootlieb, van Nieuwenhuizen, van der Graaf, Wittebol-Pose, & Willemse, 1992). The extent of visual involvement can vary by etiology or type of cerebral palsy (Guzetta, Mercuri, & Cioni, 2001). For example, premature infants may have visual impairment caused by retinopathy of prematurity. Nystagmus, a condition with involuntary oscillating eye movements, is more common in children with ataxia whereas children with hemiplegia can exhibit homonymous hemianopia, which is the loss of one part of the visual field. Strabismus is also common, and optic atrophy or delayed visual maturation may also be present. It is interesting that children with cerebral palsy are more likely to be farsighted than typically developing children (Ashwal et al., 2004; Sobrado, Suarez, Garcia-Sanchez, & Uson, 1999). As might be expected, severity of visual impairment varies with increased levels of severity on the GMFCS (Pruitt & Tsai, 2009).

Hearing Impairments

Estimates of frequency of hearing loss in children with cerebral palsy range from 30 to 40% (Pruitt & Tsai, 2009). Sensorineural (SN) hearing loss in infants shares risk factors with cerebral palsy which include pre- or postnatal exposure to viruses, bacteria or other toxins, hypoxic damage to the cochlea, intracranial hemorrhage, and neonatal hyperbilirubinemia. Premature infants, especially those weighing <1,500 grams, are particularly susceptible to these problems. Infants with these exposures should have baseline testing as soon as possible and have their hearing tested at least once per year (Herer, Knightly, & Steinberg, 2007).

Herer and colleagues (2007) report that children with cerebral palsy are at risk for chronic otitis media with effusion, and their hearing should be screened regularly. Granet, Balaghi, and Jaeger (1997) report that 6% of adults with cerebral palsy have hearing impairment.

Dental Issues

The prevalence of dental caries and other oral health issues is greater in children with cerebral palsy than in the general population (Rodrigues dos Santos, Masiero, Novo, & Simionato, 2003) and there is an increased prevalence of malocclusion in children with cerebral palsy (Franklin, Luther, & Curzon, 1996). In fact, it appears that occlusal characteristics vary with the type of cerebral palsy. Carmagnani, Goncalves, Correa, and dos Santos (2007) report that individuals with spastic cerebral palsy showed a high incidence of open bite and Class II malocclusion (overbite) whereas overbite and tooth wear were prominent in individuals with athetosis. It should also be remembered that malocclusion may affect eating efficiency and control of saliva (Schwartz, Gisel, Clarke, & Haberfellner, 2003; Tahmassebi & Luther, 2004).

Osteoporosis and Osteopenia

Some studies have indicated that bone density is reduced in almost all tested children with cerebral palsy (Henderson et al., 2002; Tasdemir et al., 2001). Increased risk of fracture can have significant implications for safety in the positioning and handling of children in school and therapy settings.

Contractures and Deformities

The term "contracture" refers to shortening of a muscle that limits joint mobility and leads to deformities such as scoliosis and hip dislocation (Pelligrino, 2007). Appropriate positioning, physical therapy, orthoses, and surgical intervention can limit the progression and severity of the deformities (Graham, 2004).

Disorders of Touch

Odding et al. (2006) reported disorders of stereognosis and two-point discrimination in children with cerebral palsy at a rate of 44 to 51%. Sensory impairments were most often seen in individuals with hemiplegia. Cooper, Majnemer, Rosenblatt, and Birnbaum (1995) found that 9 of 10 hemiplegic children showed bilateral sensory deficits, most commonly stereognosis and proprioception. However, the extent of sensory deficit did not necessarily reflect the severity of motor involvement. Nonetheless, the type and extent of sensory deficits should be considered when choosing or working with augmentative communication systems.

Behavioral Issues

McDermott et al. (1996) reported that children with cerebral palsy were over five times more likely to demonstrate behavioral problems than control subjects. Behavioral issues have been studied primarily by parental report (Brossard-Racine et al., 2012; Sigurdardottir et al., 2010). It has been found that 40 to 50% of parents characterized their child as having behavioral and emotional difficulties, whereas teachers reported an incidence of 60 to 65%. These behaviors included attention problems, aggressive behavior, anxiety, and depression. Parental distress correlated significantly with conduct problems and emotional disturbances. There is also an indication that behavioral issues persist and peer problems seem to increase with age (Brossard-Racine et al., 2013).

Along with behavioral issues, an increased frequency of sleep disorders in children with cerebral palsy has been identified. Newman, O'Regan, and Hensey (2006) reported sleep disorders in 23% of 6 to 11-year-olds with cerebral palsy, compared to 5% of typically developing peers. Among sleep problems most frequently noted were: difficulty with initiation and maintenance of sleep, sleep–wake transition, and disorders of breathing during sleep, with higher prevalence in the presence of epilepsy and among single-parent families.

In addition to the child, parents are adversely affected by caring for a child with cerebral palsy. Majnemer, Shevell, Law, Poulin, and Rosenbaum (2012) found that parents of school-aged children with cerebral palsy are likely to experience high levels of stress, increased time constraints, financial concerns, and psychological burdens. Sleep disorders and depression are also commonly seen in parents of children with cerebral palsy (Sajedi, Alizad, Malekkhosravi, Karimlou, & Vameghi, 2010; Sawyer et al., 2011; Wayte, McCaughey, Holley, Annaz, & Hill, 2012).

Autism Spectrum Disorders

In recent years, attention has been directed toward the occurrence of autism spectrum disorders in individuals with cerebral palsy. Kilincaslan and Mukaddes (2009) found 11% of their sample met the criteria for autism and 4% for pervasive developmental disorder not otherwise specified (PDD-NOS). Both disorders were more common in children with tetraplegia, hemiplegia, and mixed cerebral palsy. In addition, the presence of epilepsy, cognitive impairment, limited speech production, and family history of autism increased the prevalence. Kirby et al. (2011) reported that 8% of their large sample of 8-year-olds with cerebral palsy also showed co-occurring autism spectrum disorders, pervasive developmental disorder (PDD), or Asperger disorder.

Cans (2009) noted the difficulty in differentiating characteristics of autism spectrum disorders and intellectual impairment, from the complications of communication disorders in children with cerebral palsy. She acknowledged the need for diagnosticians to consider the possible presence of autism spectrum disorders in children with cerebral palsy.

Feeding and Swallowing Disorders

Feeding and swallowing disorders can be some of the first signs of involvement in as many as 60% of children diagnosed with cerebral palsy (Odding et al., 2006). Dysphagia has been positively related to the severity of motor impairment in cerebral palsy (Calis et al., 2008). Interestingly, parents of children with moderate to severe dysphagia tended to underestimate its prevalence. Rogers, Arvedson, Buck, Smart, and Msall (1994) reviewed the records of 90 patients, ages 1 week to 22 years, who presented with severe motor involvement and concerns regarding inadequate airway protection during feedings. Videofluoroscopic modified barium swallow (VMBS) studies showed abnormalities of both the oral and pharyngeal phases of swallow. Reduced tongue control and delayed oral phase of swallow were present in over 90% of the patients. Silent aspiration was present in 97%.

Drooling

Parkes, Hill, Platt, and Donnelly (2010) reported drooling in 20% of their population sample. Two types of drooling can be encountered in individuals with cerebral palsy. Typically, drooling is thought of as " . . . the abnormal, unintentional spilling of saliva from the mouth onto the lips, chin, neck, clothing, and environmental objects" (Arvedson & Brodsky, 2002, pp. 495–496). Posterior drooling can be even more troublesome. In this situation, secretions pool in the hypopharynx. When secretions move into the pharynx, audible breathing, coughing, gagging, vomiting, and possible aspiration can occur (Arvedson & Brodsky, 2002; Blasco, 1996). Drooling can result from a variety of factors including: mouth breathing secondary to nasal obstruction, inability to maintain a closed mouth posture, reduced sensation, difficulty with formation or control of the saliva bolus, or swallowing issues. Allaire (2001) has hypothesized that a bolus of saliva may be more difficult to control than a bolus of food because of differences in size, weight, and texture of the bolus.

Disorders of Communication

Disorders of communication include speech disorders and receptive and expressive language disorders. Individuals with cerebral palsy can demonstrate the gamut of communication disorders, from stuttering to specific language deficits, to developmental articulation disorders. Communication disorders can occur in any combination. Prevalence estimates of communication disorders in individuals with cerebral palsy vary from 30% (Pelligrino, 2007) to 80% (Odding et al., 2006). Parkes et al. (2010) studied oromotor and communication dysfunction in a large population of individuals with cerebral palsy, and reported that 33% showed motor speech involvement and 37% had some degree of communication impairment. The presence of oromotor and communication disorders correlated to the level of gross motor function and the degree of intellectual impairment.

In a study of communication disorders by type of cerebral palsy, Andersen, Mjoen, and Vik (2010) found that 92% of children with dyskinesia/athetosis, 43% of children with spastic quadriplegia, and 11% of children with hemiplegia exhibited speech disorders. These variances may relate to the differences in type and location of the underlying lesion.

The Natural History of Cerebral Palsy

With improved medical care for neonates, most children with cerebral palsy will live to adulthood. Researchers have identified some factors that affect an individual's life span. Strauss, Shavelle, and Anderson (1998) looked at survival rates by functional ability and found that mobility and feeding skills were the best functional predictors of life span. Among children with good motor and eating skills, 90% or more reached adulthood.

Early Years

Parents of infants with risk factors for cerebral palsy are generally consumed with the medical aspects of the infant's condition, and are dealing with the psychological trauma of having a child with an unexpected medical condition. This may create financial, family, and work-related stressors. Typically, unless the child's involvement is severe, a diagnosis of cerebral palsy is not usually made until 1 to 2 years of age or later.

As delays in development and other medical conditions become apparent, the family becomes increasingly involved with medical and therapy providers. Early intervention programs typically provide in-home therapy services for children until the age of 3. One of the primary concerns of most families during the early years is whether or not their child will walk. Bobath and Bobath (1975) note that severity of motor involvement and level of cognitive impairment are the primary predictors for physical abilities. These authors state that children with spasticity reach their motor development peak by 6 to 8 years of age, and children with athetosis or ataxia could see progress until the age of 15 or later. More recently, the Gross Motor Classification System has been developed, which can assist in identifying the present level of motor function and predict future levels (Palisano et al., 1997; Rosenbaum et al., 2002).

Early School Years

Once children enter school programs, therapies are provided within the framework of the school program through close collaboration between therapists and teachers. Some families seek additional therapy services outside the school system, dependent upon availability of services through the school program and needs of the child. Mobility equipment and other assistive technology may be needed as the child is growing and spending more time away from family.

Need for neuropsychological assessment usually becomes apparent as the child enters the primary grades. In most communities, mainstreaming is the preferred method of education, and accommodations, if necessary, must be made to ensure success.

Medical intervention, in the form of orthopedic surgeries, spasticity management, management of feeding issues, and/or management of seizures may impact the child's attendance and performance at school. Communication between the parents, medical providers, and school personnel is, again, key to successful school performance and medical intervention.

Later School Years and Adolescence

Adolescence is a challenging time for typically developing children, and perhaps even more so for those with cerebral palsy. Medical issues continue to demand attention and take time away from school. In many educational environments, therapy services are not as readily available as in earlier years, but caregivers continue to advocate for their child's needed services. Decisions about the direction of education, for example, academic versus vocational, need to be made. Planning for transition from school to postschool environments must begin.

Adulthood

As young adults transition from school to community, many barriers exist despite the expansion of community programs for social and vocational opportunities. Bjornson, Kobayashi, Zhou, and Walker (2011) reported that 48% of subjects, ages 19 to 21, with cerebral palsy or spina bifida were enrolled in postsecondary education and nearly a quarter of them had paid employment. Receiving physical and/or occupational therapy services during the teenage years correlated with enrollment in postsecondary educational programs, whereas social interaction and expressive language skills correlated with paid employment. However, chronic health problems have been reported that can interfere with function (Mesterman et al., 2010).

Moll and Cott (2013) reported on nine adults who had intensive habilitation services in childhood focusing on "normalizing" movement, which were withdrawn in adolescence, because their level of potential was ostensibly reached. The adults felt they lost functional abilities over time after these services were withdrawn, and frustration was expressed with lack of access to therapy services. As they age, individuals experience multiple medical conditions, including musculoskeletal issues, gastrointestinal problems, fatigue, and pain (Bohmer, Klinkenberg-Knol, Niezen-de Boer, & Meuwissen, 2000; Brunner & Doderlein, 1996; Jahnsen, Villien, Stanghelle, & Holm, 2003; Turk, Scandale, Rosenbaum, & Weber, 2001).

Speech Production

Acquisition of Speech in Typically Developing Children

Development of speech production in a typical infant is generally taken for granted and leads to the much heralded first word around 1 year of age. It is necessary to look at the development of sound production by the typical infant to better understand the nature of speech disorders in children with cerebral palsy. Netsell (1986) put forward several hypotheses regarding development of speech production, including "speech is a motor skill" and "speech motor control is an acquired motor skill" (p. 27).

The infant learns through imitation of speech patterns of the adult model.

A "sensitive period" of acquisition of speech motor control occurs during the third to twelfth months. If the infant has not matured at normal or near normal rates by this time, there is risk of delays or other abnormalities in speech production. Speech motor control during the first 24 months is devoted to development of spatial goals that yield acoustic patterns similar to the model. This involves practice with placement, shaping, and movement of the component parts. Development of spatial-temporal coordination follows this with increasing precision and timing of speech production resulting in more mature patterns. Timing of segment durations then develops and is influenced by linguistic content. Refinement continues to approximately 11 years of age, as the development of speech motor skills is a continuous and nonlinear process.

Acquisition of speech motor skills has been described by multiple authors (Boliek, Hixon, Watson, & Morgan, 1996, 1997; Netsell, 1986; Proctor, 1989; Robb & Bleile, 1994) and includes the development of the subsystems of the speech production system. Gross motor development of the infant provides the support for this development.

Respiratory and Laryngeal Systems

At birth, the respiratory and laryngeal systems are coordinated for crying. By 3 months of age, fundamental frequency varies with emotional state and there is easy onset of phonation. Consonant–vowel combinations emerge by 4 months. By 6 months of age, there is stable subglottal air pressure for up to three syllables with productions lasting 2 to 3 seconds. There is rising and falling inflection in crying and coo/babble productions. Voiced/voiceless consonants are produced indicating abductor/adductor reciprocation at the level of the vocal folds.

By 9 months of age, spontaneous phonation of greater than 3 seconds is noted. Sentence-like intonation can be heard by 14 months of age, and respiratory support is adequate for production of two-syllable words at 15 months of age. By 24 months of age, there is loudness variation within phrases and inflection for greetings and interjections are appropriate.

Velopharyngeal System

Up until approximately 3 months of age, most sound production consists of nasalized vowels. By 6 months of age, the nasal/non-nasal differentiation of /m/ and /b/ are present.

Orofacial System

At birth, most oral movement is reflexive and relates to feeding. At approximately 3 months of age, vowel production progresses from schwa variants to fronted vowels. Lip closure is achieved, and lip rounding or spreading may be seen. Velar consonants may be heard, particularly when the infant is in a supine position. By 6 months of age, there is sustained jaw position for production of prolonged vowels. Jaw, lip, and tongue movement are coordinated for consonant production, and velar and alveolar consonants are heard. Bilabial consonants are produced with synchronous lip and jaw movement.

Graded jaw movement for vowel-to-vowel transitions is present by 9 months, as is a full range of movement of the lips in consonant production. By 10 months, coordination of oral structures is adequate for production of consonant (C)–Vowel (V) or CVC combinations. By 12 months, jaw stability is seen in production of CVCV combinations, and tongue shaping is possible for /r, s, z, u/, and /ð/. By 14 months of age, babbling contains a variety of consonants. An inventory of approximately six consonants is present by age 18 months from the set /b, d, g, t, m, n, h, w, l/. By 24 months, a full range of vowels and diphthongs is present and all consonants of the primary language have been produced at least once. At this age, the consonant inventory will contain 10 to 20 consonants of the set previously noted with additions from /p, k, f, s, z, d ʒ, j/.

Acquisition of Speech in Children with Cerebral Palsy

Dysarthria is the most common speech disorder seen in individuals with cerebral palsy.

Netsell (2001) defined dysarthrias as "a group of speech disorders resulting from neural lesions that yield a variety of movement disorders of the vocal tract" (p. 415). Disturbances in speech motor control can be secondary to abnormal muscle tone,

strength, coordination, and/or endurance of the speech musculature. Affected parameters of speech production can be range,
force, speed, timing, and accuracy of movement (Duffy, 1995).
Adults with acquired dysarthria resulting either from degenerative diseases, trauma, or stroke have had some period of normal
speech production, and, therefore, have a memory of the acoustic, tactile, and kinesthetic properties of a normal model. This
differs from children with cerebral palsy who have not had such
a model, and treatment of their dysarthria should be considered
habilitation rather than rehabilitation.

Little information regarding the long-term process of development of speech production in children with cerebral palsy is
known. Differences between the diagnostic classifications are
present, and there is a general, but typical, sequence of development of speech production (Rutherford, 1944; Workinger, 2005).

Spastic Cerebral Palsy

Children who present with mild to moderate spastic diplegia or
quadriplegia develop speech along the normal developmental
sequence. Articulation skills are generally appropriate for age,
but they may demonstrate reduced loudness levels and subtle indicators of laryngeal involvement, for example, breathy
voice quality. Children with more severe motor involvement
may present more extensive involvement of all speech subsystems. A perceptual study of the dysarthrias of cerebral palsy by
Workinger and Kent (1991) showed that children with spasticity
tend to have involvement of the respiratory and laryngeal systems. Speech dimensions most characteristic of this group were
breathy voice quality, monopitch, monoloudness, hypernasality,
and voice quality changes through an utterance. Children with
spasticity show less articulation errors than those with athetosis.
Types of errors in order of prevalence were omission with vowel
errors, substitutions, and nasalization errors. Omission errors,
particularly in the final position of words or at the end of an
utterance, may relate to reduced respiratory support.

As children grow, they sometimes experience increased difficulty with laryngeal and respiratory involvement, particularly
during periods of rapid growth. For example, a first-grader may
be referred for speech therapy services, because the teacher has
difficulty hearing the child's voice over the noise of the class-

room, or the parent cannot hear the child from the back seat of the car. In adolescence, as growth and weight gain continue, children may spend more time sitting and become less active. Contractures and deformities may develop that restrict respiratory function and are reflected in regression of the laryngeal voice quality, resonant voice quality (increased hypernasality), and respiratory support (Workinger, 2005). Severely involved children may need augmentative communication systems early in the development of communication skills, and those who do develop intelligible speech may need to supplement their verbalization with amplification or alphabet boards in situations where they cannot make themselves heard.

Dyskinetic Cerebral Palsy

Children diagnosed with dyskinetic (athetoid) cerebral palsy usually present with hypotonia and may not show the movement patterns typical of dyskinesia until 18 to 24 months of age. In early years, their vocalizations may be limited to vowel production. They may not produce word approximations until 4 to 7 years of age. Depending on their motor and cognitive abilities, they may be good candidates for augmentative communication systems early in development.

As they gain body weight and stability, children with athetosis can show improved speech production. All speech subsystems tend to be involved. Workinger and Kent (1991) showed that the speech dimensions most characteristic of speakers with athetosis were slow rate, dysrhythmia, inappropriate voice stoppage or release, and reduced stress. The most frequent articulation errors for children with athetosis were substitutions, vowel errors and substitutions, then voicing errors and additions. Phrase duration for children with athetosis was two to three times longer than for children with spasticity (Workinger, 1986). Some individuals with athetosis may develop intelligible speech production as late as adolescence or early adulthood.

Childhood Apraxia of Speech (CAS)

CAS is a second neurologically based disorder of speech production seen in children with cerebral palsy, sometimes in conjunction with dysarthria. Morley (1965) defined what she called "developmental articulatory dyspraxia" as "the failure or limited ability to control and direct the movements and coordinations of the respiratory, laryngeal, and oral muscles for articulation when muscle tone is otherwise adequate" (p. vii). CAS is a disorder of motor planning rather than a disorder of basic motor control. However, some recent research has indicated that CAS may also have a phonological component (Froud & Khamis-Dakwar, 2012) with implications for language development. If a child presents with both moderate to severe dysarthria and CAS, the prognosis for significant improvement tends to be more limited than if a single disorder is present.

Speech Assessment

Tone, Posture, and Movement

Postural stability is very important in order to accomplish distal movements such as pointing or gesturing with an arm or finger, or the production of speech. The speech pathologist should make observations about the child's ability to support the trunk, shoulder, girdle, and neck, noting any structural issues that would limit range of motion. Muscle tone and any abnormal movement patterns that may influence speech production should also be noted. Observations identifying the postures in which a child spends the most time should be made. Speech production should be observed in a variety of positions to determine their effect on loudness, voice quality, and articulation. Abnormal patterns of movement, which interfere with speech production, such as extensor thrusting, should be noted. These observations differentiate the evaluation of the whole child from a typical SLP assessment which only considers the communication disorder and is more limited in scope.

Structure of the Speech Mechanism

Formal evaluation of the speech mechanism in children, particularly young children, is sometimes difficult. Besides formal examination, valuable information can be obtained through observation of play, eating, and speaking. Symmetry and structural anomalies of the face, lips, tongue, and palate should be noted. Any differences in tissue status (e.g., redness may indicate inflammation) of the mouth or face and health of the teeth should be observed. Dental occlusion should be assessed, particularly if malocclusion may impact the child's ability to achieve lip closure. Status of dental health should be noted since oral pain may negatively affect the child's willingness to participate in communication activities.

Respiratory Function

Information regarding any medical conditions affecting the child's respiratory status may be available through parent interviews or in review of medical records. This will be important in assessing adequacy of respiratory support and for treatment planning. In the clinical setting, an oral manometer can estimate subglottal air pressure for speech production in children who are able to participate in formal evaluation (Hixon, Hawley, & Wilson, 1982; Netsell & Hixon, 1978).

Informal methods include observation of rest breathing and breathing during speech production. Sustained phonation can be measured in structured tasks. Observation of spontaneous speech production or repetition of structured utterances can yield information on number of syllables produced per breath and adequacy of respiratory support and loudness through an utterance. Strength of voluntary and involuntary cough can also provide information concerning respiratory adequacy. Questions to the caregivers can also elicit information on functional performance in various settings. For example, can the child be heard and understood by the parent in the front seat of the car when the child is in the back seat with the motor running? Can the child awaken the parent at night by calling or crying without an amplifying monitor?

Laryngeal Function

Visual inspection of the larynx by an otolaryngologist or trained SLP should be accomplished via nasendoscopy or laryngoscopy if laryngeal pathology is suspected. Vocal characteristics to observe include adequacy of pitch, laryngeal voice quality, the ability to vary pitch, voice breaks, pitch breaks, extraneous vocalizations, and adductor or abductor blocks characterized by voice stoppage or rushes of air, respectively. At a very early age, voice onset should be easy and well-coordinated with breathing. Any difficulty with coordination of voicing, respiration, and articulation should be noted.

Velopharyngeal Function

Visual evaluation of soft palate movement should be made during phonation, laughter, or crying. Adequacy of resonant voice quality (e.g., hypernasal, denasal), nasal air emission on production of consonants, or nasalized vowel production should be noted. If there is improvement in building intraoral air pressure for production of bilabial plosives or fricatives with the nares occluded, this would be an indicator of velopharyngeal incompetence. If a child cooperates, the oral manometer can be used to assess velopharyngeal adequacy by having the child perform tasks with the nares open and closed to check for a difference in results. Improved performance with the nares occluded would indicate velopharyngeal incompetence.

Orofacial Function

Assessment of lip and tongue function can be made through play, observation, and in structured tasks to assess range of movement. Analysis of articulation skills can be made either with a formal articulation test, or by transcription of spontaneous speech production.

Some children, generally those with moderate to severe motor involvement, may show abnormal movement patterns, including lip retraction or pursing, jaw thrust, lack of jaw grading, tonic bite reflex, tongue retraction, and tongue thrust (Arvedson & Brodsky, 2002; Morris & Klein, 2000). Each of these can interfere with speech sound production. Any trigger for these abnormal movements and any posture in which they are elicited should be documented. For example, lip retraction and tongue retraction may be observed with extensor patterns of movement.

The clinician should make estimates of intelligibility for known material as well as unknown material, for example, counting versus a description of their room or a toy in their own words. A more formal measure of intelligibility is calculation of the percentage of consonants correct (PCC) (Shriberg, 1993; Shriberg & Kwiatkowski, 1982).

Classification Systems

Recently, two classification systems have been developed to aid clinicians in assessing communication function. To classify communication on the basis of speech–motor and language impairment, Hustad, Gorton, and Lee (2010) have proposed a system of eight speech and language profiles as seen in Table 3–1. It is being studied to determine its clinical and research use.

Hidecker and colleagues (2011) have developed the Communication Function Classification System (CFCS), which classifies

Table 3–1. Classification of Communication Function by Speech–Motor and Language Impairment Developed by Hustad, Gorton, and Lee (2010)

Profile	Speech–motor/language description
1	No clinical speech-motor impairment and no clinical language impairment
2	No clinical speech-motor impairment and clinical language impairment
3	Mild speech-motor impairment and no clinical language impairment
4	Mild speech-motor impairment and clinical language impairment
5	Moderate/severe speech-motor impairment and no clinical language impairment
6	Moderate/severe speech-motor impairment and clinical language impairment
7	Unable to produce speech (anarthria) and no clinical language impairment
8	Unable to produce speech (anarthria) and clinical language impairment

communication at the activity and participation level and is shown in Table 3–2. This system rates everyday communication into one of five levels. It can be used in conjunction with the Gross Motor Classification Scale (GMCS) and the Manual Ability Classification System (MACS) to describe functional profiles (Hidecker et al., 2012).

Use of tools such as these will aid the clinician in choosing methods and directions of treatment that will maximize resources available to each child.

Prognosis

When establishing the prognosis for functional change in speech production, the clinician must consider a number of factors. First, the natural history of the disorders should be considered. In the child with spasticity, there may be concern for periods of regression as the child ages, and perhaps a return for additional treatment. The child with athetosis may benefit from weight gain and achievement of greater stability, and, therefore, have the ability to make additional gains in speech production despite showing moderate to severe involvement initially.

Diagnostic therapy, which can be accomplished during dynamic assessment, can provide prognostic information. For example, during the evaluation of a 3-year-old with athetosis

Table 3–2. Communication Function Classification System (CFCS) Developed by Hidecker and Colleagues (2011) Classifies Communication at the Activity and Participation Level

Level	Functional description
I	Effective sender and receiver with unfamiliar and familiar partners
II	Effective but slower-paced sender and/or receiver with unfamiliar and familiar partners
III	Effective sender and receiver with familiar partners
IV	Inconsistent sender and/or receiver with familiar partners
V	Seldom effective sender and/or receiver with familiar partners

who has never had a seating system, the child may only produce a single word approximation per breath. However, by providing stability in a supportive seating system, the child may immediately be able to produce two, and sometimes three syllables per breath. This would certainly be a positive prognostic indicator.

Type and extent of associated conditions will also factor into prognosis. Cognitive impairment, attention issues, a seizure disorder, presence of other speech disorders, level of language function, and the extent of involvement of those conditions can negatively impact prognosis. Presence of sensory disorders, such as hearing or vision impairments, may also limit treatment outcomes. The ability to retain and carry over skills learned in the therapy setting and the motivation to participate in the session and practice outside the session are also indicators. Willingness of caregivers to participate in the therapy process is also a positive indicator. Availability of appropriate treatment services is a limiting factor in some areas, as are funding issues.

Treatment Planning

The ultimate treatment goal for children with all speech disorders is functional, intelligible speech production. In children with cerebral palsy, this is not always an achievable goal. In many instances, the goal could be functional communication through use of some intelligible speech production supplemented by augmentative communication.

Short-term goals should be drawn directly from the speech assessment and diagnostic therapy. For example, if the clinician achieved rapid change by modifying a seating system or by introducing a simple augmentative communication system, this should be the immediate focus of treatment. In working on speech production, focus should be placed on the lowest component that impacts speech production significantly, unless the velopharynx is involved. If the velopharynx is an issue, it should be managed first since it has a direct effect on respiratory support, voice, and articulation. Short-term goals should be achievable in a very reasonable time frame to maintain the interest of the child and the caregiver.

Conclusions

This chapter has provided an overview of the nature, causes, and types of cerebral palsy, along with associated conditions and speech disorders present in children with cerebral palsy. The goal has been to provide a framework for assessment and treatment planning while acknowledging that children with cerebral palsy are not physically typical, and their development of speech motor skills may be compromised as well as their development of fine and gross motor function.

Ten Principles for Understanding Cerebral Palsy

1. The lesion that causes cerebral palsy is static. Symptoms change over time and in response to other factors, for example, growth or development of seizures.
2. The lesion occurs before, during, or shortly after birth. This impacts development.
3. Cerebral palsy is a heterogeneous disorder. No two children present with the same set of characteristics and circumstances.
4. A number of disorders mimic cerebral palsy, and more is being understood about them. Genetic and metabolic disorders are some examples.
5. The most current classification system considers the major types of cerebral palsy to be: spasticity, dyskinesia, choreoathetosis, and ataxia.
6. There are multiple conditions seen in conjunction with cerebral palsy, and the clinician needs to be aware of those that are specific to the child being treated. A few of the most common are cognitive deficits, speech and language disorders, feeding/swallowing disorders, and visual disorders.
7. Dysarthria is the most common speech disorder in children with cerebral palsy.
8. Careful evaluation of all speech subsystems and the effect of muscle tone and movement patterns must be considered before establishing treatment goals.

9. Before establishing a treatment plan, the clinician needs to consider the prognostic indicators that pertain to the student/patient's situation.
10. Functional communication is a goal of treatment whether through speech production or augmented or alternative means.

Think Critically for Self-Study or Classroom Discussion

1. List three characteristics of the tone and movement of an individual with spastic cerebral palsy.
2. List three characteristics of the tone and movement of an individual with dyskinetic cerebral palsy.
3. Discuss the possible effects of abnormal tone and movement on the communication of an individual with cerebral palsy.
4. Discuss the influence that a seizure disorder or visual impairment could have on treatment planning.
5. List the three prognostic factors you consider to be most important and explain why.

References

Allaire, J. H. (2001). Young children and drooling: Effective swallowing interventions. *NDTA Network, 8,* 1–4.

Andersen, G., Mjoen, T. R., & Vik, T. (2010). Prevalence of speech problems and the use of augmentative and alternative communication in children with cerebral palsy: A registry-based study in Norway. *Perspectives in Augmentative and Alternative Communication, 19*(1), 12–20.

Arvedson, J. C., & Brodsky, L. (2002). *Pediatric swallowing and feeding: Assessment and management* (2nd ed.). Albany, NY: Singular.

Ashwal, S., Russman, B. S., Blasco, P. A., Miller, G., Sandler, A., Shevell, M., . . . Practice Committee of the Child Neurology Society. (2004).

Practice parameter. Diagnostic assessment of the child with cerebral palsy: Report of the quality standards subcommittee of the American Academy of Neurology and the Practice Committee of the Child Neurology Society, *Neurology*, *62*(6), 851–863.

Bax, M., Goldstein, M., Rosenbaum, P., Levion, A., Paneth, N., Dan, B., . . . Executive Committee for the Definition of Cerebral Palsy. (2005). Proposed definition and classification of cerebral palsy. *Developmental Medicine and Child Neurology*, *47*(8), 571–576.

Beckung, E., & Hagberg, G. (2002). Neuroimpairments, activity limitations, and participation restrictions in children with cerebral palsy. *Developmental Medicine and Child Neurology*, *44*(5), 309–316.

Bjornson, K., Kobayashi, A., Zhou, C., & Walker, W. (2011). Relationship of therapy to postsecondary education and employment in young adults with physical disabilities. *Pediatric Physical Therapy*, *23*(2), 179–186.

Blasco, P. A. (1996). Drooling. In P. B. Sullivan & L. Rosenbloom (Eds.), *Feeding the disabled child* (pp. 92–105). London, UK: Mac Keith Press.

Bobath, B., & Bobath, K. (1975). *Motor development in the different types of cerebral palsy*. London, UK: Butterworth-Heinemann.

Bohmer, C. J., Klinkenberg-Knol, E. C., Niezen-de Boer, M. C., & Meuwissen, S. G. (2000). Gastroesophageal reflux disease in intellectually disabled individuals: How often, how serious, how manageable? *American Journal of Gastroenterology*, *95*(8), 1868–1872.

Boliek, C. A., Hixon, T. J., Watson, P. J., & Morgan, W. J. (1996). Vocalization and breathing during the first year of life. *Journal of Voice*, *10*(1), 1–22.

Boliek, C. A., Hixon, T. J., Watson, P. J., & Morgan, W. J. (1997). Vocalization and breathing during the second and third years of life. *Journal of Voice*, *11*(4), 373–390.

Brossard-Racine, M., Hall, N., Majnemer, A., Shevell, M., Law, M., Poulin, C., & Rosenbaum, P. (2012). Behavioural problems in school age children with cerebral palsy. *European Journal of Paediatric Neurology*, *16*(1), 35–41.

Brossard-Racine, M., Waknin, J., Shikako-Thomas, K., Shevell, M., Poulin, C., . . . Majnemer, A. (2013). Behavioral difficulties in adolescents with cerebral palsy. *Journal of Child Neurology*, *28*(1), 27–33.

Brunner, R., & Doderlein, L. (1996). Pathological fractures in patients with cerebral palsy. *Journal of Pediatric Orthopedics*, *5*(4), 232–238.

Calis, E. A., Veugelers, R., Sheppard, J. J., Tibboel, D., Evenhuis, H. M., & Penning, C. (2008). Dysphagia in children with severe generalized cerebral palsy and intellectual disability. *Developmental Medicine and Child Neurology*, *50*(8), 625–630.

Cans, C. (2009). Pervasive developmental disorders in individuals with cerebral palsy. *Developmental Medicine and Child Neurology, 51*(4), 252–255.

Carmagnani, F. G., Goncalves, G. K., Correa, M. S., & dos Santos, M. T. (2007). Occlusal characteristics in cerebral palsy patients. *Journal of Dentistry for Children, 74*(1), 41–45.

Centers for Disease Control and Prevention (CDC). (2013). Retrieved March 3, 2013, from http://www.cdc.gov/ncbddd/dd/ddcp.htm

Cooper, J., Majnemer, A., Rosenblatt, B., & Birnbaum, R. (1995). The determination of sensory deficits in children with hemiplegic cerebral palsy. *Journal of Child Neurology, 10*(4), 300–309.

Duffy, J. (1995). *Motor speech disorders: Substrates, differential diagnosis, and management*. St. Louis, MO: Mosby.

Eliasson, A. C., Krumline-Sundholm, L., Rosblad, B., Beckung, E., Arner, M., Ohrvall, A. M., & Rosenbaum, P. (2006). The Manual Ability Classification System (MACS) for children with cerebral palsy: Scale development and evidence of validity and reliability. *Developmental Medicine and Child Neurology, 48*(7), 549–554.

Froud, K., & Khamis-Dakwar, R. (2012). Mismatch negativity responses in children with a diagnosis of childhood apraxia of speech (CAS). *American Journal of Speech-Language Pathology, 21*, 302–312.

Franklin, D. L., Luther, F., & Curzon, M. E. (1996). The prevalence of malocclusion in children with cerebral palsy. *European Journal of Orthodontics, 18*(6), 637–643.

Graham, J. K. (2004). Mechanisms of deformity. In D. Scrutton, D. Damiano, & M. Mayston (Eds.), *Management of the motor disorders of children with cerebral palsy* (pp. 105–129). London, UK: Mac Keith Press.

Granet, K. M., Balaghi, M., & Jaeger, J. (1997). Adults with cerebral palsy. *New Jersey Medicine, 94*(2), 51–54.

Guzetta, A., Mercuri, E., & Cioni, G. (2001). Visual disorders in children with brain lesions: 2. Visual impairment associated with cerebral palsy. *European Journal of Paediatric Neurology, 5*(3), 115–119.

Henderson, R. C., Lark, R. K., Gurka, M. J., Worley, G., Fung, E. B., Conaway, M., . . . Stevenson, R. D. (2002). Bone density and metabolism in children and adolescents with moderate to severe cerebral palsy. *Pediatrics, 110*(1 Pt. 1), e5.

Herer, G. R., Knightly, C. A., & Steinberg, A. G. (2007). Hearing: Sounds and silences. In M. L. Batshaw, L. Pellegrino, & N. J. Roizen (Eds.), *Children with Disabilities* (pp. 157–183). Baltimore, MD: Paul H. Brookes.

Hidecker, M. J., Ho, N. T., Dodge, N., Hurvitz, E. A., Slaughter, J., Workinger, M. S., . . . Paneth N. (2012). Inter-relationships of functional status in cerebral palsy: Analyzing gross motor function, manual ability, and communication function classification systems in children. *Developmental Medicine and Child Neurology, 54*(8), 737–742.

Hidecker, M. J., Paneth, N., Rosenbaum, P. L., Kent, R. D., Lillie, J., Eulenberg, J. B., . . . Taylor, K. (2011). Developing and validating the Communication Function Classification System for individuals with cerebral palsy. *Developmental Medicine and Child Neurology, 53*(8), 704–710.

Hixon, T. J., Hawley, J. L., & Wilson, K. J. (1982). An around-the-house device for the clinical determination of respiratory driving pressure: A note on making simple even simpler. *Journal of Speech and Hearing Disorders, 47*(4), 413–415.

Howle, J. M. (2002). *Neuro-developmental treatment approach: Theoretical foundations and principles of clinical practice.* Laguna Beach, CA: Neuro-Developmental Treatment Association.

Hustad, K. C., Gorton, K., & Lee, J. (2010). Classification of speech and language profiles in 4-year-old children with cerebral palsy: A prospective preliminary study. *Journal of Speech, Language and Hearing Research, 53*(6), 1496–1513.

Jahnsen, R., Villien, L., Stanghelle, J. K., & Holm, I. (2003). Fatigue in adults with cerebral palsy in Norway compared with the general population. *Developmental Medicine and Child Neurology, 45*(5), 296–303.

Kelley, R. I. (2008). Metabolic diseases and developmental disabilities. In P. Accardo (Ed.), *Caputo & Accardo's neurodevelopmental disabilities in infancy and childhood* (3rd ed., pp. 115–146), Baltimore, MD: Paul J. Brookes.

Kilincaslan, A., & Mukaddes, N. M. (2009). Pervasive developmental disorders in individuals with cerebral palsy. *Developmental Medicine and Child Neurology, 51(4)*, 289–294.

Kirby, R. S., Wingate, M. S., Van Naarden Braun, K., Doernberg, N. S., Arneson, C. L., Benedict, R. E., . . . Yeargin-Allsopp, M. (2011). Prevalence and functioning of children with cerebral palsy in four areas of the United States in 2006: A report from the Autism and Developmental Disabilities Monitoring Network. *Research in Developmental Disabilities, 32*(2), 462–469.

Kwong, K. L., Wong, S. N., & So, K. T. (1998). Epilepsy in children with cerebral palsy. *Pediatric Neurology, 19*(1), 31–36.

Majnemer, A., Shevell, M., Law, M., Poulin, C., & Rosenbaum, P. (2012). Indicators of distress in families of children with cerebral palsy. *Disability and Rehabilitation, 34*(14), 1202–1207.

McDermott, S., Coker, A. L., Mani, S., Krishnaswami, S., Nagle, R. J., Barnett-Queen, L. L., & Wuori, D. F. (1996). A population-based analysis of behavior problems in children with cerebral palsy. *Journal of Pediatric Psychology, 21*(3), 447–463.

Menkes, J. H., & Flores-Sarnat, L. (2006). Cerebral palsy due to chromosomal anomalies and continuous gene syndromes. *Clinics in Perinatology, 33*(2), 481–501.

Mesterman, R., Leitner, Y., Yifat, R., Gilutz, G., Levi-Hakeini, O., Bitchonsky, O., . . . Harel, S. (2010). Cerebral palsy—long-term medical, functional, educational, and psychosocial outcomes. *Journal of Child Neurology, 25*(1), 36–42.

Moll, L. R., & Cott, C. A. (2013). The paradox of normalization through rehabilitation: Growing up and growing older with cerebral palsy. *Disability and Rehabilitation, 35*(15), 1276–1283.

Morley, M. (1965). *Development and disorders of speech in childhood.* (2nd ed.). Baltimore, MD: Williams & Wilkins.

Morris, S. E., & Klein, M. D. (2000). *Pre-feeding skills: A comprehensive resource for mealtime development* (2nd ed.). San Antonio, TX: Therapy Skill Builders.

Netsell, R. (1986). *A neurobiologic view of speech production and the dysarthrias.* San Diego, CA: College-Hill Press.

Netsell, R. (2001). Speech aeromechanics and the dysarthrias: Implications for children with traumatic brain injury. *Journal of Head Trauma Rehabilitation, 16*(5), 415–425.

Netsell, R., & Hixon, T. J. (1978). A non-invasive method for clinically estimating subglottal air pressure. *Journal of Speech and Hearing Disorders, 43*(3), 326–330.

Newman, C. J., O'Regan, M., & Hensey, O. (2006). Sleep disorders in children with cerebral palsy. *Developmental Medicine and Child Neurology, 48*(7), 564–568.

Nordmark, E., Hagglund, G., & Lagergren, J. (2001) Cerebral palsy in southern Sweden II. Gross motor function and disabilities. *Acta Paediatrica, 90*(11), 1277–1282.

Odding, E., Roebroeck, M. E., & Stam, H. J. (2006). The epidemiology of cerebral palsy: incidence, impairments and risk factors. *Disability Rehabilitation, 28*(4), 183–191.

Palisano, R., Rosenbaum, P., Walter, S., Russell, D., Wood, E., & Galuppi, B. (1997). Development and reliability of a system to classify gross motor function in children with cerebral palsy. *Developmental Medicine and Child Neurology, 39*(4), 214–223.

Parkes, J., Hill, N., Platt, M. J., & Donnelly, C. (2010). Oromotor dysfunction and communication impairments in children with cerebral palsy: A register study. *Developmental Medicine and Child Neurology, 52*(12), 1113–1119.

Pelligrino, L. (2007). Cerebral palsy. In M. L. Batshaw, L. Pellegrino, & N. J. Roizen (Eds.), *Children with disabilities* (6th ed., pp. 387–408). Baltimore, MD: Paul H. Brookes.

Proctor, A. (1989). Stages of normal non-cry vocal development in infancy: A protocol for assessment. *Topics in Language Disorders*, *10*(1), 26–42.

Pruitt, D. W., & Tsai, T. (2009). Common medical comorbidities associated with cerebral palsy. *Physical Medicine and Rehabilitation Clinics of North America*, *20*(3), 453–457.

Robb, M. P., & Bleile, K. M. (1994). Consonant inventories of young children from 8 to 25 months. *Clinical Linguistics and Phonetcs*, *8*(4), 295–320.

Rodrigues dos Santos, M. T., Masiero, D., Novo, N. F., & Simionato, M. R. (2003). Oral conditions in children with cerebral palsy. *Journal of Dentistry for Children*, *70*(1), 40–46.

Rogers, B., Arvedson, J., Buck, G., Smart, P., & Msall, M. (1994). Characteristics of dysphagia in children with cerebral palsy. *Dysphagia*, *9*(1), 69–73.

Rosenbaum, P. L., Walter, S. D., Hanna, W. E., Palisano, R. J., Russell, D. J., Raina, P., . . . Galuppi, B. E. (2002). Prognosis for gross motor function in cerebral palsy: Creation of motor development curves. *Journal of the American Medical Association*, *288*(11), 1357–1363.

Rutherford, B. R. (1944). A comparative study of loudness, pitch, rate, rhythm, and quality of the speech of children handicapped by cerebral palsy. *Journal of Speech and Hearing Disorders*, *9*, 263–271.

Sajedi, F., Alizad, V., Malekkhosravi, G., Karimlou, M., & Vameghi, R. (2010). Depression in mothers of children with cerebral palsy and its relation to severity and type of cerebral palsy. *Acta Medica Iranica*, *48*(4), 250–254.

Sawyer, M. G., Bittman, M., La Greca, A. M., Crettenden, A. D., Borojevic, N., Raghavendra, P., & Russo, R. (2011). Time demands of caring for children with cerebral palsy: What are the implications for maternal mental health? *Developmental Medicine and Child Neurology*, *53*(4), 338–343.

Schenk-Rootlieb, A. J., van Nieuwenhuizen, O., van der Graaf, Y., Wittebol-Pose, D., & Willemse, J. (1992). The prevalence of cerebral visual disturbance in children with cerebral palsy. *Developmental Medicine and Child Neurology*, *34*(6), 473–480.

Schwartz, S., Gisel, E. G., Clarke, D., & Haberfellner, H. (2003). Association of occlusion with eating efficiency in children with cerebral palsy and moderate eating impairment. *Journal of Dentistry for Children*, *70*(1), 33–39.

Shriberg, L. D. (1993). Four new speech and prosody-voice measures for genetics research and other studies in developmental phonological disorders. *Journal of Speech and Hearing Research, 36,* 105–140.

Shriberg, L. D., & Kwiatkowski, J. (1982). Phonological disorders II. A procedure for assessing severity of involvement. *Journal of Speech and Hearing Disorders, 47,* 256–270.

Sigurdardottir, S., Eiriksdottir, A., Gunnarsdottir, E., Meintema, M., Arandottir, U., & Vik, T. (2008). Cognitive profile in young Icelandic children with cerebral palsy. *Developmental Medicine and Child Neurology, 50*(5), 357–362.

Sigurdardottir, S., Indredavik, M. S., Eiriksdottir, A., Einarsdottir, K., Gudmundsson, H. S., & Vik, T. (2010). Behavioural and emotional symptoms of preschool children with cerebral palsy: A population-based study. *Developmental Medicine and Child Neurology, 52(11),* 1056–1061.

Sobrado, P., Suarez, J., Garcia-Sanchez, F. A., & Uson, E. (1999). Refractive errors in children with cerebral palsy, psychomotor retardation, and other non-cerebral palsy neuromotor disabilities. *Developmental Medicine and Child Neurology, 41*(6), 396–403.

Strauss, D. J., Shavelle, R. M., & Anderson, T. W. (1998). Life expectancy of children with cerebral palsy. *Pediatric Neurology, 18*(2), 143–149.

Surveillance of Cerebral Palsy in Europe. (2002). Prevalence and characteristics of children with cerebral palsy in Europe. *Developmental Medicine and Child Neurology, 44,* 633–640.

Tahmassebi, J. F., & Luther, F. (2004). Relationship between lip position and drooling in children with cerebral palsy. *European Journal of Paediatric Dentistry, 5*(3), 151–156.

Tasdemir, J. A., Buyukavci, M., Akcay, F., Polat, P., Yildiran, A., & Karakelleoglu, C. (2001). Bone mineral density in children with cerebral palsy. *Pediatrics International, 43*(2), 157–160.

Turk, M. A., Scandale, J., Rosenbaum, P. F., & Weber, R. J. (2001). The health of women with cerebral palsy. *Physical Medicine and Rehabilitation Clinics of North America, 12*(1), 153–168.

United Cerebral Palsy (UCP). (2013). Retrieved March 3, 2013, from http://ucp.org/

Wayte, S., McCaughey, E., Holley, S., Annaz, D., & Hill, C. M. (2012). Sleep problems in children with cerebral palsy and their relationship with maternal sleep and depression. *Acta Paediatrica, 101*(6), 618–623.

Workinger, M. S. (1986). *Acoustic analysis of the dysarthrias in children with athetoid and spastic cerebral palsy.* (Unpublished doctoral dissertation). University of Wisconsin, Madison.

Workinger, M. S. (2005). *Cerebral palsy: Resource guide for speech-language pathologists*. Clifton Park, NY: Thomson Delmar Learning.

Workinger, M. S., & Kent, R. (1991). Perceptual analysis of the dysarthrias in children with athetoid and spastic cerebral palsy. In C. A. Moore, K. M. Yorkston, & D. R. Beukelman (Eds.), *Dysarthria and apraxia of speech: Perspectives on management* (pp. 109–126). Baltimore, MD: Paul H. Brookes.

Yeargin-Allsopp, M., Boyle, C., Braun, K. V., & Trevathan, E. (2008). The epidemiology of developmental disabilities. In P. Accardo (Ed.), *Capute & Accardo's neurodevelopmental disabilities in infancy and childhood* (3rd ed., pp. 61–104). Baltimore, MD: Paul H. Brookes.

CHAPTER 4

Feeding the Whole Child Using NDT

Fran Redstone

Introduction

Many of my friends agree that eating is one of the most enjoyable activities in life. The tastes, smells, and social interactions that occur around the feeding experience are described in books and portrayed in movies. In addition, eating is one of the two necessary functions for survival (Arvedson & Brodsky, 2002). As SLPs we think of eating as an oral–motor activity but it is so much more. Now consider how this experience may be affected by the sensorimotor deficits associated with cerebral palsy.

The prevalence of feeding disorders in children with cerebral palsy has been reported to be as high as 80% (Rogers, Arvedson, Buck, Smart, & Msall, 1994). Although there may be controversy over the influence of feeding on speech development, the fact that these young children with cerebral palsy need help is not controversial. Neurodevelopmental treatment (NDT) provides the framework for successful feeding intervention by treating the "whole child."

Terms like "whole child" and "holistic" sound so faddish and new age but are appropriate for NDT feeding because the NDT feeding therapist looks at the child from head to toe. We look beyond the mouth and the head, to the pelvis and feet, and acknowledge their influence on oral functioning for feeding. The feeding therapist addresses all of these components. But the good feeding therapist addresses them within a pleasurable mealtime experience.

Development of Feeding Skills

Infants are born to suck. They are hard-wired for this skill. This is not true for the skills needed to eat a steak dinner with a nice glass of cabernet sauvignon. The infants' facial structures will grow, their nervous systems will mature, and they will gradually gain control over their oral mechanism for safe feeding. This, however, assumes normal motor and sensory systems. Alexander (1987) discusses the reciprocity between oral–motor and gross motor development. Neonates are born with passive physiological flexion. Over the first year the infant develops active extension starting at the head. Active flexion develops slightly later than extension. This development facilitates greater feeding control and safety and is, in turn, reinforced by feeding movements.

In addition, typical children encounter many sources for oral experiences well before any solid foods are expected to be processed and swallowed. Although developmental milestones do not usually include hand-to-mouth or object-to-mouth skills, they play a significant role throughout the typical child's first 2 years. These experiences modify sensitivity and allow for adaptive movements based on the different sensations (Alexander, Boehme, & Cupps, 1993). Many feeding milestones are based on these early mouthing activities.

A number of ill or premature infants may later be diagnosed with cerebral palsy (Pelligrino, 2007). These infants are typically floppy and have decreased movements including hand-to-mouth movements. Older infants and children with cerebral palsy may exhibit abnormal muscle tone, an asymmetrical tonic reflex (ATNR), or other abnormal patterns that involve their arms and hands for hand-to-mouth activities. This is one example of the impact of a congenital neuromotor disorder on later development. In addition, many feeding milestones are based not only on structural and neural maturation, but on the oral experiences offered to the child as well. If the child had no experience with a spoon, cracker, or cup, the child is unlikely to develop the skill within the expected time line.

Neonate to 3 Months

The newborn does not have volitional motor control to find food, take it in, and swallow. However, the neonate is influenced by physiological flexion and a small intraoral space giving oral structures their stability. These, along with strong oral reflexes, make bottle or breast feeding safe. The reflexes that ensure food finding and safety are rooting, suckle/suck, bite, and gag. Throughout this book the concept of increasing the child's movement options is emphasized. However, this is the one time in life when providing the fewest options for movement is the best option for function. This will change as the child develops motor control.

By 3 months of age the typical child has developed extension in the upper trunk, and the infant lifts the head and bears weight on forearms in prone (Alexander et al., 1993). Weight shift and some reaching begin. At this point we see changes in oral reflexes. Rooting is less important because the infant has some head control. The initial physiological flexion has decreased so that lip closure is looser. More movement options are being created.

Four to Six Months

A flexor component in the upper thorax results in midline orientation with hands together and hands to knees. Extension is continuing its development down the spine, and head control is established. In addition, weight bearing is seen in prone on extended arms by 6 months. This balance of flexion and extension allows reaching in all positions along with rolling.

When an object is found, it typically goes in the mouth. There is further change in oral reflexes, which become less obligatory. The infant's motor control has developed and is reflected in the increase in oral movement options.

This is the period in which spoon-feeding is introduced. It is a new experience and one for which the infant must learn skills in order to be successful. A strategy that is often seen is one that the infant has used in the past: the child sucks the food off a spoon using the forward–backward tongue movement of suckling (Alexander et al., 1993). It is interesting that the child triggers this with hand-to-mouth movement. A feeder usually needs to scrape food back into the child's mouth since the tongue often pushes food out. By 6 months the child often has been given solids for biting because of the beginning of teething. A great variety of movements are seen that include suckling and munching using a rhythmic bite reflex pattern.

Arvedson and Brodsky (2002) discuss the possibility that this is the critical period for changing textures. New textures often lead to gagging for a short while. However, the continued processing of textures leads to the ability to handle them.

Seven to 9 Months

During the beginning of the second half of the first year, the infant is very active. The many movement options available to an infant this age are evident by watching the ways the child attains a desired object and explores it. The infant may creep, crawl, long sit, side sit, and pull up to stand. The child is also stable in sitting due to dissociation and the balance between extension and flexion of the trunk and pelvis. This variety is reflected orally as well.

Suckling has changed to a well-coordinated suck pattern on the bottle or breast with longer sequences, smaller jaw excursions, tighter lip closure, and an up–down tongue pattern. However, the cup is typically introduced during this period, and suckling along with wide jaw excursions may be present with attempts to drink from it. This "regression" occurs as a new oral experience is introduced. This is "normal" and will stabilize with greater exposure to the novel item. The child has gained experience with the spoon and now actively takes food off with lips and propels it posteriorly with the tongue as seen in Figure 4–1. Of course, this depends on when the spoon was introduced. Further experience with biting and chewing continues. An early chewing pattern is munching, which is rhythmical up–down jaw movement. Tongue lateralization may also be seen but is not functionally used during feeding.

Ten Months to 1 Year

The child is now exploring in an upright position and transitioning to upright in a myriad of ways that reflect increased strength, grading, and dissociation. The child may weight shift and begin to cruise around furniture while holding on with two hands. However, by 1 year the child attempts standing and even moving by holding just one hand. Then there are the first steps. However, crawling is typically the preferred method for rapid movement

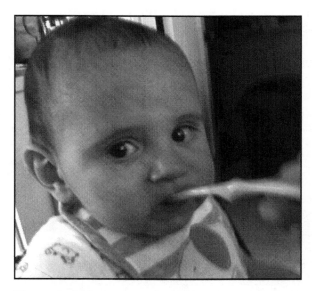

Figure 4–1. Active spoon feeding in a 7 to 9-month-old.

through the environment. Again, it is the increase in movement options that is dazzling.

While moving, children are experimenting with oral control in different positions. However, we may see a loss of oral control during periods requiring greater neural resources for equilibrium, as in unstable standing and ambulation. Alexander et al. (1993) note oral posturing for stability during these times along with drooling.

Weaning from the bottle often occurs at 1 year as cup drinking increases. There is less fluid loss during cup drinking, but jaw excursions are still apparent, and the tongue may be positioned forward, or even under the cup, to provide stability. Finger feeding of a cracker occurs with better grading of bite-taking and a rotary component during chewing as seen in Figure 4–2. Now tongue lateralization is functional and food is shifted to the chewing surfaces.

One to 2 Years

During this period the child begins walking and balance improves. Cup drinking is independent and successful through external

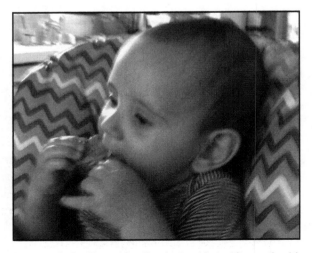

Figure 4–2. Finger-feeding in the 10- to 12-month-old.

jaw stabilization on the rim of a cup at 18 months of age. Internal jaw stability is demonstrated during cup drinking by age 2. There is a minimal loss of food during chewing due to increased dissociation of the oral structures. In addition, the bolus can be moved across midline.

Atypical Feeding Development—Cerebral Palsy

Children with cerebral palsy have a neurological impairment affecting motor control, and their sensorimotor experiences are influenced by this. Because motor control underlies successful feeding, it is not unexpected that children with cerebral palsy will have feeding problems. Some of the factors that directly influence oral functioning for feeding include the alignment, stability, and dissociation, which have been discussed in Chapter 1.

Early feeding problems are often a "soft" sign of neurological damage. In fact, the sucking behavior of children in a neonatal intensive care unit (NICU) has been considered a "barometer of central nervous system organization" (Tsai, Chen, & Lin, 2010, p. 67). These feeding problems often persist into childhood (Barlow, Poore, Zimmerman, & Finan, 2010). Some premature infants demonstrate dysfunctional sucks suggesting their underlying neurological problems. And some infants demonstrate a disorganized suck initially but may become more normal as their systems mature. However, if the disorganized suck persists, there is a greater risk of later developmental delays (Tsai et al., 2010).

Compensations that interfere with later development may accompany attempts at movement. Bly (1983) has referred to these as "blocks." A neck block leads to head hyperextension, which directly affects the child's feeding safety and efficiency. It also leads to mouth opening, vocal fold abduction, and misalignment of the oral structures. A pelvic block's influence on feeding is less direct but just as detrimental. It leads to an unstable pelvic area which, in turn, results in poor head/trunk alignment and head hyperextension.

Some of the characteristics of feeding that may develop in children with cerebral palsy involve muscle tone and head extension. An open mouth pattern from extensor tone is typical. Oral reflexes may be weak initially, and as muscle tone develops these reflexes may develop abnormally. Some children attempt to compensate by using an abnormal pattern such as the asymmetrical tonic neck reflex (ATNR) to self-feed. Other children with spasticity have limited range of motion influencing tongue movements for manipulation of food and may use hyperextension to propel food posteriorly. Children with athetoid cerebral palsy lack grading of the jaw for bite-taking, spoon feeding, and cup drinking. It is imperative to determine the cause of the abnormal functioning and to identify which component is missing. Will this interfere with future development of feeding?

Assessment

The main purpose of the assessment is to determine if there is, in fact, a problem. Typically, if the parent thinks there is a problem, there is. However, an evaluation should also indicate the direction of therapy. Noting areas of strength is important because these can facilitate treatment planning. When an evaluation is completed, can you determine the one improvement that will make the biggest impact on the child's functioning? Because children with cerebral palsy often have multiple problems, prioritizing goals is important.

There are several feeding evaluation protocols that are worthwhile, but the World Health Organization reminds clinicians to target participation and context. We can evaluate the integrity of the oral structures along with muscle tone. We can also assess maximum strength, but the most important component of the assessment is evaluating the actual behavior in context. Much of an evaluation can be observed informally or during a mealtime, but some parts need to be dynamically assessed through direct manipulation of the feeding experience by the feeding therapist. This will indicate the potential for change. The assessment process involves information gathering, observation, and handling. This section targets the most important feeding issues for the child with cerebral palsy.

Information Gathering

In addition to an interview, reading a recent medical report can give you valuable information related to feeding history, safety, and comfort of swallowing. The right questions can facilitate a better understanding of the underlying problem. Beecher and Alexander (2004) instruct us to gather information regarding gastrointestinal issues, surgeries, bouts of coughing and choking, and histories of pneumonia, vomiting, and infections. If the child coughs, it should be noted whether the cough is strong and clears the airway. Pinder and Faherty (1999) indicate that children with cerebral palsy often have weak or delayed cough reflex. This knowledge is most important prior to initiating any feeding and may indicate a need for referral for an instrumental feeding.

In general, sensory issues are more difficult to assess than motor issues, because there are no norms for the former. Some questions related to textures and ease of transitioning to new foods will give important diagnostic information about sensory issues. Another important question is the length of a meal. Many new parents are unaware of how quickly a typical child eats. A meal lasting more than 30 minutes is considered "prolonged" (Eicher, 2007, p. 486). Remember that if your information was derived through a questionnaire or report, you need to determine whether there have been changes since the time of the original information gathering. This is typically done during the interview. In addition, this is a good opportunity to have the family describe its goals for the child. These items are listed in Table 4–1.

Observation and Handling

It is important for SLPs to use all their senses during observation and handling: Look, listen, and feel. The items to be assessed are the same during the observation of a parent feeding the child, as they are when the SLP is doing the feeding. Note the length of time a meal takes. If the meal is long, fatigue may lead to changes in tone and patterns. Although the assessment typically highlights areas of need, it is also important to note all positive aspects throughout the assessment.

Table 4–1. Questions for a Parent Interview or Questionnaire Related to the Child's Safety and Comfort During Feeding, the Possible Underlying Feeding Problem, Indications of Sensory Issues, and Intervention Planning

Safety and Comfort *Have there been . . .*	Underlying Problem *Is there a history of . . .*	Sensory Issues *Does your child . . .*	Therapy Plan *What . . .*
problems such as reflux?	a medical diagnosis?	enjoy bathing	position does your child like for eating?
chronic constipation?	prematurity?	put hands over ears or eyes?	is the length of a typical meal?
any oral surgeries?	an immature or atypical suck?	have favorite foods?	other therapies does your child receive?
vomiting, gagging, or choking?	seizures, cardiac, or respiratory issues?	like only foods of one texture?	has been attempted in the past?
chronic fussing during meals?	allergies or medications?	transition easily to new foods?	are you child's favorite activities?
change in respiration or color during meals?	delay of developmental milestones?	tolerate face wiping?	are your goals?

Observations

Observation in both a feeding and a nonfeeding context is desirable because more comprehensive information regarding parent handling and interaction can be obtained. This will aid in the determination of the difficulty of the feeding context compared to other activities.

Motor Observation

Movement of the oral structures and coordination of these structures are influenced by muscle tone and posture. It is imperative that these be evaluated. Other professionals can help the SLP, but it is the responsibility of the SLP to determine how a child's posture influences feeding and swallowing. Stability and head posture impact swallow safety. Is the head position part of a total body pattern? If the head is extended, is it due to low tone, which results in the head falling back? Or is it due to high tone and part of an extensor pattern affecting other parts of the body? SLPs can observe muscle tone, posture, alignment, and movement during informal assessment when the child is playing or interacting with parents.

Nonfeeding Motor Observations and Implications for Oral Functioning

- Does the child creep, crawl, cruise, or walk?
  - □ These are indications of a balance of extension and flexion, weight bearing, and dissociation.
- Does the child sit independently? Is there pelvic stability? Anterior or posterior pelvic tilt?
  - □ These are indications of head/trunk alignment.
- What is the typical head posture? Extended? Is it related to total body patterns? Related to pelvic stability?
  - □ Head posture influences alignment of oral structures for feeding safety and efficiency.
- Can the child bear weight on arms? Does the child use the arms and hands functionally?
  - □ This is an indication of shoulder stability for head control.

Observation of Structures

All SLPs have taken courses that include protocols for assessing oral structures. First, it is important to determine what structures are working atypically and if they compromise function. If abnormality is present, the clinician needs to be a detective and determine its cause. Then it is our job to apply this knowledge to improve functionality.

Begin the observation of oral structures when the child walks or is carried in, and continue this assessment during feeding.

Remember, the jaw is the base of function for the other oral structures. The jaw should not be depressed and lead to an open-mouth posture. This is not typical. Is the oral posture due to an extended head position, lack of stability, or low tone? Is the open mouth due to some obstruction of the child's nasal area? Or does the child have a cold?

Reasons for Open-Mouth Posture

- Extended head posture from generalized hypo- or hyper-tonicity
- Lack of pelvic stability leading to lack of head/trunk alignment
- Hyperextension of the jaw from extensor hypertonicity
- Low tone in the jaw musculature
- Nasal obstruction
- Upper respiratory infection

When the child initiates movement or vocalization does the jaw thrust forward? Does the jaw deviate to one side, and do you see this asymmetry in other parts of the body? Typically, if the jaw is correctly positioned, the lips will be well positioned at rest. However, if tone is high we may see lip retraction. Many times parents describe these children as "smiley." These observations need to be made at rest and during feeding.

The tongue is the next important structure to evaluate since sucking, swallowing, and chewing depend on its movements. When the child comes in, can you see the tongue? Is it positioned forward on the lower lip? Again, this is probably due to low tone. However, if the head is back, gravity will influence a hypotonic tongue and lead to tongue retraction. Do you see this hypotonia in other parts of the body? An interesting feature noted in some children with hypotonia is a "fixing" of the tongue on the roof of the mouth as a compensation for a floppy tongue. Forward tongue movement on stimulation may also be an indication of low tone or a retention of the suck–swallow pattern. On the other hand, a forceful tongue thrusting indicates hypertonia, which is rarely isolated to the oral area. Additional observations could reveal positive aspects such as lateral lingual movements to both sides.

Abnormal Tongue Positions

- Forward tongue posture from low tone
- Lingual fixing on the palate
- Retracted tongue from low tone due to head in extended position
- Forceful forward movements (thrusting) from hypertonus seen in other parts of the body

The child's vocalizations give us a clue to the position of the tongue and lips. If you hear /b, p, m/ you know lip closure is possible. If you hear /g, k/ posterior lingual movements are being made, whereas /d, t/ indicate anterior lingual movement. It is important to use all our senses to gather information and then integrate this information into what we know about movement, development, and the child's history.

Observation During Feeding

It is desirable to have the parent feed the child a meal. The food and setting should resemble a typical meal. This is best done in the child's home using the child's chair and equipment. Also, the timing of the assessment should conform to the child's regular schedule. Of course, timing and setting need to be considered but the ideal is not always possible.

After the child is seated, the initial observations relate to head position, trunk stability, and alignment during the various tasks of feeding: bottle or cup drinking, spoon feeding, or chewing solids. Since seating influences stability and alignment, note if the child is fed in the parent's lap or in a chair. Is the seating age-appropriate? Does it provide enough support and stability for distal oral structures to move in a coordinated manner? This is not an activity for the child to work on balance and trunk control. It should be comfortable and stable. Because we are looking at the child in a holistic manner, we need to relate the oral movements observed to the rest of the child's body.

We've all studied the stages of a normal swallow during a dysphagia course. Typically, children with cerebral palsy have abnormal muscle tone and coordination that interfere with the movements for processing food orally, the retention of food, and the safe transport of the bolus posteriorly. I have just described the oral preparation and oral stages of swallowing. These are volitional and will be influenced most by the child's muscle tone, head posture, method of bringing food to the mouth, and the texture of food.

The pharyngeal and esophageal stages are reflexive. These may be delayed or abnormal in children with cerebral palsy. In addition, the safety of the reflexive swallow depends on the ability of the vocal folds to adduct quickly which, in turn, is influenced by head posture. An extended head predisposes the vocal folds to abduct. Remember, when CPR is administered the head is pushed into an extensor posture so that the airway is open. Neutral head position or a chin tuck posture is safest as they facilitate vocal fold closure and breathing coordination.

Head posture needs to be assessed throughout the meal. Does feeding begin with a neutral head position that is then lost? The most typical abnormal pattern is head extension. Observe if there is a pattern. Does this happen only when the spoon approaches? Only for certain textures? Is it related to loss of pelvic stability? Some children use head extension as a compensation for lack of tongue movement to propel the bolus posteriorly. Does this lead to coughing or gagging? Or is the child successful? Another variable is the amount of self-feeding the child attempts. Often, this leads to an increase in muscle tone and loss of oral coordination. It may also trigger an ATNR with head extension and jaw thrusting. However, the attempt is an indication of independence and should be noted.

Bottle Drinking

Many very young infants for whom bottle or breast feeding is appropriate may have been treated for feeding in the NICU. Others may be referred due to difficulty gaining weight or because feeding is taking too long. Some infants fall asleep or just stop sucking. This may result from weak or abnormal reflexes. Often, infants referred for therapy have previously discontinued breast-feeding since bottle feeding is easier (Wolf & Glass, 1992). An assessment should note the position of the infant, size of the bottle, and type of nipple. Does the milk drip slowly or too fast? Has the size of the nipple been changed? Note the rate and rhythmical quality of the child's suck. This is described fully in Chapter 5. Are there any signs of distress such as body extension or fast rate of breathing? This may indicate discomfort from reflux or a general feeling of fullness that often accompanies constipation.

Spoon Feeding

As stated previously, infants are not hard-wired for spoon feeding. It is learned and takes time to master. Therefore, determine when the child began spoon-feeding. Again, observing the child's position is essential. The feeder's position is also important. Is the feeder standing with the child gazing upward with head extension? How does the feeder approach with the spoon? Does the feeder scrape food on the roof of the mouth? The foods and type of spoon used should be recorded. Is the size of the spoon appropriate? Is it commercially available or is it a "special spoon?"

Observe whether the child anticipates the spoon by opening the mouth. Is the jaw movement graded so that the opening is just large enough to accommodate the spoon? Tongue position should be noted at that moment. Once the spoon enters the oral area, is there clamping on the spoon? Also, many children do not use their lips to clear the spoon and may push food out with their tongue. This may be due to inexperience, retention of the suck reflex, or it may be part of a thrusting pattern. Is food retained with the lips? Is there coughing? It is important to note positive aspects such as well-coordinated, graded movements of the structures along with favorite foods.

Solids

Does the child self-feed? Where is the food placed? Does placement on the tongue trigger a suckle? It is important to inquire when the child was first introduced to solids. The suckle may be an indication of inexperience and is being used as a strategy to move the food. Note the texture and the size of the food along with the attempts to bite. It is also important to note mandibular elevation and how the child bites off a piece of food. Some strategies involve head extension. Using hyperextension may lead to a total pattern of extension throughout the body. After a bite is taken is there tongue lateralization for chewing? This would be a positive item to note especially if it occurs on both sides. If tongue thrusting is observed, it indicates hypertonicity. Remember, there is development of chewing skills that begins with munching and ends with a rotary component. At what stage is the child?

Cup Drinking

Cup drinking is the most difficult feeding skill to master. Fluid moves quickly and a great deal of oral/respiratory coordination is required for a safe swallow. In addition, when the toddler is holding the cup, coordination between fine-motor and oral-motor systems is essential. Typically, coughing may occur during initial attempts but should not be consistent. Of course, a strong cough is worthy of a positive notation as it indicates clearing of the laryngeal area.

To be successful lip closure is required on the cup rim. Are there attempts to draw fluid in using the lips? This would be indicated by upper lip movement. Do you see the tongue moving forward in an attempt to suckle? Also note the breathing pattern. If the child is out of breath after cup drinking, it may be an indication of breath-holding or a long apneic period. The most typical patterns present in children with cerebral palsy are poor lip closure and wide jaw excursions. Biting the rim of the cup may be the child's attempt to stabilize the jaw. This may be considered a positive indication of external jaw stability. If, however, it interferes with drinking, it may be abnormal clamping due to hypertonicity which should be evident by observing the rest of the body.

Behavioral Observation

In general, is mealtime pleasurable? This is as important for the success of intervention as it is for the development of feeding skills. Are mealtime behaviors similar to those observed during other activities? During nonfeeding activities some children enjoy novel items and activities whereas others need several exposures before actively participating. It is important to note these behavioral characteristics because they may aid in intervention planning. If negative behaviors are observed, the SLP must determine the source of these behaviors.

Some observable behaviors that may be related to physical discomfort include extension, fussiness, vomiting, and respiratory rate changes. Are these specific to the feeding situation? For example, oral hypersensitivity or reflux may lead to food avoidance through using negative behaviors. It is typically thought that head extension seen in a child with cerebral palsy is a result of abnormal patterns and muscle tone. However, discomfort may lead to this as well. The medical history or parent questionnaire may give an indication of these issues. If not, a medical referral is appropriate. The history may also describe past medical interventions that were necessary, or therapies provided with the best of intentions, but which may have been the source of the oral aversion.

However, head extension may also be a signal that the child is bored or finished eating. Parents of children with cerebral palsy have been found to be more directive and less responsive to their children's signals (Hanzlik & Stevenson, 1986; Pennington & McConaghie, 1999), which may be influencing feeding behaviors.

Handling for the Feeding Assessment: Dynamic Assessment

Now it is finally time for the SLP to feed the child. Always begin in the child's comfort zone. This typically means continuing whatever the parent has been doing. By this time the SLP might already have some idea of the initial functional goal or the next developmental step for the child. A dynamic assessment of the child's feeding might involve changing the child's position to improve stability, altering the texture of the food, or providing a utensil. Then, any improvement in the child's functioning should be noted. The items to be observed during a dynamic assessment are the same as those presented previously. They include structures and their movements for efficiency and safety of feeding, and behaviors during presentation of feeding stimuli. However, because the SLP is now doing the feeding, muscle tone can be felt and oral structures observed more closely.

This is the opportunity for the SLP to test oral reflexes. It is also important to determine if the child's response is age appropriate. When the child is stimulated, is the response a normal one or is it influenced by abnormal muscle tone? The methods of stimulating for oral reflexes and possible responses are noted in Table 4–2. Testing the gag reflex is not a pleasant experience for the child. However, before intervention, the SLP needs to test this reflex in order to determine the risk of aspiration. The discomfort can be mitigated by close observation of any nasal flaring or eye widening that often occurs prior to a full gag. If the tester removes the finger quickly and closes the mouth, the gag is active but the child's full response can be interrupted.

Although sensitivity can be inferred from observing feeding behaviors with the parent and from the child's history, direct testing will give more specific information. The gag reflex is often related to sensitivity. Is the gag reflex elicited in the anterior portion of the mouth? Can the faucial pillars be touched without a response? This would be an indication of inactive gag reflex. How does the child react to tactile stimulation of the trunk or extremities? Another confusing variable is the possibility of a

Table 4–2. Characteristics of Oral Reflexes

Reflex	Age	Elicited	Normal Response	Atypical Response
Rooting	To 4 mos.	Stroking cheek	Head turning	Absent
Suck/ swallow	Suckling to 6 mos.; nonobligatory suck to 12 mos.	Finger on anterior tongue	Rhythmical forward/ backward, up/ down tongue movement	Absent, weak, wide jaw excursions, tongue protrusion, thrusting
Bite	Integrated into munching at 7 mos.	Rubbing on lateral gum ridge	Rhythmical opening and closing of jaw	Absent, weak, clenching
Gag	Lifetime but elicitation moves posteriorly	Finger on the posterior tongue	Gagging	Absent, elicited anteriorly

mixed sensitivity. It is possible for the child to be hyposensitive periorally but hypersensitive intraorally. SLPs should not assume that a child with hypotonicity (or hypertonicity) is also hyposensitive (or hypersensitive).

Some hypersensitivity during feeding may appear inconsistent and may have been a learned behavior. If there are indicators of hypersensitivity but the cause of it is questionable, testing of sensitivity should be attempted during a nonfeeding activity like book reading. This will provide important information and perhaps present a starting point for therapy.

Checklist for Feeding Observation and Handling

- Position of child
  - ☐ Upright or reclining
  - ☐ Seating
    - Lap or chair
    - Pelvic stability
    - Foot support
- Head position
  - ☐ At the beginning of feeding
  - ☐ As food approaches
  - ☐ At different stages of feeding
  - ☐ At self-feeding attempts
- Position of feeder
- Equipment
  - ☐ Bottle, nipple, spoon, cup
    - Typical commercial type
    - Special adaptive size
- Food
  - ☐ Texture
  - ☐ Variety
- Process
  - ☐ Feeding time
  - ☐ Structures-grading
    - Jaw-grading
    - Tongue-range, lateralization, protrusion, retraction
    - Lip-active, retraction

□ Self-feeding
■ Behaviors
   □ Fussiness
   □ Hyperextension
   □ Physical-respiratory rate, coughing
■ How long does the meal take?
   □ Is alignment adequate throughout?
   □ Are behaviors similar throughout?
■ Sensitivity
   □ Oral
      • Hypersensitive
      • Hyposensitive
   □ Trunk
   □ Extremities
■ Oral reflexes-age appropriate, retained, atypical
   □ Rooting
   □ Suck/swallow
   □ Bite
   □ Gag

The next section presents some techniques that are suggested for feeding intervention but may also be used during dynamic assessment.

Feeding Intervention

There are a number of important guidelines when treating children. These apply to any type of intervention including NDT. First, the parent must play an active part in the intervention program. A therapist may be able to see a child several times a week for feeding therapy, but children may be fed three to six times a day. Therefore, the parent needs to feed the child in an enjoyable context and pleasant setting, hopefully, in a way that maximizes change but, minimally, in a way that achieves safety. The parents need to understand why a change is being made or a technique is being used. This approach has been referred to as parent coaching and has been encouraged in the development of communication skills (Pennington, Goldbart, & Marshall, 2004). In addition, it is important that parents feel competent and realize that what they are doing is important for the child's development. If this does not happen, the parent will not comply with the program and will revert to what had been successful in the past. This may be exactly what you are attempting to change. This is as true of NDT as any other approach.

Feeding therapy by the therapist and daily feedings by a parent should not look the same. It is expected that the parent provide safe feedings at a level that is nonthreatening and comfortable. The skills being repeated and practiced daily are those that the SLP initially attained in therapy. It is the SLPs job to "push" and bring the child to the next level. Only when the child is comfortable, and requires fewer supports to be fully functional, should the new skill be introduced for daily use with the parent. This is a process that is theoretically supported by the dynamic systems theory (Kamm, Thelen, & Jensen, 1990; Thelen, 1991). The therapist provides the new experience and necessary supports for the development of a new movement to accomplish a task, whereas the parent provides practice for the development of a stable pattern.

The World Health Organization emphasizes the importance of function and participation. If the tongue's range of motion, strength, or the child's postural control improves, they are only worthwhile if reflected in a function such as feeding (or speech). Feeding therapists cannot get so focused on the movement specifics and techniques that they ignore the big picture. In addition, feeding intervention will not be successful without enhancing trust and making the feeding experience pleasurable. It is not a worthwhile therapy session if the child is crying and not participating actively. On the other hand, just playing or having fun without accomplishing any goals is not worthwhile either. The ability to provide therapy that improves function in a context that is enjoyable for the child is the "art" of therapy.

NDT Feeding Therapy-Postural Control

Feeding intervention using an NDT approach for a child with cerebral palsy follows directly from the assessment. The SLP is armed with information about the child's strengths and areas of need. However, the SLP also has the knowledge of typical feeding development along with information about the motor bases of that development. Mature oral skills are based on postural control that includes pelvic stability, head and trunk alignment, and head control. Although most SLPs would agree that head control is necessary for the oral movements for a safe swallow (Arvedson & Brodsky, 2002; Larnert & Ekberg, 1995; Redstone & West, 2004; Seikel, King, & Drumright, 2000; West & Redstone, 2004), it needs to be emphasized that "trunk control is fundamental to head control" (Mohr, 1990, p. 1), and trunk control depends on stability of the pelvis (Herman & Lange, 1999; Zemlin, 1998). Children with cerebral palsy lack this stability, which then leads to poor development of jaw stability (Alexander et al., 1993; Hall, 2001; Redstone & West, 2004). In turn, lip and tongue movements that depend on mandibular stability (Daniels, Brailey, & Foundas, 1999; Seikel et al., 2005; Tamura, Mizukami, Ayano, & Mukai, 2002) do not develop well.

This, then, is the SLP's first and primary strategy for improving oral motor control for feeding. The NDT therapist addresses trunk control through movement and handling at nonfeeding times, prior to feeding, and positioning for feeding. Again, a dual-track approach is worthwhile. Parents can be trained to recognize situations that occur daily to encourage postural control and they can be taught appropriate handling skills for their child. So many times throughout the day there are opportunities to encourage head/trunk alignment and experiences for improving trunk control. For example, parents can be taught to pick up, carry, diaper, and play with their child in a manner that encourages trunk elongation with a flexor component and a neutral head posture.

Something as simple as giving the child the time to weight shift and reach for a toy without total extension can lead to important changes that will be reflected during feeding if done regularly. Attaining head and trunk alignment gives the child the possibility of a chin-tuck position and mouth closure. This is an efficient intervention since the SLP gets appropriate mouth posture without ever touching the oral area.

Positioning for Feeding

Once head and trunk alignment, symmetry, and as normal muscle tone as possible have been attained, the goal of positioning should be to maintain that posture during feeding. Although very young children are fed in a parent's lap, most children are seated in chairs. The best starting position for intervention for an oral–motor function like feeding is upright posture with 90-degree flexion at the hips, knees, and ankles. This provides the greatest stability for oral functioning. When positioned for bottle feeding the infant should be upright with neck flexion. However, it is very important for the feeder to be able to see the infant's face for any indications of stress. This is often difficult to attain in the lap. Feeding chairs, car seats, or the use of a wedge as seen in Figure 4–3 can be used to provide face-to-face upright posture with head support.

The same principles apply to high chairs for older infants and children. Items that will facilitate stable positioning are seat belts

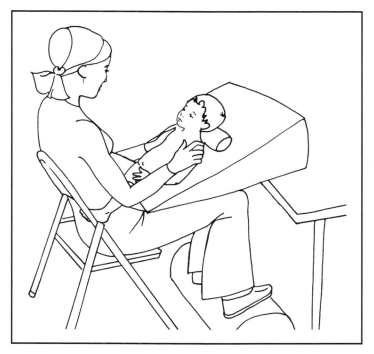

Figure 4–3. Face-to-face positioning on a wedge for an infant. (Illustration by Barbro Salek as seen in Connor, F. P., Siepp, J. M., & Williamson, G. G. [1978]. *The program guide for infants and toddlers with neuromotor and other developmental disabilities.* New York, NY: Teachers College Press.)

for pelvic stability, lateral supports so the child does not fall over to one side, trays for upper extremity weight bearing, and well-placed foot rests as seen in Figure 4–4.

Preschoolers and school-aged children sit in chairs at tables in schools or centers. The 90-degree flexion principle applies here as well. SLPs often neglect foot stability because their primary focus is head control for oral functioning. However, foot support contributes to the ability to function at high levels orally. If the child's feet do not reach the floor for support, place a foot stool or similar item under the child's feet until a more permanent solution is found. This can also be accomplished by the use of a commercially available adaptive chair.

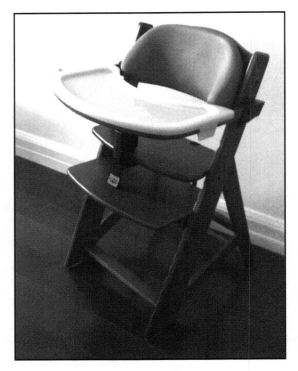

Figure 4–4. Seating for feeding with foot support for stability, tray for upper extremity weight-bearing, and a seat belt for pelvic stability.

Although this dates me, I had typically used the 5-inch-thick Manhattan telephone book for foot stability when working in NYC many (many) years ago. Then I moved to Colorado. When positioning a child in the preschool where I was working, I suggested using a phone book to address this need. However, as this was a rather small city in Colorado, the phone book was only a half-inch thick!

The feeding therapist is fortunate in that there are many companies that meet the needs for appropriate positioning for functioning. However, adaptive equipment is expensive and may take months to fund. Therefore, SLPs need to be creative in order to enhance the child's functioning by using household items like pillows, wedges, towels, and stools. In addition, just because a high chair is expensive does not necessarily mean it will work for the child. Moreover, will it still address the child's needs after a few months of use?

Children's therapy centers and hospitals often have departments that can make inexpensive equipment for children with special needs. These departments work with feeding therapists so that each piece of equipment is highly individualized for a specific child. Materials used have included triwall corrugated cardboard, which is relatively inexpensive and is easy to work with. Children can use the equipment until they outgrow it or it is no longer needed. Hulme and her associates (1987) developed seating devices using NDT principles (Bergen & Colangelo, 1985) and found improved drinking and feeding skills.

NDT-Feeding Procedures

It is always best to begin with whatever the child is presently using. The goal is safe and efficient intake of food that is age appropriate. Changes in food, utensils, and process should be based on assessment and direction of intervention. The SLP should always have a rationale for any changes made.

Spoon-Feeding: Utensils, Foods, and Procedure

Spoon-feeding begins by 6 months of age so it is an early developing skill. The child should be well positioned before starting, and the mouth closed, unless there are structural issues. The food on a spoon should be a uniform consistency that is thick enough to remain on the spoon without running off. The food chosen depends on the child's food preferences but is often fairly bland. Sugars and acids are typically avoided because they increase saliva production, which then is more difficult for the child to handle orally.

If the spoon is going to be needed to control the tongue, the bowl of the spoon should fit in the child's mouth comfortably without causing a gag but should also cover a significant portion of the surface of the tongue. The spoon should be shallow and smooth so that the child is more likely to successfully remove food. The amount of food on the spoon should be determined by the child's needs. For example, a small amount placed near the tip of the spoon increases the possibility for success, but some children with hyposensitivity require more mass in their mouths.

The feeder should be sitting and approach with the spoon at the child's eye level or below so that head hyperextension does not occur. The expected response from the child is to open the mouth enough to accept the spoon. If this does not occur, the feeder can model opening. This often occurs automatically. Touching the chin gently may also help by providing a sensory input. The clinician should note the quality of the grading of the jaw throughout the feeding. In general, a least-to-most prompting order during feeding includes modeling, gentle sensory input, and oral control.

The feeder then places the *spoon in, down on the tongue . . . WAITS . . . and pulls the spoon straight out*. Waiting, or time delay, is a useful therapy technique in feeding, as well as other areas of intervention, because the child with cerebral palsy often has a delayed response. Also, modeling of mouth closure by the feeder or the use of a sensory stimulus can be used. The child may not get food off the spoon initially because of lack of lip movement or inexperience. However, modeling lip movement and providing more flexion are strategies that can be effective. Remember, spoon-feeding is learned and often takes a physically typical child about a month to be successful. The clinician must also be attuned to subtle attempts at new strategies.

Solid Foods: Foods, Utensils, and Procedure

To begin bite-taking and chewing, the child and feeder should be well positioned. For the early stages of therapy, easily dissolvable, finger-sized foods should be used. This is safest for the child and easiest for placement by the feeder. Mouth opening should be graded and the food placed on the chewing surfaces of the teeth on the child's better side. This may be the side that has better sensation or movements. The food should not be placed on the tongue because that is likely to trigger suckling. Again, *wait,* because the bite should be initiated by the child. If this does not occur, modeling, a gentle tactile reminder, or oral control can be attempted. When the child closes the mouth, the feeder may help the child take a bite by providing a slight tug as the jaw is closed. The next bite should be presented to the other side of the mouth so that both sides are stimulated equally.

The feeder should observe tongue movement as well as the pattern of chewing. This is a functional activity that can be used to foster tongue lateralization. In addition, it may also be part of a sensitivity program.

Cup Drinking: Liquids, Cups, and Procedures

Cup drinking is the most difficult feeding skill for both the child and the feeder. This is due to the speed at which liquid moves. Often, it is suggested that thickened liquids be used. This can be done using naturally thick foods such as nectars or milk shakes, but remember, sweets and acids increase saliva production. This may also be useful for children who are just beginning to hold a cup themselves, or for a parent who is having trouble controlling the flow of fluid. During direct feeding therapy, the clinician should be able to facilitate successful cup drinking using a free-flowing liquid.

The cup should be small enough for the child's comfort and the feeder's ease of manipulation. The sensory input from the rim of the cup may assist in lip closure. Cut-out cups have been popular; they are easier for the feeder and help to maintain a chin-tuck position when the fluid is low. If the child has a favorite cup that is not cut-out, use it. However, the cup will need to be fairly full so that head hyperextension does not occur.

To begin cup drinking, the child needs to be *very well positioned* with mouth closure initiated. The feeder needs to observe the child's lips, the rim of the cup, and the flow of the fluid. The cup should be placed between the child's lips, and the fluid needs to be brought up to the child's lips. The feeder needs to *wait* for movement of the upper lip, indicating the attempt to draw fluid in. The feeder should not pour fluid into the child's mouth. Modeling, along with stimulation of the upper lip, are sensory strategies to encourage this lip movement.

It is important to take note of the child's respiratory pattern. If there are indications of breath-holding, take the cup away from the child's face. The child may only be able to take one sip/swallow between breaths. Consecutive swallows require successful coordination of breathing with swallowing, which may require stability and experience. Often, children who do not require oral control for other feeding activities may need it for cup drinking, because of its complexity and speed.

Other NDT Feeding Techniques

Postural control and positioning for postural control are the most important strategies to use for intervention with children with cerebral palsy with feeding disorders. However, this group is highly heterogeneous, and this may not be enough for all children. The next sections will present additional NDT techniques that may be used *when needed*. The SLP should have a rationale for the use of any technique and should evaluate its usefulness regularly.

Oral Control

When performed correctly by the SLP, oral control will increase movement options for the child with cerebral palsy. It is an NDT technique that was first published by Mueller (1972) when it was called "jaw control." It is therapeutic handling of the oral area and can be used to facilitate mouth closure and jaw, tongue, and lip movements for feeding (Arvedson & Brodsky, 2002; Hall, 2001; Mueller, 2001).

Oral control from the side, as seen in Figure 4–5A, is typically used for children with more severe oral motor issues. While sitting on the child's side, the clinician uses one hand for oral control while the other is employed for feeding. The arm of the hand being used for oral control must go around the back of the client's head. This hand is supinated so that the elbow is high and can assist in alignment of the head and trunk. The index finger of this hand is then placed midway between the lower lip and the bottom of the chin, and the middle finger is placed under the chin. There is a balance that must be reached between these fingers so that just enough control is provided to maintain jaw posture and movements. If too much pressure is applied, the child may hyperextend or may demonstrate negative behavior if there is restriction of movement causing this experience to be unpleasant.

Oral control can be provided from the front, as seen in Figure 4–5B, by sitting at eye level with the child and placing the thumb on the chin while the middle finger is under the chin, midway between the prominence of the chin and the neck. This position permits eye contact but offers less control than side oral control. It is best used with infants in a feeding seat or with older children who have been in feeding therapy and may just need a sensorimotor reminder.

Since 1972, this technique has been published by therapists and researchers who trained with Mueller (Morris & Klein, 2000; Pinder & Faherty, 1999; Redstone & West, 2004) and those who studied interventions for preterm infants (Boiron, Da Nobrega, Roux, Henrot, & Saliba, 2007; Einarsson-Backes, Deitz, Price, Glass, & Hays, 1994; Hill, Kurkowski, & Garcia, 2000).

Remember, oral control is used *only when necessary*. Improving postural control will often result in better oral functioning without addressing the mouth directly. This would eliminate the need for oral control. If oral control is used, it is only provided for function within a specific context such as feeding (Sheppard, 2008). Oral control should be considered as a type of scaffold or prompt. And like any prompt, oral control should be faded.

NDT Sensitivity Programs

If the child's assessment indicates that atypical sensitivity interferes with feeding, a program should be tailored specifically for

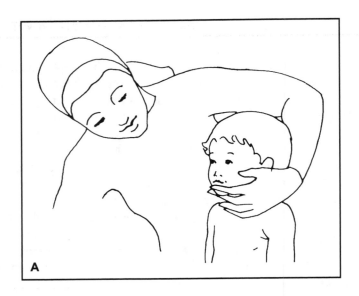

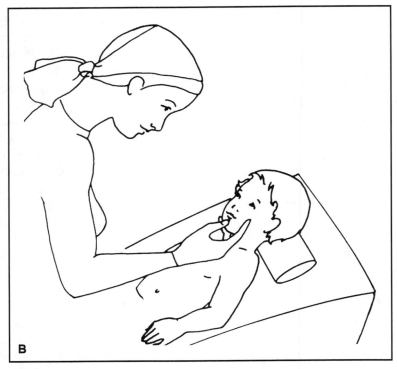

Figure 4–5. Oral control from the side (**A**) and from the front (**B**). (Illustration by Barbro Salek as seen in Connor, F. P., Siepp, J. M., & Williamson, G. G. [1978]. *The program guide for infants and toddlers with neuromotor and other developmental disabilities.* New York, NY: Teachers College Press.)

that child. It may include oral tactile stimulation, graded input of new textures, and/or toothbrushing (Arvedson & Brodsky, 2002; Pinder & Faherty, 1999). The goal is to increase the possibility of a more normal motor response through manipulation of the sensory environment (Alexander, 1987).

The program may include arm and hand movements to facilitate hand-to-mouth and object-to-mouth activities. These activities can be performed throughout the day by parents. However, these movements need to be facilitated without increasing muscle tone and abnormal patterns. Daily activities that can be taught to parents include methods of face wiping and toothbrushing. Often these daily activities are performed in a way that leads to disorganization and discomfort. But they need to be accomplished in a way that children can tolerate and help them to mitigate their sensitivity issues. For example, while cleaning a child's face, a parent can provide firm pressure to a specific area, then move to a different section. This would avoid taking broad swipes, which could disorganize the child and be upsetting.

Every child with a tooth should brush that tooth every day. This does provide strong sensory input, but if it is done well, it can provide excellent stimulation and an opportunity to teach children to swallow their saliva. This will reduce drooling (Pinder & Faherty, 1999). However, oral control may be needed to facilitate and maintain mouth closure. The parent or therapist needs to allow for spitting or swallowing, ridding the mouth of the extra saliva produced during toothbrushing. Initially, brushing should be accomplished without toothpaste. First, the outside of the teeth are brushed as intraoral sensitivity is typically greater, and the child may not be able to tolerate brushing inside the mouth.

Toothbrushing as Part of a Sensitivity Program

1. Position the child correctly.
2. Monitor mouth closure. Oral control may be necessary.
3. Place toothbrush at the midline of the outside of the teeth. Start on the upper section of the better side.

4. Brush the way the teeth grow, down on the top and up on the bottom.
5. Brush from the front to back, and return the same way, back to front.
6. Remove the brush and wait for a swallow.
7. Brush the teeth on the bottom on the same side.
8. Brush the outside of the teeth on opposite side of the mouth.

Depending on the child's needs, the stimulation during toothbrushing can be modified. The child who is hyposensitive may need lighter, faster, stimulation whereas a hypersensitive child will need firm, slower stimulation. In addition, the actual feeding context can be used to improve oral sensitivity. Making incremental changes in the texture of the child's foods can improve sensitivity.

NDT courses teach "normalizing oral tactile sensitivity" (Mueller, 1972, p. 297). This includes the same type of stimulation just described, but the therapist's finger is used to adjust the input based on the child's sensitivity and response to the stimulation. In addition, the intraoral area is targeted as well. Commercially available instruments and vibrators can also be used to provide stimulation. However, their inputs cannot be individualized for each child. The response to any stimulation needs to be monitored closely. Remember, oral stimulation increases saliva production. If the child's mouth is open, and if swallowing is not facilitated during the activity, this may lead to drooling.

NDT Oral Muscle Tone Programs

Handling and positioning that normalize muscle throughout the body will be reflected in the oral area. For the child with hypotonicity, involving weight-bearing and pushing can increase muscle tone. Wheelbarrow walking or pushing a weighted chair or wagon across the room have been used to improve tone in the extremities and trunk. In NDT tapping techniques are taught that target the lips and tongue muscles. Likewise, oral tug-of-war games may increase strength in the mandible. Instruments such as the Iowa Oral Performance Instrument (IOPI) have been reported in the literature to improve swallow function in adults, but have not been studied with children.

Children with hypertonicity require movement to reduce muscle tone. Gross motor movements that reduce tone proximally and in the extremities such as reaching, laterally flexing, and rotating are examples of movements that can be incorporated into play and daily routines. These will influence the oral area for feeding. NDT techniques that are taught in postgraduate continuing education courses include having the clinician provide a slow stretch with two fingers, along with fine vibration to the cheek or tongue. However, they are only used after other less invasive handling techniques have been attempted.

Behavioral Programs and Weaning from Tube Feeding

Many children with cerebral palsy have had discomfort associated with feeding. This may have resulted from the motor disorder, sensory deficit, reflux, or even some therapy or medical interventions. Consequently, food aversion may be present (Fraker & Walbert, 2011; Palmer, 1998) or other behavioral issues that need to be addressed within a feeding program. Toomey and Ross (2011) describe a feeding aversion as a learned avoidance from either physically being unable to perform or from discomfort.

If the child experienced severe reflux, was diagnosed as "failure-to-thrive," demonstrated signs of aspiration, or had severe oral–motor issues, a gastrostomy tube (G-tube) may have been placed. Once a child is medically and nutritionally stable and has gained sufficient oral motor skills through therapy, a program to wean the child from a G-tube to oral feeding is typically recommended. Although the child may now be better nourished and experience less discomfort, negative behaviors and aversions may still exist due to past unpleasant experiences associated with feeding.

Programs that address weaning to oral feeding and food avoidance have several principles in common. Both emphasize the need for pleasant feeding experiences. They acknowledge the child's preferences, do not force the child to eat, and make incremental changes that the child can tolerate. The SLP providing feeding therapy for a child with cerebral palsy needs to address these principles as well as the child's oral–motor skills.

Conclusions

Because so many children with cerebral palsy exhibit feeding problems, it is essential that the SLP treating these children be cognizant of both the swallowing issues and the motor deficits involved. It is crucial for the SLP to understand that the motor component directly influences the development of safe, functional feeding skills.

The NDT approach presented emphasizes the need to assess and treat several systems of the developing child within a functional context; not just the oral system by itself. NDT was one of the first approaches that stressed early intervention (The Telegraph, 2001) and a team approach. All of these principles are essential when treating children with cerebral palsy who exhibit feeding disorders.

Ten Items for Improving Intervention

1. Assess and treat the whole child.
2. The child's head control is essential for oral–motor control for feeding.
3. Successful feeding relies on gross-motor stability.
4. Addressing postural control is the first step in feeding intervention.
5. Maintaining postural control is the goal of positioning.
6. Oral closure and improved functioning may occur automatically with improved postural control with no need for direct oral intervention.
7. Feeding therapy begins at the level the child is functioning at comfortably.
8. A dual treatment approach implies that feeding therapy is different from the parent's daily feeding of the child.
9. There must be a rationale for using an intervention technique or making a change in the child's foods, utensils, or feeding procedure.
10. All procedures and techniques need to be performed in a manner that allows interaction and an enjoyable feeding experience.

Think Critically for Self-Study or Classroom Discussion

1. List three items from typical feeding development that you can use in treatment.
2. Discuss three reasons why pelvic stability influences feeding.
3. List three reasons why a clinician might use oral control.
4. How does reflux influence feeding? How can the SLP address this?
5. How should the SLP address the child's extended head when it is being used to compensate for lack of tongue movement to propel the bolus posteriorly?

References

Alexander, R. (1987). Oral-motor treatment for infants and young children with cerebral palsy. *Seminars in Speech and Language, 8,* 87–100.

Alexander, R., Boehme, R., & Cupps, B. (1993). *Normal development of functional motor skills.* San Antonio, TX: Therapy Skill Builders.

Arvedson, J. C., & Brodsky, I. (2002). *Pediatric swallowing and feeding: Assessment and management* (2nd ed.). San Diego, CA: Singular.

Barlow, S. M., Poore, M. A., Zimmerman, E. A., & Finan, D. S. (2010, June 8). Feeding skills in the preterm infant. *The ASHA Leader.* Retrieved from http://www.asha.org/Publications/leader/2010/100608/Feeding-Skills-Infant.htm

Beecher, R., & Alexander, R. (2004). Pediatric feeding and swallowing: Clinical examination and evaluation. *Perspectives in Swallowing and Swallowing Disorders, 13,* 21–27.

Bergen, A. F., & Colangelo, C. (1985). *Positioning the client with central nervous system deficits: The wheel chair and other adaptive equipment* (2nd ed.). Valhalla, NY: Valhalla Rehabilitation.

Bly, L. (1983). *The components of normal movement during the first year of life.* Oak Park, IL: Neurodevelopmental Treatment Association.

Boiron, M., Da Nobrega, L., Roux, S., Henrot, A., & Saliba, E. (2007). Effects of oral stimulation and oral support on non-nutritive sucking and feeding performance in preterm infants. *Developmental Medicine & Child Neurology, 49,* 439–444.

Daniels, S. K., Brailey, K., & Foundas, A. L. (1999). Lingual discoordination and dysphagia following acute stroke: Analyses of lesion localization. *Dysphagia, 14*, 85–92.

Eicher, P. S. (2007). Feeding. In M. L. Batshaw, L. Pelligrino, & N. J. Roizen (Eds.), *Children with disabilities* (pp. 479–498). Baltimore, MD: Paul H. Brookes.

Einarsson-Backes, L. M., Deitz, J., Price, R., Glass, R., & Hays, R. (1994). The effect of oral support on sucking efficiency in preterm infants. *The American Journal of Occupational Therapy, 48*, 490–498.

Fraker, C., & Walbert, L. (2011). Treatment of selective eating and dysphagia using pre-chaining and food chaining therapy programs. *Perspectives on Swallowing and Swallowing Disorders, 20*, 75–81.

Hall, K. D. (2001). *Pediatric dysphagia: Resource guide.* San Diego, CA: Singular, Thomson Learning.

Hanzlik, J. R., & Stevenson, M. B. (1986). Interaction of mothers with their infants who are mentally retarded, retarded with cerebral palsy, or nonretarded. *Journal of Mental Deficiency, 90*, 513–520.

Herman, J. H., & Lange, M. L. (1999). Seating and positioning to manage spasticity after brain injury. *NeuroRehabilitation, 12*, 105–117.

Hill, A. J., Kurkowski, T. B., & Garcia, J. (2000). Oral support measures used in feeding the preterm infant. *Nursing Research, 49*, 2–10.

Hulme, J. B., Shaver, J., Acher, S., Mullette, L., & Eggert, C. (1987). Effects of adaptive seating devices on the eating and drinking of children with multiple handicaps. *The American Journal of Occupational Therapy, 41*, 81–89.

Kamm, K., Thelen, E., & Jensen, J. L. (1990). A dynamical systems approach to motor development. *Physical Therapy, 70*, 763–775.

Larnert, G., & Ekberg, O. (1995). Positioning improves the oral and pharyngeal swallowing function in children with cerebral palsy. *Acta Pediatrica, 84*, 689–692.

Mohr, J. D. (1990). Management of the trunk in adult hemiplegia: The Bobath concept. *Topics in Neurology, In-Touch series*, Lesson 1, 1–11.

Morris, S. E., & Klein, M. D. (2000). *Pre-feeding skills: A comprehensive resource for feeding development.* San Antonio, TX: Therapy Skill Builders.

Mueller, H. (1972). Facilitating feeding and prespeech. In P. H. Pearson & C. E. Williams (Eds.), *Physical therapy services in the developmental disabilities* (pp. 283–310). Springfield, IL: Thomas.

Mueller, H. (2001). Feeding. In N. R. Finnie, *Handling the young child with cerebral palsy at home* (3rd ed., pp. 209–221). Boston, MA: Butterworth-Heinemann.

Palmer, M. M. (1998). Weaning from gastrostomy tube feeding: Commentary on oral aversion. *Pediatric Nursing, 24*, 475–478.

Pelligrino, L. (2007). Cerebral palsy. In M. L. Batshaw, L. Pelligrino, & N. J. Roizen (Eds.), *Children with disabilities* (pp. 387–408). Baltimore, MD: Paul H. Brookes.

Pennington, L., Goldbart, J., & Marshall, J. (2004). Interaction training for conversational partners of children with cerebral palsy: A systematic review. *International Journal of Language & Communication Disorders, 39*, 151–170.

Pennington, L., & McConachie, H. (1999). Mother-child interaction revisited: Communication with non-speaking physically disabled children. *International Journal of Language & Communication Disorders, 34*, 391–416.

Pinder, G. L., & Faherty, A. S. (1999). Issues in pediatric feeding and swallowing. In A. J. Caruso & E. A. Strand (Eds.), *Clinical management of motor speech disorders in children* (pp. 281–318). New York, NY: Thieme.

Redstone, F., & West, J. F. (2004). Postural control for feeding. *Pediatric Nursing, 30*, 97–100.

Rogers, B., Arvedson, J., Buck, G., Smart, P., & Msall, M. (1994). Characteristics of dysphagia in children with cerebral palsy. *Dysphagia, 9*, 60–73.

Seikel, J. A., King, D. W., & Drumright, D. G. (2005). *Anatomy and physiology for speech, language, and hearing* (4th ed.). Clifton Park, NY: Delmar, Cengage.

Sheppard, J. J. (2008). Using motor learning approaches for treating swallowing and feeding disorders: A review. *Language, Speech, and Hearing Services in Schools, 39*, 227–236.

Tamura, F., Mizukami, M., Ayano, R., & Mukai, Y. (2002). Analysis of feeding function and jaw stability in bedridden elderly. *Dysphagia, 17*, 235–241.

The Telegraph. (March 29, 2001). Mary Quinton obituary. Retrieved from http://www.telegraph.co.uk/news/obituaries/1328204/Mary-Quinton.html

Thelen, E. (1991). Motor aspects of emergent speech: A dynamic approach. In N. Krasnegor (Ed.), *Biobehavioral foundations of language acquisition* (pp. 339–362). Hillsdale, NJ: Erlbaum.

Toomey, K. A., & Ross, E. S. (2011). SOS approach to feeding. *Perspectives on swallowing and swallowing disorders, 20*, 82–87.

Tsai, S., Chen, C., & Lin, M. (2010). Prediction for developmental delay on Neonatal Oral Motor Assessment Scale in preterm infants without brain lesion. *Pediatrics International, 52*, 65–68.

West, J. F., & Redstone, F. (2004). Alignment during feeding and swallowing: Does it matter? A review. *Perceptual and Motor Skills, 98*, 349–358.

Wolf, L. S., & Glass, R. P. (1992). *Feeding and swallowing disorders in infancy: Assessment and management.* Tucson, AZ: Therapy Skill Builders.

Zemlin, W. R. (1998). *Speech and hearing science: Anatomy and physiology* (3rd ed.). Boston, MA: Allyn & Bacon.

CHAPTER 5

Feeding in the NICU

Marjorie M. Palmer

Introduction

Speech-language pathologists (SLPs) play a significant role in the neonatal intensive care unit (NICU) especially concerning the assessment and treatment of feeding skills of infants and the education of team and family members (ASHA, 2004). SLPs first provided NICU services in the 1980s, before ASHA became involved in feeding and swallowing. The clinicians who worked in this environment were typically NDT certified because they had the knowledge, skills, training, and experience of working with young infants. They did not, however, have a background in premature infant development, because in the 1980s the very young or sick infants usually did not survive. But research, technology, medical science, and training have all changed since those early days, and premature infants born at 23 weeks are now able to survive.

Improved technology and medical advances in the NICU have led to a significantly increased survival rate of premature and medically fragile infants. However, as the survival rate has increased, so has the rate of developmental disabilities. Prematurity or low birth weight is associated with 40 to 50% of the cases of cerebral palsy. Early feeding problems can be the first symptom of a later disability (Katsumi & Veda, 2005), and many of these infants have feeding problems that persist into early childhood (Barlow, Moore, Zimmerman, & Finan, 2010), which may be due to the fact that successful feeding is dependent on motor stability (Ross, 2013). Because early sucking is an important oral–motor function, it has been hypothesized that a delay or disorder of this skill is correlated with later delays in other motor skills (Slattery, Morgan, & Douglas, 2012). However, not all premature infants with delay in the development of suck and swallow will necessarily have later motor problems. They just need time to mature neurologically and develop adequate respiratory support for successful oral feeding. We must learn to differentiate these populations in order to provide the best interventions for optimal functional outcomes.

Typical full-term newborns are anatomically and physiologically prepared to feed orally. The infant first experiences the extrauterine environment through the mouth or "oral sensorium" (Bosma, 1975, p. 4). Such nomenclature derives from the vast number of sensory receptors on the tongue, rendering the oral cavity one of the most sensitive areas of the body. This explains the full-term infant's good adaptability to changing circumstances of feeding.

Anatomy and Physiology of the Newborn's Oral Area

The mouth of the full-term infant is completely filled by the tongue as seen in Figure 5–1. The tongue contacts all of the lateral borders and the palate when the mouth is closed and the tongue is at rest. There is no buccal cheek cavity because the elasticity in the cheek is stretched tightly over the sucking pads or fat pads in the buccal area. In addition, the mandible is small. Because the oral structures in the newborn are vertically compressed at birth, the soft palate approximates the epiglottis, and the tongue tip is anatomically positioned against the alveolar ridge at rest. This tongue position is anatomically determined. It is only when the tongue moves away from the palate as the mouth is opened which signals that the infant is ready to eat.

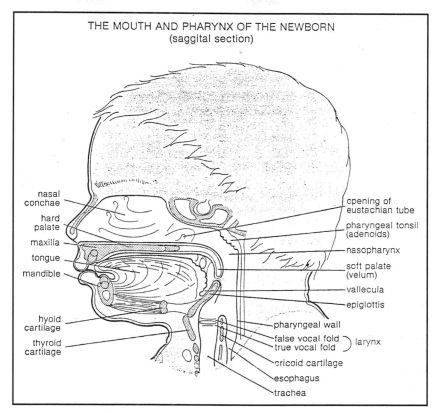

THE MOUTH AND PHARYNX OF THE NEWBORN
(saggital section)

nasal conchae

hard palate

maxilla

tongue

mandible

hyoid cartilage

thyroid cartilage

opening of eustachian tube

pharyngeal tonsil (adenoids)

nasopharynx

soft palate (velum)

vallecula

epiglottis

pharyngeal wall

false vocal fold
true vocal fold ⎞ larynx

cricoid cartilage

esophagus

trachea

Figure 5–1. Diagram of the mouth and pharynx of the newborn. Proportions differ from the infant at 6 months. (From: *The normal acquisition of oral feeding skills* by Suzanne Evans Morris. Published by Therapeutic Media 1982. Reprinted with permission.)

Primitive Oral Reflexes

The full-term infant enters the world equipped with a repertoire of primitive oral reflexes to ensure survival in the extrauterine environment. Obviously, if the infant is born too early these primitive oral reflexes may not yet be present. The most familiar ones are the rooting reflex, gag reflex, transverse tongue reflex, phasic bite, and non-nutritive and nutritive suck are described below. Another significant feature of these primitive reflexes is that they provide us a window into the functioning of the cranial nerves and alert us to the level of functioning in the infant (Bingham, 2009).

Rooting Reflex

The rooting reaction consists of a sequential series of four steps. The first is a sensory step that occurs as a tactile stimulus touches the mouth. The infant must be able to differentiate this as the source of the stimulus. Then there is a motor response with the infant's head turning toward the stimulus. The third step involves both sensory and motor components as the infant latches on to the nipple. The last step involves the infant actually initiating sucking.

Although the rooting reaction has been reported in the literature as occurring well before term at 28 weeks postconceptual age (PCA) (Nyquist, Sjoden, & Ewald, 1999), it was not divided into four sequential steps. This sequence became clear to me after 30 years of observation. Because of the lack of this division the rooting reaction was reported as occurring earlier than it would have been had all four steps been considered. In the full-term infant the rooting reaction has often been interpreted as a cue for readiness-to-feed. This is only true if the infant completes the four-step rooting sequence. The rooting reflex, however, is not a cue for readiness-to-feed in the premature or sick newborn.

Gag Reflex

The gag reflex is protective in nature for infants 6 months and older. It involves head and jaw extension, rhythmic protrusions of the tongue, and contractions of the pharynx. In the newborn and preterm infant, it is the cough reflex that protects the airway. However, we may also gain information from this reflex. If the gag is absent in the premature or sick newborn, it may indicate an absent cough reflex as well. Therefore, oral feeding is frequently not advised when the gag reflex is absent. Be aware that the gag reflex is state-dependent and should be rechecked if it is absent initially. It provides us with a window into the level of functioning of the cranial nerves in the term neonate and the premature infant.

Transverse Tongue Reflex

This reflex is demonstrated by the horizontal shifting of the tongue toward a touch pressure stimulus as seen in Figure 5–2. This stimulus is applied to the lateral tongue border on the anterior third of the infant's tongue (Weiffenbach & Thach, 1972). This reflex does not play an active role in early feeding but becomes important later as mastication develops. Without this reflex we cannot chew solids.

Phasic Bite

This reflex is seen as a series of consecutive jaw openings and closings that occur in response to a touch pressure cue that is applied to the lateral gum tissue. The jaw movement is fluid and easy to elicit, and the mandible neither clamps shut nor hangs open (Morris & Klein, 1987).

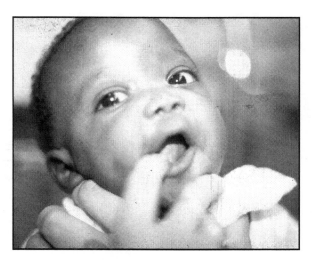

Figure 5–2. Transverse tongue reflex. (From: *NOMAS Certification Course Instructor's Manual.* Reprinted with permission.)

Non-nutritive Suck

A non-nutritive suck is a suck on a pacifier that does not deliver any nutrient as seen in Figure 5–3. The rate is about two per second, which is twice as fast as the nutritive suck. Jaw excursions are short and rapid, and the tongue is cupped around the nipple, forming a central tongue groove. The lips do not play a role in neonatal sucking. This suck does not require a great deal of coordination with pharyngeal swallow or respiration, and many infants may suck quite well on a pacifier while being unable to feed orally.

Nutritive Suck

The suck that occurs when liquid is transferred into the baby's mouth from an external source is a nutritive suck. This suck requires coordination of suck, swallow, and respiration, and it occurs more slowly than the non-nutritive suck, usually at the rate of one suck per second. There are two types of normal,

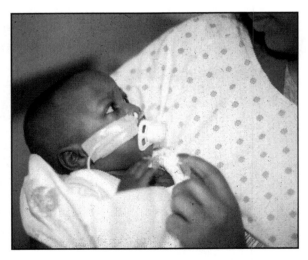

Figure 5–3. Non-nutritive suck (NNS) on a pacifier. (From: *NOMAS Certification Course Instructor's Manual.* Reprinted with permission.)

nutritive suck patterns. The *mature* suck pattern is usually not seen in the infant until close to term, at about 37 to 38 weeks PCA. This is the only sucking pattern that has all three components of suck, swallow, and respiration during a sucking burst which occurs at 10 to 30 sucks per burst (Gryboski, 1975). Sucks occur at the rate of one per second, and the average ratio of suck to swallow to respiration is 1:1:1 (Bu'Lock, Woolridge, & Baum, 1990). Reportedly, this rhythmic stability is established by term (Qureshi, Vice, Taciak, Bosma, & Gewolb, 2002). The ratio of suck to swallow to respiration may be influenced by the choice of nipples. For example, when offered a firmer nipple the infant may need to suck two or three times to extract a sufficient volume of liquid to trigger the pharyngeal swallow. As long as the infant is able to demonstrate a specific pattern with a consistent ratio for the first 2 minutes of the feeding, the suck is considered normal (Braun & Palmer, 1985; Palmer, 1993; Palmer, Crawley, & Blanco, 1993).

The second type of normal nutritive suck pattern is the *immature suck*. This may be present in a premature infant who does not yet have adequate respiratory support or the neurological maturation to suck like an infant at term. Although it differs from the suck of the typical neonate, it is not pathological. The sucking bursts are short, consisting of three to five sucks per burst, followed by a pause of equal duration during which the breathing and/or swallow may occur. Some infants demonstrate a pattern with suck/swallow, suck/swallow, suck/swallow, and then pause for 3 seconds to breathe. Other infants may suck for 3 seconds and then pause to swallow and breathe for 3 seconds. Either of these patterns would be considered to be within normal limits for younger infants (Gryboski, 1975).

In neonatal reflexive sucking the tongue is proximal to the jaw and is responsible for all that happens during the oral phase of swallow. This phenomenon changes with the anatomical growth of the oral mechanism and the transition from reflexive to volitional movement that occurs by 6 months of age. As the mandible grows the anatomical position of the tongue moves away from the palate. At this stage tongue tip elevation must occur for a normal swallow. This is possible since the typical 6-month-old has developed some jaw stability along with some independent and dissociated movements of the lips, tongue, and jaw. Tongue tip elevation is now possible. However, the child with cerebral palsy does not make the transition from reflexive to volitional movement of the oral musculature and, therefore, does not develop bilabial closure or tongue tip elevation for a swallow. This child continues to move in a reflexive pattern that will soon be identified as abnormal.

Normal Nutritive Suck Patterns

- Mature suck
  - □ 10 to 30 sucks per burst
  - □ one suck per second
  - □ suck/swallow/breathe ratio of 1:1:1
  - □ breathing and swallowing occur during the burst
- Immature suck
  - □ short sucking bursts of 3 to 5 sucks
  - □ burst–pause pattern
  - □ bursts and pauses of equal duration
  - □ breathing and/or swallowing occur during the pause

Characteristics of Infants in the NICU

The cranial nerves located in the brainstem are responsible for both sensory and motor control of the mouth, pharynx, and esophagus (Bosma, 1975). Some feel that this is to ensure that even the most neurologically compromised infants will survive (Katsumi & Veda, 2005). For example, even anencephalic infants born without a cortex will have the ability to suck and swallow during this early reflexive period. Sometimes with severe cases of neurological insult such as the infant with hypoxic-ischemic encephalopathy, neonatal reflexive feeding is their optimal behavior. The degree of disability does not become obvious until the infant ages and develops. Occasionally, the opposite occurs. Those infants who do not suck and are sent home from the NICU on a gastrostomy tube may later be able to manage pureed foods and soft solids. Each infant is different. According to Bosma, "an infant's suck is as individual as his fingerprint" (personal communication, June 4, 1976). Remembering this should help us to view each infant as a unique individual.

The premature or sick infant in the NICU may have experienced negative oral input from interventions that involved suctioning and placement of tubes through the mouth or nose. From the moment of birth this infant may have been subjected to a variety of life-saving procedures directed to the orofacial area that altered his orofacial and intraoral sensory awareness and perception. This stimulation often leads to a hypo- or hypersensitivity resulting in diminished oral responses.

The full-term neonate or preterm infant has a limited repertoire of oral movements secondary to the specific anatomy of the infant's oral mechanism (Bosma, 1975). The infant's oral structures change between 3 and 6 months of age. This change is reflected in the infant's suck. It has been reported that the normal term infant develops a stronger suck at 3 months of age, which is attributable to the growth of the mandible and active tongue and jaw movements (Tamura, Matsushita, Shinoda, & Yoshida, 1998). By 6 months of age muscle function must take the place of the earlier protective nature of the small, vertically compressed oral structures. It is at this time that some infants who had fed adequately orally earlier in development may begin to demonstrate feeding difficulties. Some may even require the placement of feeding tubes because of aspiration.

Assessment

In general, the preterm infant or infant under 6 months of age usually does not require a modified barium swallow study unless a structural abnormality, neuromuscular, or neurological issue is suspected that would impact the pharyngeal phase of swallow and cause aspiration. However, it is important for the feeding specialist in the NICU to recognize differences in sucking. But to do this, special training is required. Typically, this is obtained through continuing education courses after the master's degree.

Observations Prior to Feeding

Because the anatomy of the oral mechanism in the neonate is well prepared to take nutrition orally and oxygen nasally, the typical infant at rest will be a comfortable nasal breather while maintaining bilabial closure. When oral feeding is being considered, we need to observe whether the infant is capable of breathing comfortably through the nose. If the infant's mouth is consistently held in an open position with the tongue postured forward, as seen in Figures 5–4A and B, the infant may not be a good candidate for oral feeding.

The open resting posture of the oral cavity may be an indication of orofacial hypotonia, poor respiration, structural anomaly, or some other underlying medical problem. In this case a pacifier could be introduced in order to observe the infant's response to having the oral cavity occluded. If an infant is not able to breathe comfortably through the nose while at rest, the coordination of suck/swallow with respiration will be far too difficult for successful feeding. Remember, for successful oral feeding there must be a well-coordinated relationship between the pharyngeal swallow and respiration (Gewolb & Vice, 2006). When these two functions are not synchronous, deglutition apnea may occur that may lessen or resolve with maturation as suck/swallow/breathe coordination improves. This usually takes place around 37 weeks PCA (Hanlon et al., 1997).

Non-nutritive Suck—Perseveration and Habituation

The non-nutritive suck (NNS) can help to rule out a sensory issue such as perseveration or habituation. Before feeding an infant in the NICU, it is important to evaluate the NNS. The normal NNS is a burst–pause pattern. We should observe the first sucking burst, the first pause, and then the second sucking burst. This will rule out both perseveration and habituation. Pay particular attention to NNS bursts that exceed 20 sucks or last longer than 7 seconds. This may be indicative of more subtle sensory differences (Sameroff, 1973). Some infants will easily initiate the NNS on a pacifier but demonstrate only one long continuous burst with no pauses. Caregivers often explain this away by saying,

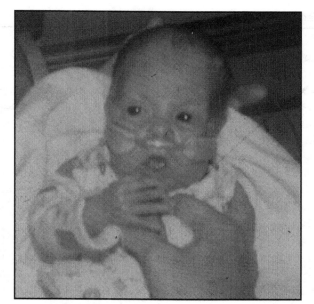

A

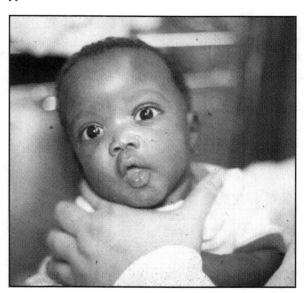

B

Figure 5–4. A. An infant with an open mouth due
to bronchopulmonary dysplasia (respiratory issues).
B. This infant has an open mouth posture due to Arnold
Chiari malformation, spina bifida, and orofacial hypo-
tonia. (From: *NOMAS Certification Course Instructor's
Manual.* Reprinted with permission.)

"he is really hungry and is trying to get milk out of the nipple." When an NNS does not occur in a burst–pause pattern it is considered to be deviant. This continuous nonstop sucking is known as perseveration and occurs when the infant responds to the initial stimulus of the pacifier being placed into the mouth but is unable to stop sucking, even when the pacifier is removed. This perseverative non-nutritive suck is an oral sensory issue and may be indicative of later problems that have a sensory basis.

Observation of the first non-nutritive burst, the first pause, and the second burst may help us rule out habituation, which is another sensory-based issue observed during this early reflexive period of sucking. Habituation occurs when the infant is only able to respond to the initial and novel stimulus. Once the novelty wears off, the sucking activity ceases. This infant's non-nutritive suck is often explained by saying, "sometimes he forgets that the nipple is in his mouth." In this situation a shake or jiggle of the nipple often serves to reactivate the sucking activity because it provides a new and novel stimulus.

Observation of NNS

- Normal Term Infant
  - □ bursts of 5 to 20
  - □ burst–pause pattern
  - □ burst not lasting more than 7 seconds
  - □ two sucks per second
  - □ short jaw excursions
  - □ cupped tongue
- Perseveration
  - □ continuous burst of more than 20 sucks
  - □ burst lasts longer than 7 seconds without a pause
  - □ may indicate sensory issues
- Habituation
  - □ suck is initiated but then stops after first burst
  - □ unable to sustain burst–pause pattern
  - □ does not initiate sucking after the pause
  - □ may reinitiate sucking with new stimulus

Infants who demonstrate perseveration or habituation during NNS may have been exposed to seizure medication or intrauterine drug exposure. Many times, however, there is no known explanation for the deviant sensory response.

Nutritive Suck—Poor Adaptability

Another type of deviant sensory response may occur with nutritive sucking when an infant is unable to adjust to changes in caregivers, nipples, or formulas. This is referred to as poor adaptability. It is a concern because sucking responses are sensitive to alterations in feeding contingencies, and sensory-motor coordination is necessary for infants to adapt their responses (Lipsitt, 1977). Sucking can provide valuable insights into the integrity of the central nervous system (Katsumi & Veda, 2005).

Readiness-to-Feed

Determining readiness-to-feed with infants in the NICU is not an easy task. The full-term, healthy infant in an alert state will root when a nipple is placed near the mouth at feeding time. This is easy to interpret. However, the touch pressure cue that is typically used to elicit the rooting reaction may be far too subtle a cue to be perceived by premature or sick-term infants in the NICU because of the desensitization from invasive orofacial procedures performed to save their lives.

The NNS is reported to occur in utero at 16 weeks PCA, so it is certainly expected to be present at birth. However, it is often absent in sick neonates and premature infants due to an injury that occurred in utero, perinatal asphyxia, a brain difference, or, again, to excessive negative input to the orofacial area. When a pacifier is placed into the infant's mouth, an adverse reaction or no reaction at all may be seen. So the NNS may not be an indicator of readiness-to-feed in this very special population.

Premature infants do not always give us easily identifiable cues for readiness-to-feed. It is necessary to be a good observer and note subtle signs. For example, you might notice the infant bringing his hands to mouth, putting hands together at midline, or opening his eyes and looking around. These are the signs of an alert, awake, and aware infant who may be developmentally ready to try a first feeding.

Infant Characteristics Prior to First Feeding

There are important characteristics of the infant that should be observed prior to starting a feed. These relate to respiration, state, and medical status.

Questions to Ask and Answer Prior to Feeding

1. What is the infant's color? Is it pink, pale, dusky, or mottled?
   □ Before feeding, the infant should be pink.
2. What is the infant's state? Is the infant awake and looking around, sleepy, irritable, drowsy?
   □ The infant should be awake and looking around.
3. What is the infant's medical status? Is the infant medically stable, unstable; does he have medical clearance for oral feeding?
   □ The infant should be medically stable with clearance for oral feeding.
4. What is the infant's respiration? Is the infant on room air, supplemental oxygen by nasal cannula, CPAP, or a ventilator?
   □ It is preferable for the infant to be on room air, but infants can often be fed while receiving supplemental oxygen from a nasal cannula.
5. What is the status of the infant's gastrointestinal (GI) tract? Does the infant have gastroesophageal reflux, allergies, constipation, diarrhea?
   □ Determine and know the implications of all GI issues before you begin feeding.
6. What are the infant's sleep–wake cycles? Does the infant sleep every few hours, sleep better at night; does he wake for feeding?

☐ The infant's sleep/wake cycle is individual. Work on the infant's schedule. Feeding should occur during those times when the infant is the most awake and alert.
7. What medications is the infant taking? What is the type and dosage?
☐ Become aware of those prescribed medications that the infant is currently taking and understand any side effects that may impact oral feeding.

Do not consider feeding until all the characteristics of the infant are known and considered. Remember, feeding should be, and usually is, a satisfying and pleasurable experience for the infant. A term infant with a mature pattern sucks effortlessly with complete coordination of suck/swallow/breathe as seen in Figure 5–5.

However, the preterm or sick neonate is often surviving because of modern medical technology. The miracle is that they have survived at all! What we have learned in the last 30 years is that before these infants are expected to orally feed, their neurological systems need to mature, and they need to have adequate respiratory support.

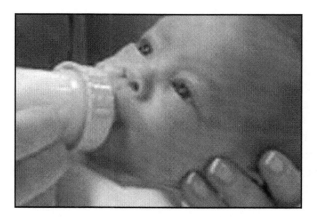

Figure 5–5. Feeding an infant with a normal suck. (From: *NOMAS Certification Course Instructor's Manual.* Reprinted with permission.)

The First Feeding

Since the mid-1980s and the development of the Neonatal Oral–Motor Assessment Scale (NOMAS) (Braun & Palmer, 1985; Palmer, 1993; Palmer, Crawley, & Blanco, 1993; Palmer & Heyman, 1999) the trained professional has been able to differentiate among normal, disorganized, and dysfunctional suck patterns. An accurate diagnosis of the suck enables appropriate treatment to be implemented.

Once you have established that the infant is medically stable with adequate respiratory status and you have obtained sufficient information about the GI tract, sleep/wake cycles, medication, allergies, and there is a medical order to begin oral feeding, you can proceed with caution.

Checklist to Determine Readiness-to-Feed

☐ Medical clearance
☐ Medical stability
☐ Adequate respiratory status
☐ GI information
☐ Sleep/wake cycles
☐ Medications
☐ Allergies

The first feeding should begin with the pacifier so that the caregiver can get a glimpse of the intraoral sensory awareness. An infant who demonstrates a burst–pause pattern with a rate of two per second is the infant whose sensory system is most likely to be intact. Next, we dip the pacifier into the formula or breast milk, allowing the infant to sample a taste and enabling you to view the tongue configuration, oral transit, and pharyngeal swallow coordination. You can do all this with just a drop of liquid on the tongue. Upon contact with the liquid the tongue should form a trough with a central tongue groove, curling up on the sides. The tongue begins to move in an extension–elevation–retraction pattern although you may be able to view only the extension–retraction. This is the wave-like pattern of sucking that infants use to transport the bolus from the oral cavity to the pharynx for swallow (Bu'Lock et al., 1990). If we see choking, gagging, coughing, or gasping for air, the infant may not be ready for bottle feeding. Most infants, however, will manage this first drop easily and effortlessly. You may then proceed to introduce the bottle.

Bottle Feeding

Introduction of the first nipple feeding should proceed carefully because there is the risk of silent aspiration. This may result from caregivers attempting to feed infants before they are ready in order to discharge them from the hospital. It is recommended that you observe the infant for the first 2 minutes of the nutritive suck in order to determine the coordination of suck/swallow/ breathe. The normal suck patterns have already been described. Now is the time to differentiate between the disorganized and dysfunctional suck patterns (Palmer, 1993; Palmer, Crawley, & Blanco, 1993; Palmer & Heyman, 1999).

Disorganized Suck

The disorganized suck was first defined as a lack of rhythm of the total sucking activity (Crook, 1979). Suck/swallow/breathe coordination is not reported to be present until 37 weeks PCA (Bu'Lock et al., 1990), and younger infants are not able to self-regulate (VandenBerg, 1990). Breathing appears to be the last function integrated into a successful feeding experience, and young preterm infants may be unable to inhibit respiration during swallow. This is indicative of immaturity and can easily result in aspiration (Vice & Gewolb, 2008). Infants may continue to attempt respiration during swallow, or they may exhibit deglutition apnea (Hanlon et al., 1997). This occurs when an infant stops breathing to swallow and is not able to reinitiate respiration. The characteristics of a disorganized suck according to the

NOMAS are based on the arthythmic jaw and tongue movements noted. There are three presentations of an arthythmic/disorganized suck with bottle feeding.

The first demonstrates too much *variability* in the number of sucks per burst. You can count the number of sucks by focusing on the jaw excursions at the point of the chin. With the mature pattern there are 10 to 30 sucks per burst with swallowing and breathing occurring in a consistent ratio. With a normal, immature suck pattern that might be present in a preterm infant, there are three to five sucks per burst with breathing and/or swallowing taking place during the pause. When the infant demonstrates sucking bursts with sucks in both of these categories, it is considered to be disorganized.

Another type of disorganized suck is called the *transitional* suck. This is demonstrated when the infant's sucking bursts contain between 5 to 10 sucks per burst. This is an indication that respiration is not well coordinated.

An *inconsistent* suck/swallow/breathe ratio also demonstrates a disorganized suck pattern. When all sucking bursts for the first 2 minutes of nutritive sucking on the bottle contain more than 10 sucks, it is important to examine the suck/swallow/breathe ratio. The normal suck's suck/swallow/breathe ratio is consistent for the first 2 minutes. An *inconsistent* ratio is demonstrated when the ratio changes from 2:1 or 3:1. When you observe an infant during the first 2 minutes and the infant has a normal continuous burst pattern, you can actually snap your fingers to the sucking rhythm. The finger-snapping rhythm is broken when the suck/swallow/breath pattern is changed.

Types of Disorganized Suck

■ *Variability* in the number of sucks per burst with some sucks over 10 and some under 10.
■ *Transitional*—sucking bursts contain between 5 to 10 sucks per burst.
■ *Inconsistent* suck/swallow/breathe ratio during continuous sucking bursts.

Infants with the diagnosis of a disorganized suck based on the NOMAS have difficulty with the coordination of respiration and may consequently exhibit signs of stress as seen in Figure 5–6. These signs include head turning, widening of eyes, elevation of eyebrows, finger splays, arms extended, nasal flaring, and/or labored breathing. If an infant exhibits any of these signs, special care must be taken to eliminate stress and make him comfortable during feeding. Infants who experience stress in the NICU during feeding are more likely to develop a sensory-based oral feeding aversion at 3 to 6 months of age.

Infants with a disorganized suck may be unable to sustain a suck for 2 minutes. This inability may be due to poorly coordinated respiration. An infant may also have audible gulping of the liquid and be at risk for aspiration. Another reason for an inability to sustain a suck may be fatigue with the infant falling asleep. A third reason is habituation which occurs when the sensory receptors in the mouth only perceive the initial novel stimulus. Subsequently, the stimulus is no longer perceived

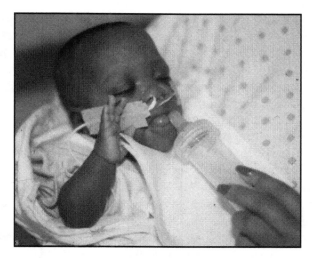

Figure 5–6. This is an example of sensory feeding aversion. Note the infant's tongue protrusion to stop the bottle from entering the mouth as well as a "stop" sign with the right hand. (From: *NOMAS Certification Course Instructor's Manual.* Reprinted with permission.)

and the sucking behavior diminishes. As mentioned previously, this may be secondary to such conditions as intrauterine drug exposure or a seizure disorder. Habituation may be due to congenitally decreased intraoral sensory awareness (Dubignon & Cooper, 1980). Future research may indicate its predictive value for later developmental problems.

Some infants who demonstrate habituation to the nipple may also have characteristics of a dysfunctional suck on the NOMAS. These infants may later be diagnosed with both motor and sensory-based problems associated with cerebral palsy.

Dysfunctional Suck

The diagnosis of a dysfunctional suck on the NOMAS is characterized by one or more abnormal movements of the tongue and jaw. These are movements that are never observed in the infant with a normal or disorganized suck (Braun & Palmer, 1985; Palmer, 1993; Palmer et al., 1993; Palmer & Heyman, 1999). Whenever an infant presents with a dysfunctional suck, there is abnormal orofacial tone. Typically, these infants have a neurological issue or may have an underlying condition that has not yet been identified such as cerebral palsy. Reflexive neonatal sucking provides a glimpse into the functioning of the cranial nerves and may also provide a gateway to brain function (Bingham, 2009). Young infants who may develop symptoms of cerebral palsy at a later time may have abnormal oral-motor patterns in early infancy that change as they grow older.

Sometimes, there are "excessively wide excursions that interrupt the intra-oral seal on the nipple" (Palmer, 1993, p. 68). This occurs often in infants who demonstrate an orofacial hypotonia. As the jaw moves downward, the degree of excursion is so wide that the anterior seal on the nipple between the tongue and the palate is interrupted. The suction component is compromised and negative pressure may not be sufficient to draw liquid out of the nipple. These infants may suck vigorously but are unable to transfer an adequate volume of fluid from the nipple. Frequently present is a tongue that is "flaccid; flattened with absent tongue groove" (Palmer, 1993, p. 68). The tongue is unable to cup around the nipple and hold it firmly against the palate. The jaw will drop excessively, as seen in Figure 5–7, and the feeding is inefficient.

When an infant's orofacial tone is hypertonic, a different jaw movement is observed. In this case there is a restriction of movement at the temporomandibular joint limiting the degree of downward depression of the jaw. This is often referred to as clenching (Palmer, 1993). The jaw excursion is short leading to poor negative pressure, which compromises the suction component. The tongue is often retracted with posterior humping against the palate and anterior flattening. This tongue configuration is also not conducive to efficient sucking.

If clenching and a retracted tongue are seen, other clinical signs should be considered to confirm a dysfunctional suck. One of these signs would be the movement of the jaw backward toward the ear instead of downward. Another sign is the upward movement of the jaw occurring at a faster rate than the downward movement. This may be due to the tongue's abnormal posture, and spurting of liquid may also occur. In this case the liquid is forced out of the mouth during the extension phase of sucking. It is not just a trickle, a drip, or a leak but appears to be pushed with force out of the mouth. These are all confirmatory signs of a dysfunctional suck.

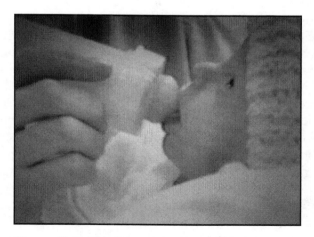

Figure 5–7. This is an example of wide jaw excursions and a flaccid tongue. (From: *NOMAS Certification Course Instructor's Manual.* Reprinted with permission.)

When assessing jaw clenching, the most important component is the degree of downward jaw depression. This is the basis of the diagnosis of a dysfunctional suck. Without jaw clenching, the clinical signs noted above do not indicate dysfunction. Not all infants with neurological issues have a dysfunctional suck.

Another characteristic of a dysfunctional suck is the "excessive protrusion beyond the labial border before or after nipple insertion" (Palmer, 1993. p. 68). This perseveration is observed when the infant continues to suck after the nipple has been removed and suggests that intraoral sensory awareness is poor. The infant does not realize that the nipple has been removed, and both motor and sensory problems are in evidence. The prognosis is guarded, and the child may be diagnosed with cerebral palsy at a later date.

The absence of movement in a full-term infant is also considered to be dysfunctional. Prior to 40 weeks PCA, however, the absence of a suck would not be diagnosed as such. In some nurseries, infants may be fed as young as 30 weeks PCA. This is before the age at which the sucking reflex is expected to be present. In such cases a diagnosis of dysfunctional suck would clearly be inappropriate. When this is observed in a NICU, it is advisable to report to the neonatologist and the team that the infant is too young to have a suck reflex and is not yet ready to feed.

A dysfunctional suck is also characterized by the lack of rate change between the non-nutritive and nutritive suck. When an infant is unable to differentiate between a nipple that delivers fluid and one that does not, it is an indication of decreased intraoral sensory perception and suggests the possibility of both sensory and motor problems. This is of concern in both the premature and full-term infant as early sucking and swallowing predict neurodevelopmental outcomes. Infants who demonstrate a lack of rate change are, therefore, at greater risk of developing cerebral palsy (Slattery, Morgan, & Douglas, 2012).

Breastfeeding

The diagnosis of a dysfunctional suck at the breast is not difficult and follows the same guidelines that have been used for bottle feeding. You will be able to observe the same abnormal movements of tongue and jaw during breastfeeding. The greatest challenge for a professional who is evaluating an infant during breastfeeding is the differentiation between normal and disorganized sucking. Because there are so many variables inherent in breastfeeding, the infant with a normal suck is able to literally "go with the flow." When infants go to the breast they may encounter a strong milk flow, a trickle of milk, or no milk at all. Infants with good adaptability will adjust easily to the changes that occur and will alter their sucking pattern accordingly. They may suck non-nutritively at the rate of two per second, demonstrate several sucks prior to the swallow, and change the number of sucks that precede the swallow frequently; or they may exhibit variability in the number of sucks per burst. All this is an indication that the infant is adapting successfully to the variables within the breastfeeding situation. The diagnosis of a disorganized suck at the breast is based solely on the coordination of suck/swallow/breathe. When an infant demonstrates nasal flaring, labored respiration, or other stress cues during breastfeeding, it is usually an indication that the pharyngeal swallow and respiration are not well coordinated.

Therapeutic Interventions

Background

In the 1980s nurses were the primary professionals feeding infants in the NICU. Therapists working in the NICU were usually NDT certified. They used feeding techniques available at the time that were primarily developed by Mueller (1975) for children with cerebral palsy and were based on NDT principles. It was thought that the feeding problems of the preterm infant stemmed from hypotonia and weak oral musculature. During this early period, infants were placed on a fast flow nipple to reduce their effort. In addition, the feeder's hand was placed under the chin to provide support for the hypotonic musculature. This technique was known as jaw control and was developed in the late 1950s for use with older children who had cerebral palsy. Now, however, we have a much larger base of information.

What We Have Learned

The feeding problems of the preterm infant are more complex than previously thought. They do not all result from hypotonia or a weak suck. These problems are secondary to a lack of neurological maturation and adequate respiratory support for the coordination of the pharyngeal swallow and respiration (Gewolb, Vice, Schweitzer-Kennedy, Taciak, & Bosma, 2001). Simply stated, these infants are too young to feed. Given time to mature, they will do well unless, of course, there are neurological deficits or injuries. It is our responsibility to differentiate between an infant who is born prematurely, or is ill, and the infant who has a damaged nervous system or cerebral palsy. They are not the same.

Plasticity of the central nervous system allows infants to overcome many adverse situations and conditions. Infants born prematurely are in a class by themselves. They are not just younger children. They need to be treated differently. We want infants in the NICU to develop their own rhythm of sucking. We need interventions to be individualized and distress-free (Lemons & Lemons, 1996). Unless the infant has a structural defect or neurological issue, there is probably no dysphagia. The typical concern for the preterm or sick full-term infant is with the *coordination* of the pharyngeal swallow and respiration, not the swallow itself.

Interventions for a Disorganized Suck

Once a disorganized suck has been determined, there are a few basic interventions to attempt with this infant. Change the nipple if the infant is having a particularly difficult time coordinating suck/swallow with respiration. Perhaps a nipple with a slower flow would be beneficial. On the other hand, if the infant seems to suck well but is unable to transfer an adequate amount of liquid, perhaps a faster flow nipple would be beneficial.

Also, you might consider changing the feeding position. For example, sidelying provides a neutral position against gravity and can often help to avoid pharyngeal pooling of liquid. Positioning the infant on your lap in sidelying also provides the caregiver with a clear view of the oral musculature, particularly underneath the nipple.

Additionally, the suck/swallow/breathe pattern can be regulated for the younger preterm infant by limiting the length of each sucking burst to three sucks. The infant may suck and swallow three times consecutively. Whenever the infant swallows, respiration ceases. Therefore, 3 seconds is long enough. If longer, it may result in deglutition apnea (Hanlon et al., 1997). Regulation is systematic and teaches the infant to anticipate the pauses for breathing (Palmer, 1993). It is usually implemented for the first minute of the feeding and then continued as needed. It is most successful when used with younger infants who are just starting oral feeding and who are not yet able to coordinate the suck/swallow/breathe triad.

The techniques used to regulate the infant's suck/swallow/breathe coordination vary and are specific to each infant. One method is to remove the nipple completely from the mouth after three nutritive sucks and swallows. Wait 3 seconds to facilitate coordinated respiration and reinsert the nipple. Another method is to tip the nipple up to break the suction seal but not remove the nipple from the mouth. This is preferred for those infants who do not initiate sucking actively a second time once the bottle has been removed. Then tip the nipple back down so that the liquid once again fills the nipple. Also, the baby can be tipped by gently rolling the infant laterally from a 45-degree reclined angle into sidelying, or from a 45-degree reclined position forward to sitting. This will serve to empty the fluid from the nipple. After a 3-second pause the infant may gently be rolled back into the original position.

External pacing is another method to help the infant regulate suck/swallow/coordination. This was developed in the 1980s when caregivers began to notice that infants were stressed during bottle feeding. Feeders in the NICU would remove the bottle from the mouth when an infant appeared stressed. Once the infant had calmed, the bottle was reinserted. Primarily, these infants were stressed because of their inability to coordinate respiration and swallow. It should be noted that this technique is most successful for those older infants who demonstrate longer continuous sucking bursts and who do not need to learn when to breathe. They just need periodic breaks for some "catch-up" breathing.

Interventions for a Disorganized Suck

- Nipple change
- Position change
  - ☐ Sidelying
- Regulation
  - ☐ Remove nipple
  - ☐ Tip nipple
  - ☐ Tip baby
- External pacing
  - ☐ Bottle removed to relieve stress
  - ☐ Bottle reinserted once infant recovers

There are a variety of commercially available products on the market that can be used for regulation. Also, remember that the specific technique may be of secondary importance. What is most critical is that you accurately identify the infant who is having difficulty feeding because he cannot breathe, coordinate breathing, or regulate suck/swallow/breathe. This infant needs your help and the technique implemented should be selected by the team, which may include the feeding therapist, nurse, parent, and most importantly, the infant.

Interventions for a Dysfunctional Suck

These techniques closely parallel the strategies employed for an older child with cerebral palsy. Using the concepts of NDT the caregiver attempts to change the movement pattern of the jaw and tongue during active sucking to facilitate more normal movement patterns. There are four suggested intervention strategies for the infant with a dysfunctional suck.

Jaw Support

For the neonate with excessively wide excursions of the jaw, the technique of jaw support can be used to maintain both the jaw and the tongue in closer proximity to the nipple during active sucking, as seen in Figure 5–8. This is the least invasive of the "hands-on" techniques and can be very successful in assisting the infant with a dysfunctional suck pattern.

Cheek Support

This technique, as shown in Figure 5–9, is a compensatory strategy for the infant who has either a flaccid or a retracted tongue. In both cases the suction component is poor because the tongue is unable to form the central tongue groove necessary for maintaining the nipple against the palate during active sucking. When pressure is applied to the cheeks in an inward/forward direction during sucking, this action serves to change the placement of the anterior seal on the nipple. With cheek support, the lips can be brought forward onto the nipple to create a seal. Once the suction component has been increased, the nipple may need to be changed in order to protect the infant from aspiration. This technique must be implemented with caution because an infant with a dysfunctional suck will have neurological issues and may already be at risk. This technique is more invasive than jaw support, and although it may serve to increase suction, it may also cause apneic spells.

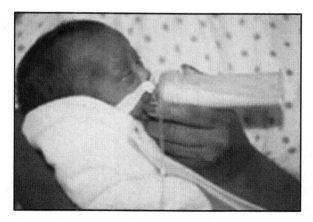

Figure 5–8. Use of jaw support for an infant with excessively wide jaw excursions during nutritive sucking. (From: *NOMAS Certification Course Instructor's Manual*. Reprinted with permission.)

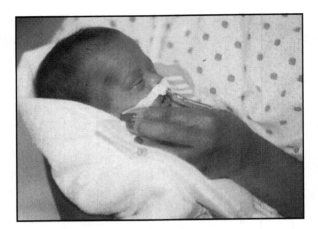

Figure 5–9. An example of cheek support for an infant with a dysfunctional suck. (From: *NOMAS Certification Course Instructor's Manual.* Reprinted with permission.)

Perioral Stimulation

For this technique, a quick stretch is applied to the cheek cavity at the rate of one per second during active sucking. This will slow the rate for those infants who do not have a rate change between the non-nutritive and nutritive suck. The goal is to slow the suck on the nipple to one per second during nutritive sucking. This provides time for respiration and helps to eliminate choking and aspiration that often occurs when sucking is too rapid.

Facilitation of a Central Tongue Groove

This can be accomplished with your finger using tubing or a commercially available product. When the tongue is flattened and a tongue groove is absent, apply downward pressure to the central tongue blade. As the infant nutritively sucks, the tongue can be maintained in the proper position within the lingual cavity. If the tongue is retracted, pressure would be applied further back to bring the tongue down and away from the palate. Because of the infant's abnormal muscle tone, the hands of the caregiver must always be prepared to facilitate more efficient feeding patterns. Once the feeder's hands are removed, the pattern often reverts back to abnormal. The prognosis for these infants is guarded because they often develop pervasive motor deficits such as cerebral palsy.

Summary of Interventions for Dysfunctional Suck

- Jaw support—for wide jaw excursions
- Cheek support—for flattened or retracted tongue
- Perioral stimulation—for rate change between NNS and NS
- Facilitation of central tongue groove—for flattened or retracted tongue

---

Conclusion

The suck pattern of the neonate may present as normal, disorganized, or dysfunctional. It is important that the NICU feeding specialist be trained to identify the differences among these patterns in order to plan appropriate treatment strategies. Treatment must be infant-specific. There is no one right answer or right technique. Each clinician and caregiver must become a partner with the infant in order to discover what makes that infant most comfortable and how best to introduce oral feeding.

The clinician also needs to remember that there are anatomical differences in the infant under 6 months of age. For example, the distance is short between the oral cavity and the upper esophagus. Additionally, there may be incoordination of suck/swallow/respiration, and the feeder needs to be familiar with neonatal development and the respiratory requirements of the preterm infant who is being fed orally. Infants under 37 weeks PCA are not expected to self-regulate the suck/swallow/breathe pattern. If this infant is fed, the feeder should be prepared to regulate this rhythm in order to prevent aspiration and to teach the infant to pause for breathing. If the infant is over 37 weeks PCA and demonstrates a disorganized suck pattern, external pacing may be the preferred intervention. Moreover, the infant who presents with a dysfunctional suck pattern will require treatment techniques that are implemented through handling. This group of infants will most likely be those who have a developmental delay (Tsai, Chen, & Lin, 2010) and may later be diagnosed with cerebral palsy. If these infants can be safely maintained as oral feeders during their early reflexive stage of feeding development, they will benefit greatly and you will have done your job well.

It is important that an infant's early feeding experience be a positive one, and one in which he is comfortable and respiration is well coordinated. We want the infant to experience satiation without stress. Early feeding is a learning experience, and the context in which the infant is fed will have a lasting influence on later development. It is up to the caregiver to provide the appropriate feeding environment for this, one in which the infant is stabilized in a midline position, comfortable, and safe for oral feeding.

Ten Items for Improving Intervention

1. Examine medical records for information about allergies, gastrointestinal tract issues, cardiac and/or lung problems, and neurological status.
2. Carefully observe the infant's respiration at rest, when awake, and when stimulated.
3. Note the infant's oral resting posture prior to feeding.
4. Introduce a pacifier, breast, or finger for NNS and note the infant's response.
5. Rule out perseveration and habituation during NNS.
6. Stimulate olfaction by allowing the infant to smell formula or breast milk.
7. Note the infant's response when you introduce a drop of formula or breast milk on the pacifier, infant's hand, or finger for tasting.
8. Position the infant in a neutral position.
9. Carefully select an appropriate nipple. It is best to begin with a slow flow nipple.
10. Be sure to have a medical order to begin oral feeding before proceeding.

Think Critically for Self-Study or Classroom Discussion

1. Infants are people, too, and you need to establish relationships with them. What is the infant saying to you about the way he feels? How do you know?
2. How would you feel if the roles were reversed and you were the infant? Imagine liquid coming into your mouth too rapidly, no time to catch your breath, suffocating, drowning, pleading for help while no one listens. And later, you hate eating. Why?
3. How can you create a situation in which the infant is an active team member during feeding, instead of a victim who simply has things done to him or her?
4. Be creative. Think outside the box. Does an infant have to drink from a bottle? Can you think of five other utensils that can be used to feed an infant? (Answer: spoon, finger, cup, clinic dropper, syringe, etc.)
5. The feeding relationship is between you (the caregiver) and the infant you are feeding. Each relationship is unique and based on a comfort level that is best for both of you. How would you go about finding this comfort level TOGETHER?

References

American Speech, Language, and Hearing Association. (2004). *Roles of speech-language pathologists in the neonatal intensive care unit: Position statement* (Position statement). Retrieved April 1, 2013, from http://www.asha.org/policy/PS2004-00111/

Bingham, P. (2009). Deprivation and dysphagia in premature infants. *Journal of Child Neurology, 24*, 743–749.

Bosma, J. F. (1975). Anatomic and physiologic development of the speech apparatus. In D. B. Tower (Ed.), *The nervous system: Human communication and its disorders* (pp. 469–481). New York, NY: Raven Press.

Braun, M. A., & Palmer, M. M. (1985). A pilot study of oral-motor dysfunction in "at risk" infants. *Physical and Occupational Therapy in Pediatrics, 5,* 13–15.

Bu'Lock, F., Woolridge, M. W., & Baum, J. D. (1990). Development of co-ordination of sucking, swallowing, and breathing: Ultrasound study of term and preterm infants. *Developmental Medicine and Child Neurology, 32,* 669–678.

Crook, C. K. (1979). The organization and control of infant sucking. *Advances in Child Development and Behavior, 14,* 209–252.

Dubignon, J., & Cooper, D. (1980). Good and poor feeding behavior in the neonatal period. *Infant Behavior and Development, 3,* 395–408.

Gewolb, I. H., & Vice, F. L. (2006). Maturational changes in the rhythms, patterns, and coordination of respiration and swallow during feeding in preterm and term infants. *Developmental Medicine and Child Neurology, 48,* 589–594.

Gewolb, I. H., Vice, F. L., Schweitzer-Kennedy, E. L., Tociak, V. L., & Bosma, J. F. (2001). Developmental patterns of rhythmic suck and swallow in preterm infants. *Developmental Medicine and Child Neurology, 43,* 22–27.

Gryboski, J. (1975). Gastrointestinal problems in the infant. *Major problems in clinical pediatrics, XIII.* Philadelphia, PA: W. B. Saunders.

Hanlon, M. B., Tripp, J. H., Ellis, R. E., Flack, F. C., Selley, W. G., & Shoesmith, H. J. (1997). Deglutition apnea as indicator of maturation of suckle feeding in bottle-fed preterm infants. *Developmental Medicine and Child Neurology, 39,* 534–542.

Katsumi, M., & Veda, A. (2005). Neonatal feeding performance as a predictor of neurodevelopmental outcome at 18 months. *Developmental Medicine and Child Neurology, 47,* 299–304.

Lemons, P. K., & Lemons, J. A. (1996). Transition to breast/bottle feedings: The premature infant. *Journal of American College of Nutrition, 15,* 126–135.

Lipsitt, L. P. (1977). Taste in human neonates: Its effects on sucking and heart rate. In J. M. Weiffenbach (Ed.), *Taste and development: The genesis of sweet preference* (pp. 125–142). Bethesda, MD: DHEW Publication No. (NIH) 77-1068.

Morris, S. E., & Klein, M. D. (1987). *Pre-feeding skills.* Tucson, AZ: Therapy Skill Builders.

Mueller, H. (1975). Feeding. In N. R. Finnie, *Handling the young cerebral palsied child at home* (2nd ed., pp. 113–132). New York, NY: E.P. Dutton & Co.

Nyquist, K. H., Sjoden, P. O., & Ewald, U. (1999). The development of preterm infants' breastfeeding behavior. *Early Human Development, 55,* 247–264.

Palmer, M. M. (1993). Identification and management of the transitional suck pattern in premature infants. *Journal of Perinatal and Neonatal Nursing, 7,* 66–75.

Palmer, M. M., Crawley, K., & Blanco, I. A. (1993). Neonatal Oral-Motor Assessment Scale: A reliability study. *Journal of Perinatology, 13,* 28–35.

Palmer, M. M., & Heyman, M. B. (1999). Developmental outcome for neonates with dysfunctional and disorganized sucking patterns: Preliminary findings. *Infant-Toddler Intervention, 9,* 299–308.

Qureshi, M. A., Vice, F. L., Taciak,V. L., Bosma, J. F., & Gewolb, I. H. (2002). Changes in rhythmic suckle feeding patterns in term infants in the first month of life. *Developmental Medicine and Child Neurology, 44,* 34–39.

Sameroff, A. J. (1973). Reflexive and operant aspects of sucking behavior in early infancy. In J. F. Bosma (Ed.), *Fourth symposium on oral sensation and perception: Development in the fetus and infant* (pp. 135–151). DHEW Publication No. (NIH) 75-546. Bethesda, MD: U.S. Department of Health, Education, and Welfare.

Slattery, J., Morgan, A., & Douglas, J. (2012). Early sucking and swallowing problems as predictors of neurodevelopmental outcome in children with neonatal brain injury. *Developmental Medicine and Child Neurology, 54,* 796–806.

Tamura, Y., Matsushita, S., Shinoda, K., & Yoshida, S. (1998). Development of perioral muscle activity during suckling in infants: A cross-sectional and follow-up study. *Developmental Medicine and Child Neurology, 40,* 344–348.

Tsai, S. W., Chen, C. H., & Lin, M. C. (2010). Prediction for developmental delay by Neonatal Oral-Motor Assessment Scale in preterm infants without brain lesion. *Pediatrics International, 52,* 65–68.

VandenBerg, K. A. (1990). Nippling management of the sick neonate in the NICU: The disorganized feeder. *Neonatal Network, 9,* 9–16.

Vice, F. L., & Gewolb, I. H. (2008). Respiratory patterns and strategies during feeding in preterm infants. *Developmental Medicine and Child Neurology, 50,* 467–472.

Weiffenbach, J. M., & Thach, B. T. (1972). Elicited tongue movements: Touch and taste in the mouth of the neonate. In J. F. Bosma (Ed.), *Fourth symposium on oral sensation and perception: Development in the fetus and infant* (pp. 232–244). DHEW Publication No. (NIH) 75-546. Bethesda, MD: U.S. Department of Health, Education, and Welfare.

CHAPTER 6

Respiratory Control

Fran Redstone

Introduction: Respiration

Breathing is one of those things we never think about (Ferrand, 2001). It just happens. And that's the way it should be. We breathe for life; to exchange gasses (Freed, 2012); CO_2 out, O_2 in. The exchange takes place in the lungs at the alveoli. Quiet breathing is also known as tidal breathing or vegetative breathing. Air is taken in when our diaphragm contracts. Contraction leads to an increase in the size of the thoracic cavity. The lungs are attached to the thorax via the pleural lining. Therefore, the volume in the lungs increases, but the air pressure diminishes compared to atmospheric pressure, and air rushes into the lungs. This is inhalation.

During exhalation, gas exchange occurs in the lungs, and air is expelled that is high in CO_2. This occurs when the diaphragm relaxes leading to a decrease in the vertical dimension of the thorax. Because the lungs are still attached to the thorax, they also decrease in volume. Again, we get a change in air pressure. This time the change leads to an increase in the air pressure in our lungs compared to atmospheric pressure and air rushes out. *Voilà*, exhalation! Then we need more oxygen again and the cycle repeats. This typically occurs 12 to 18 times a minute for adults and 40 to 70 times for neonates (Seikel, King, & Drumright, 2005).

Air provided by our respiratory system is the foundation for phonation. Our respiratory pattern changes for speech. Simply put, while vegetative breathing is fairly passive, breathing for speech is active. Children learn to use the muscles of their trunk, over the first several years of life, to control exhalation for speech production. Length of utterance, loudness, and phonemic distinctions influence respiratory needs for speech. Although this will be discussed further in Chapter 7, it is important to note that dissociated muscle control is required, as well as coordination between the subsystems of speech production.

Ferrand (2001) reminds us that the respiratory system is involved in swallowing as well as in quiet breathing and speech breathing. Like speech, feeding also requires adjustment of the respiratory pattern in order for a safe swallow to occur. Again, this is something we do not think about. However, haven't we all had occasional coughing while eating? When this happens we are usually talking, distracted, or dealing with something unusual in our mouths. If respiration continues and the airway remains open during chewing and bolus transport, we are at risk for aspiration.

Anatomy and Physiology of Respiration

When we think of the framework of our respiratory system, the rib cage with the 12 pairs of ribs, the sternum, and the vertebral column come to mind. However, the system actually begins at the nose and mouth. It then continues through the larynx to the trachea and into the lungs (Redstone, 1991). These various parts have been divided and classified by several authors. Hoit (1995) divides the system into the pulmonary and chest-wall systems, which can then be further subdivided into upper and lower respiratory systems. Zemlin (1998) notes that the larynx is the dividing point between the upper and lower tracts.

In addition, we also need to consider the shoulder and pelvic girdles. After all, we have so many options to increase the volume of the thorax and thereby improve our expiratory capacity for speech. The muscles that allow this to occur are attached to structures other than the rib cage. And then there are the nasal, oral, pharyngeal, and laryngeal structures for passage of air in and out of the system.

The diaphragm is the major muscle of inspiration (Ferrand, 2001). This muscle along with the external intercostals increases the size of the thoracic cavity. However, the levator and serratus muscles of the spine also help elevate the rib cage. Then there are the accessory muscles of the neck and shoulders that may also be involved, especially to stabilize the shoulder girdle. The muscles of inspiration, however, are primarily those of the thorax (Seikel et al., 2005).

Exhalation for speech requires more muscles than tidal breathing. Muscles of the abdominal area are particularly active during exhalation. The latissimus dorsi stabilizes the abdominal wall while the rectus, transverse, and obliques all help to compress the abdomen to force more air out for speech. Trunk musculature is used for both respiration and for postural control (Redstone, 1991; Zemlin, 1998).

Although the larynx is associated with phonation, and the oral-nasal-pharyngeal areas with speech, we must consider them to be part of the respiratory system because air passes through these areas during both tidal and speech breathing. Adjustments must be made by the laryngeal muscles in order to abduct the vocal folds and allow the passage of air during tidal breathing. Partial adduction of the vocal folds must occur for phonation and full adduction for safety during feeding. In fact, Zemlin (1998) calls the larynx an "intrinsic component of the respiratory system, and as such it functions as a protective device" (p. 101). We need to remember that food and air share the oral area and pharynx (Redstone, 1991).

Respiratory Coordination for Feeding

Respiration during feeding and swallowing in typical adults has been investigated by several authors (Edgar, 2003; Huckabee, 2009; Matsuo, Hiiemae, Gonzales-Fernandez, & Palmer, 2008).

Arvedson and Brodsky (2002) note that the cerebral cortex is not essential to the pharyngeal swallow. Huckabee (2009) agrees that breathing and swallowing coordination is primarily under brainstem control. She goes on to investigate cortical control for voluntary and nonvolitional swallows. Her results indicate that cortical control influences volitional swallows.

It is felt that aspiration is prevented in adults by the inhibition of respiration during bolus formation in the oropharynx. The typical pattern of coordinative control is to swallow and then exhale (Edgar, 2003; Huckabee, 2009). It is felt that this respiratory pattern prevents inhalation or aspiration of food into the trachea. Matsuo and colleagues (2008) hypothesize that the downward pull of the diaphragm during inhalation makes laryngeal elevation more difficult. Therefore, swallowing during exhalation may facilitate laryngeal elevation for improved safety.

Children over 1 year (Huckabee, 2009; Kelly, Huckabee, Jones, & Frampton, 2007; McPherson et al., 1992) coordinate feeding with respiration by initiating the swallow in a pattern similar to adults. The swallow occurs at the peak of inspiration with expiration occurring postswallow.

Development of Respiratory Coordination

The child's first year is characterized by immense growth of the complex breathing mechanism (Boliek, Hixon, Watson, & Morgan, 1996). The development of respiratory control depends on neural maturation, anatomical growth, and experience. Changes that occur include the number of alveoli in the lungs. The newborn has about 25 million alveoli, whereas an adult has 300 million (Seikel et al., 2005). Therefore, a neonate's respiration is quite rapid allowing it to meet metabolic needs. The rate of breathing decreases steadily during the first year. The thoracic cavity increases in size and becomes more stable and less compliant (Boliek et al., 1996). The myelination of neural pathways is also increasing.

The infant's physical framework differs from the adult's with the infant's rib cage riding high. This means that it takes up only about one-third of the trunk. The influence of gravity and upright posture leads the adult rib cage to be angled downward and take up about half of the trunk. As typical children develop a balance between extension and flexion in the trunk, they are able to hold themselves upright. Even at 3 months of age, scapular stability is present with decreased shoulder elevation. This facilitates the descent of the rib cage.

Early weight shifting during the first 6 months of infancy strengthens the trunk musculature, which enhances the performance of respiration. Trunk control in the second part of the first year is reflected in the child's ability to crawl, rotate, and manipulate toys. In addition, by 1 year, the child has been working against gravity. Head and trunk alignment has been established, and now pelvic stability is apparent in the child's ability to stand. This stability influences respiration and respiratory control. The BPM has decreased from about 70 at birth to 40, and there is greater variety in the sounds and suprasegmentals of vocalizations. But always remember, the structures of the upper respiratory system are shared by the functions of gas exchange, sound production, and feeding.

Development of Respiratory Coordination for Feeding

When infants suck from the bottle or breast, significant coordination is required between the muscles of breathing and feeding (Miller & Kiatchoosakum, 2004). The typical infant is anatomically and neurologically prepared to avoid aspiration during feeding. This results from the restricted oral space and intact oral reflexes. The infant's oral structures provide a small space to provide stability for efficient movements for sucking. Wolf and Glass (1992) describe this as positional stability. However, the infant's anatomy changes due to growth and upright positioning. The increased pharyngeal space is less safe for feeding. This arrangement is more likely to allow food to penetrate the larynx, unless there is adequate muscular coordination, because the structures need to move greater distances to protect the airway. We need to keep in mind that the major function of the pharynx is air passage (Beecher & Alexander, 2004). Food passage may jeopardize airway protection.

In the same way that changes are seen in the infant's anatomy in the first year, there are modifications in reflex control as well. These reflect gains in voluntary control. Kelly et al. (2007) also suggest that the disappearance and modifications evident in some of some the oral reflexes by 6 months is due to cortical inhibition but that the numerous oral experiences during feeding contribute to this. Typical children by age 5 coordinate breathing for feeding in a manner that is similar to adults. This results from their intact nervous systems that support motor control along with sensory and feeding experiences.

Huckabee's (2009) research suggests that full-term infants are "hard-wired" (p. 22) for control over the apneic duration during swallows. In Chapter 5 of this book, Palmer describes this as a mature suck, which is typically present in infants who are born at 37 weeks postconceptual age. The infant born prior to this time may demonstrate an immature suck, lacking in adequate respiratory support, and coordination.

Very early in development the healthy, full-term infant has a respiratory swallow pattern that is close to the adult pattern, which is expiration after swallow. Kelly et al.'s (2007) research suggests that this occurs after the first week and becomes more evident in the second 6 months during volitional swallows. After the second day of life, infants demonstrate a tendency to swallow at the "inspiratory-expiratory cusp" (Huckabee, 2009, p. 22). Expiration after swallowing is typical of infants in the second half of the first year, which is also the typical pattern in adults. It appears that the infant is protected by brainstem control of breathing and swallowing, but cortical modulation increases for voluntary swallows throughout the infant's first year until it quite adult-like (Huckabee, 2009).

Respiration and Children with Cerebral Palsy

A great deal has been written about the respiration of children with cerebral palsy. Most of the descriptive literature was published before the 1980s whereas most of the intervention information has been provided since the 1980s by many SLPs who were neurodevelopmental treatment (NDT) certified and trained by Helen Mueller.

Always remember that cerebral palsy is a disorder of muscle coordination (Bobath, 1972; Healy, 1983) and abnormal muscle tone palsy (Bartlett & Palisano, 2000; Finnie, 2001). Because respiration for the functions of feeding and speech require muscle coordination, it is not unexpected that children with cerebral palsy often have difficulty with respiratory muscle control. In fact, respiratory issues have long been recognized as common in this group of children (Solomon & Charron, 1998).

The respiratory issues seen in children with cerebral palsy may be due to hypotonia or muscle weakness in the thoracic muscles resulting in flared ribs (Redstone, 1991) and flexion of the spine making expansion of the chest difficult (Davis, 1987). Weakness may also account for the inward movement of the sternum that is often observed in children with cerebral palsy. It is suspected that this is caused by the strength of the diaphragm's contraction (Davis, 1987; Redstone, 1991) during the early period of development. This contraction has pulled the sternum inward.

The pattern of decreased movement may also be due to rigidity of the chest wall from hypertonicity. It diminishes the ability to maintain and coordinate air moving through the larynx for speech. A fast rate of breathing may be required that can interfere with communication and lead to incoordination with swallowing. In addition, children with cerebral palsy lack stability/mobility, extension/flexion balance, and dissociation of the musculature of the trunk required for coordinated function (Davis, 1987). Due to lack of stability, the shoulders of the child with cerebral palsy are often elevated to support the head. This may be exacerbated by pulmonary issues that lead to head extension for an open airway. In turn, head/trunk alignment is compromised and rib cage expansion is hindered (Eicher, 2007) causing a decrease of inspired air. The lack of stability may be due to hypotonicity, which leads to a greater compliance of the abdominal wall as well as a limited expansion of the upper thorax.

Achilles' (1955) survey indicated rib-flaring, thoracic-abdominal opposition, and shallow breathing in the review of case records of clients with cerebral palsy from 2 to 22 years of age. However, this study included an unusually large percentage of individuals with athetoid cerebral palsy, therefore making inferences to the cerebral palsy population difficult. Hardy's early study (1964) on pulmonary function used nonspeech respiratory tasks and found that the capacities and rates of children with cerebral palsy varied significantly from typical children.

Mueller described the respiration of children with cerebral palsy as "shallow and irregular and is often blocked by intermittent spasm" (1972, p. 291). It has been reported that at least 50% of individuals with cerebral palsy have decreased vital capacity (McPherson et al., 1992). It is interesting that whereas Redstone and West (2004) found position influenced the respiration of 4 to 5-year-old children with cerebral palsy, Hardy (1964) found that position did not affect the respiration of older subjects with cerebral palsy. He attributed this to the inflexibility of these children's respiratory systems.

Clearly, this literature acknowledges that the respiratory systems of children with cerebral palsy differ from the respiration of typical children. This then affects the functions that rely on respiratory control: speech and feeding. However, the functional problems we see with respiration for children with cerebral palsy are less a matter of capacities than of coordination.

Respiratory Coordination for Feeding in Cerebral Palsy

Neural reflexes are required for swallowing control and coordination with breathing. The infant who may be diagnosed with cerebral palsy has a different underlying neurological system than that of a typical infant. Because the newborn's coordination between breathing and swallowing is controlled by neural input from the brainstem, the child with cerebral palsy, who has a compromised nervous system, may show problems from the beginning. Huckabee (2009) suggests that there may be a critical period for the development of protective coordination of respiration and swallowing. This may have implications for premature, ill, or neurologically impaired infants. Many of these infants are those who may be diagnosed with cerebral palsy.

Conversely, there may be adequate brainstem control to provide protection in the early months while the structures are small and the oral–pharyngeal space is restricted. However, the cortical control needed for coordination during volitional swallowing in later infancy may not be adequate. This is often the case in children with cerebral palsy.

In addition, abnormal muscle tone leading to a fast rate of breathing will influence the coordination of breathing with swallowing. Anything that influences head posture can compromise this coordination. As noted previously, abnormal muscle tone and lack of stability will influence head/trunk alignment. The typical pattern seen in children with cerebral palsy is hyperextension of the head. This leads to an open airway and a greater risk of aspiration.

There also appears to be a reciprocal relationship between these two important functions. Poor respiratory function leads to feeding issues (Beecher & Alexander, 2004; Miller & Willging, 2007). This may occur in cases of airway obstruction as well as in the premature. Children with cerebral palsy may have medical conditions that contribute to poor respiration (Workinger, 2005). These conditions may lead to greater effort during breathing which, in turn, may lead to head postures to open the airway during feeding (Eicher, 2007).

Placing food in a child's mouth may occlude easy air passage. On the other hand, poor feeding skill from oral-motor problems that are typical in children with cerebral palsy may lead to respiratory problems. This may result from the child's inability to form and control the bolus safely through the oropharynx. Both of these situations may occur in children with cerebral palsy.

Respiratory coordination for feeding was investigated by McPherson et al. (1992) who compared 5- to 12-year-old children with cerebral palsy to a group of age-matched children without cerebral palsy. These authors found that apnea occurred earlier in the participants with cerebral palsy. Breathing was halted even before oral transit began. In addition, there was a high incidence of inhalation at the end of a swallow, even for liquids, which differed greatly from the typical children. This pattern may be dangerous because inhalation may lead to penetration of food into the laryngeal area. These children tend to have a high threshold for initiation of a cough, and weakness may make the cough less effective. Additionally, the children with cerebral palsy had a breathing pattern that McPherson et al. (1992) described as "not unlike that seen in infants" (p. 585).

Assessment of Respiratory Function

When assessing children with cerebral palsy, the SLP not only needs to know typical respiratory patterns and development of these patterns, but also needs to determine if they are due to abnormal muscle tone or due to lack of head/trunk alignment influencing the breathing. This type of problem solving is one of the unique attributes of NDT.

Workinger (2005) notes that respiratory function is often assessed with various instruments in research studies. But these are not available to most clinicians who must rely on perceptual evaluations. This means that the SLP needs to look, listen, and feel respiratory movements. This last component is not one that SLPs are typically comfortable with. However, after assessing just a few children, you will realize how easy it is to gain a great deal of information. Hixon and Hoit (1999, 2000) suggest a close examination of the rib cage and abdomen, but their protocols are somewhat unwieldy for clinicians and impractical for evaluating children. However, their suggestions regarding use of a checklist and observation of the chest wall are worthwhile.

Structural deformities, asymmetries, and the region of predominant movement during breathing should be noted (Redstone, 1991). One measurement that is easy to obtain is the rate of breathing, which can be determined by placing hands on the child's torso and counting while using a stopwatch. Figure 6–1 includes a checklist of respiratory attributes for the speech pathologist that can be incorporated into a clinical evaluation. These characteristics are based on the clinician's ability to observe and feel the child's trunk and also listen to the child's breathing and vocalizations.

Assessment of Respiration—Speech

It is difficult to discuss respiration for speech without including phonation. Therefore, in Chapter 7, the role of respiration, phonation, and speech production will be discussed in greater detail.

Checklist of Attributes to Guide Respiratory Assessment

Visual	Auditory	Tactile
☐ Deformities such as flaring ribs or depressed sternum	☐ Breathing rate	☐ Breathing rate
☐ Asymmetry of thorax	☐ Quality of vocalizations	☐ Depth of breathing
☐ Region of predominant movement in different positions	☐ Duration of vocalizations	☐ Rhythm of breathing
☐ Nasal/oral breathing	☐ Audible breathing	☐ Region of predominant movement
☐ Breathing rate		☐ Asynchronous movement between rib cage and abdomen
☐ Depth of breathing		☐ Increased tonus during speech
☐ Rhythm of breathing		
☐ Asynchronous movement between rib cage and abdomen		
☐ Abnormal movement patterns such as head extension or shoulder elevation to initiate phonation		
☐ Increased tonus during speech		
☐ Incoordination between breathing and other activities		

Figure 6–1. Checklist of respiratory attributes for assessment. (Table 2–1 Checklist of Attributes to Guide Respiratory Assessment, by F. Redstone. From *Neurodevelopmental strategies for managing communication disorders in children with severe motor dysfunction* [p. 41], by M. B. Langley and L. J. Lombardo [Eds.], 1991, Austin, TX: Pro-Ed. Copyright 1991 by Pro-Ed, Inc.).

Again, the emphasis is on the use of our senses during an evaluation. Begin observing when the child comes into the room. We should *observe* any muscle imbalance in the trunk that will influence breathing for speech when the child begins walking or sits with weight on one side. This can also be done during other aspects of the evaluation such as assessment of language and play.

Listen carefully when the child makes sounds, because this will allow us to make inferences about respiration. Are the sounds made on inspiration (stridor)? Are the phonations short? Low volume? Are all utterances monosyllabic? If so, is this due to respiratory capacity or linguistic issues? In addition, the child's position should be compared to these variables: Is there a position in which phonations are longer, louder, have more variety and better quality? Please refer to Chapter 7 for more information on the role of respiration for phonation and speech.

Assessment of Respiration—Feeding

Chapter 4 in this book addresses the feeding of the child with cerebral palsy. However, it is important to remember that respiratory coordination is an aspect of the feeding experience. We often take it for granted and assume it is adequate until it is NOT. Although we know that vital capacity for children with cerebral palsy is reduced (McPherson et al., 1992), there is no standardized test we can administer and score regarding *coordination* of breathing and swallowing. Instead, we will obtain information from our senses and use our problem-solving skills to determine the missing components needed for improved functioning. These will constitute our intervention plan.

Observation

The single best way to assess is to observe respiration during feeding. This will reveal how successful the child will be at protecting the airway. Arvedson and Brodsky (2002) tell us that the child's posture is strongly related to the coordination between respiration and swallowing during feeding. There is strong agreement between clinicians and researchers that the alignment of the head, neck, and trunk is the vital issue to note (Arvedson & Brodsky, 2002; Beecher & Alexander, 2004) because this will influence the coordination of respiration with feeding. However, it is also important to record the equipment being used during feeding to aid in alignment and stability.

It is imperative that we watch the head and neck during feeding. This will give us information about oral alignment and provide clues from the child as to whether something is wrong. Hyperextension of the neck, so commonly seen in cerebral palsy, places children at high risk for aspiration (Arvedson & Brodsky, 2002). Open mouth posture is another typical characteristic of children with cerebral palsy. This may be due to extensor hyperonus, a floppy head due to hypotonus, or it may result from nasal congestion or an obstruction. Careful evaluation of the reasons for open mouth posture is required (Pinder & Faherty, 1999).

As noted in Chapter 4 of this book, mouth closure is important for efficient feeding movements. However, prior to initiating mouth closure, we need to be sure that the child can switch to nasal breathing easily. If head position is an issue, further examination of alignment and stability is needed. It is not enough to state that "the child exhibits open mouth posture" without further explanation as to its cause.

Stability is required for efficient movement. However, too much stability will only cause immobility. We are looking for a balance between stability and mobility (Davis, 1987; Morris, 1987). Where are the child's hips? If the child is sitting with posterior pelvic tilt, which looks like he is sitting on his tailbone, the neck is likely to be in hyperextension (Pinder & Faherty, 1999). This will compromise respiratory coordination during feeding. A stable base at the pelvis will enhance alignment, stability, and control (Boehme, 1990) for coordinating oral functioning with respiration. Is the child struggling to get food to the mouth? The effort of self-feeding may interfere with the coordination of respiration.

In addition, it is critical to note any grimacing, change of color, or negative behaviors from the child because they may be due to difficulty in breathing or the child's fear of not being able to breathe. If this is the case, be cautious and make a medical referral.

Listening

Listen to the child's breathing. You can correlate what you hear to inspiratory and expiratory movements by placing a hand on the child's trunk at the junction of the rib cage and abdomen. Note what phase of respiration occurs right after the child's swallow. Exhalation is the safest. In addition, listen to the quality of the child's vocalization after swallows. This will indicate if the child has cleared the airway. Gasping after swallowing may be a sign of breath holding or that the child is unable to coordinate breathing with swallowing.

Handling During Feeding Assessment

Dynamic assessment is most worthwhile in this situation. It may give us a picture of the *potential* for change (ASHA, 2013). The evaluator makes a systematic change and assesses the child's response, how quickly the child learns, and how much support the child needs to be successful. For example, an evaluator might change the child's posture and then observe any changes in the child's alignment, assessing whether this led to better coordination between breathing and swallow.

Other variables that may be changed and then evaluated could be external pacing or giving the child food with time in between to adjust the breathing pattern. This requires careful observation on the part of the feeder. It is a strategy that has been successfully used to improve the respiratory coordination of premature children.

Treatment

The coordination for breathing during functions such as speech and feeding is influenced by things we take for granted: muscle tone, stability, and alignment. Children with cerebral palsy need help to attain these precursors for functioning. SLPs cannot change the neural maturation or skeletal framework of the respiratory system, but they can address the type of input and facilitate the child's response to that input. NDT provides this type of functional, developmental support through positioning, handling, movement for stability, and dissociation for improved functioning. In this section, we are focusing on the enhancement of respiration for feeding.

Direct Therapy Handling to Improve Trunk Stability—Prefeeding Activities

SLPs provide direct therapy to children. Therapeutic handling is an NDT technique used during direct therapy. It has been covered previously in this book. The goal of handling is the development or improvement of a specific function. In terms of what we are discussing now, the goal would be coordinated breathing and swallowing through the facilitation of stability and alignment.

For respiratory coordination we need to address stability first. An increase in trunk stability will be the most likely method to improve respiratory-swallow coordination, because the trunk includes most of the structures for respiration. In addition, a stable trunk is essential for good head control so that hyperextension of the neck is less likely to occur. The framework of the respiratory system includes the spine and the rib cage. Improved trunk control leading to stability of the spine will allow better rib mobility for efficient breathing (Arvedson & Brodsky, 2002). This principle of stability for mobility has been discussed extensively by several authors (Bahr, 2001; Davis, 1987; Redstone, 2012).

We need to remember that many of the muscles of respiration are also trunk muscles used for flexion, lateral flexion, and rotation. In addition, when they are used for functions like bending, weight shift, or reaching across midline, they are being used in a dissociated manner, which is what is needed for respiratory control. Trunk stability can be improved through naturally occurring daily activities and through direct handling during therapy. One example might be an SLP facilitating trunk rotation for improved muscle control for respiratory support during therapy as seen in Figure 6–2. Typically, this would occur within the context of a simple, play activity.

An SLP would not facilitate rotation or lateral flexion while feeding a child, because the coordination of respiration with swallowing along with oral preparation and transit of food is

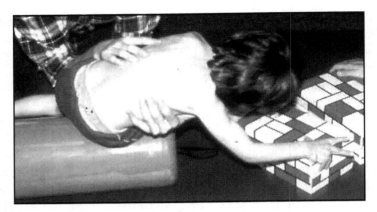

Figure 6-2. Facilitation of respiratory muscle through trunk movement and rotation during therapy.

already placing great demands on the child's system. However, a play activity activating the trunk musculature could precede feeding. Vocabulary such as "up," "high," and "over there" can be employed along with the facilitation of movements in an activity devised to bring about the elongation of the trunk. But always remember to maintain a flexor component in the neck and upper torso so that a total extensor pattern is avoided while facilitating dissociation of body parts.

Other therapeutic suggestions are given in Chapter 7 although they are presented in the context of respiration for phonation. Still, these can be used as preparatory activities. In addition, there are continuing education courses that include worthwhile clinical information on mobilizing and handling the rib cage to improve respiratory function.

Direct Therapy Positioning for Feeding

Sitting is a static position that is appropriate to use during a function such as feeding to maintain the muscle tone, alignment, and symmetry that was attained through active movement and handling. This is discussed in Chapter 4 of this book. The child needs a safe, stable position, which can be maintained with minimal effort. This is the guiding principle of finding a good position for feeding. Typically, we start with 90 degrees of flexion at the hips, knees, and ankles. This provides the stability needed to facilitate coordination between breathing and swallowing (Bergen & Colangelo, 1982; Morris, 1985; Redstone & West, 2004).

Although an infant is often fed in the parent's lap, this may, or may not, provide the best head alignment for a safe swallow. For example, it is often difficult to maintain neck flexion in upright while bottle feeding due to the shape of the bottle. However, using an angled bottle is one simple solution to improve safe transit. It is particularly important for the position chosen to allow careful, constant inspection of the child's face for any indication of respiratory stress. If the swallow is compromised by continued hyperextension of the head during feeding, better preparation through handling and movement prior to feeding is suggested (Wolf & Glass, 1992) along with the development of other seating arrangements. If pathology is seen during feeding that increases the likelihood of aspiration, it needs to be addressed immediately. In general, the goal is to have just enough support and stability through positioning to provide for safe, efficient functioning.

Indirect Therapy—Daily Activities

When working with young children and infants, SLPs must consider the integration of goals into family activities. SLPs may only be able to see the child one to three times a week, but caregivers can incorporate trunk stability into daily activities. This can provide the benefit of having a skill practiced many times in different contexts. There are many activities throughout the day that may contribute to the improvement of trunk musculature control.

**Daily Activities to Encourage
Trunk Control for Respiration**

1. Carrying the child upright with the head and upper torso supported on the adult's shoulder while maintaining head alignment.

2. Carrying the infant like a football in a sidelying position with trunk rotation provided by having the upper leg rotate over the lower leg.
3. Diapering the infant and maintaining alignment while encouraging flexion of the abdominals by raising the infant's legs.
4. Dressing with elongation of the trunk, neck flexion, and dissociation of legs and arms.
5. Picking up the child by saying "up," waiting for the child to move the arms in conjunction with elongation of the trunk, indicating a desire to go up.
6. Stimulating the child with toys to encourage reaching with lateral flexion or rotation while the child is in sitting, prone, or supine positions.
7. Having the child sit with just enough support while moving up-and-down or side-to-side to music.
8. Placing pictures on an easel and having the child reach up for extension (elongation), to the side for lateral flexion, or across midline for rotation.

Conclusions

There is a difference in the coordination of breathing for speech and feeding. However, both functions require coordinated muscular activity involving the oral, pharyngeal, laryngeal, and respiratory subsystems. Efficient respiration for speech develops over several years, and its development is closely related to the needs of the child's growing linguistic system. Breathing coordination for feeding is initially controlled by reflexes and supported anatomically because the consequences of incoordination are so serious.

Maturation and growth lead to the need for greater coordination during feeding because anatomical safeguards are fewer. The child with cerebral palsy requires improved stability and alignment to achieve the greatest possibility of a coordinated swallow. Providing successful therapy necessitates a thorough working knowledge of the alignment necessary for respiratory coordination of the swallow with respiration and its development. The NDT SLP has this knowledge along with the skills to attain this alignment through proper handling, and then to maintain it by good positioning.

Ten Items to Remember to Improve Intervention

1. Respiration involves dissociated, coordinated muscle activity of the trunk.
2. Trunk muscles used for respiration are also used for gross motor functions.
3. Air and food share the same space in the oral and pharyngeal areas.
4. The development of respiratory coordination requires stability.
5. Assessment requires making observations while the child is functioning, listening to the child, and feeling any changes in muscle tone.
6. Neck hyperextension is a pattern often seen in children with cerebral palsy. This may lead to aspiration.
7. Poor respiratory coordination of the child with cerebral palsy may cause aspiration.
8. Upright positioning with head and trunk alignment and stability are essential for safe feeding.
9. Incorporation of alignment and trunk movements into therapy and daily activities will enhance respiratory control.
10. Equipment should be used for feeding when it enhances positioning. It should be evaluated frequently.

Think Critically for Self-Study or Classroom Discussion

1. Discuss how speech breathing differs from tidal breathing.
2. Discuss how the pattern of breathing changes during feeding.
3. How does the development of upright positioning affect respiration?

4. Describe two techniques you can use to enhance respiratory coordination during feeding.
5. Discuss techniques you might suggest to families that will enhance respiratory coordination.

References

Achilles, R. (1955, Sept.–Oct.). Communicative anomalies of individuals with cerebral palsy. *Cerebral Palsy Review*, pp. 15–24.

American Speech, Language, and Hearing Association. (2013). *Dynamic assessment*. Retrieved from http://www.asha.org/practice/multicultural/issues/Dynamic-Assessment.htm

Arvedson, J. C., & Brodsky, I. (2002). *Pediatric swallowing and feeding: Assessment and management* (2nd ed.). San Diego, CA: Singular.

Bahr, D. C. (2001). *Oral motor assessment and treatment: Ages and stages*. Needham Heights, MA: Allyn & Bacon.

Bartlett, D. J., & Palisano, R. J. (2000). A multivariate model of determinants of motor change for children with cerebral palsy. *Physical Therapy, 80*, 598–614.

Beecher, R., & Alexander, R. (2004). Pediatric feeding and swallowing: Clinical examination and evaluation. *Perspectives in Swallowing and Swallowing Disorders, 13*, 21–27.

Bergen, A. F., & Colangelo, C. (1982). *Positioning the client with central nervous system deficits: The wheelchair and other adaptive equipment* (2nd ed.). Valhalla, NY: Valhalla Rehabilitation.

Bobath, B. (1972). *Neurodevelopmental treatment syllabus*. Chicago, IL: Neurodevelopmental Treatment Association.

Boehme, R. (1990). *The hypotonic child: Treatment for postural control, endurance, strength, and sensory organization*. Tucson, AZ: Therapy Skill Builders.

Boliek, C. A., Hixon, T. J., Watson, P. J., & Morgan, W. J. (1996). Vocalization and breathing during the first year of life. *Journal of Voice, 10*, 1–22.

Davis, L. F. (1987). Respiration and phonation in cerebral palsy: A developmental model. *Seminars in Speech and Language, 8*, 101–105.

Edgar, J. D. (2003). Respiration and swallowing in healthy adults and infants. *Perspectives in Swallowing and Swallowing Disorders, 12*, 2–6.

Eicher, P. S. (2007). Feeding. In M. L. Batshaw, L. Pelligrino, & N. J. Roizen (Eds.), *Children with disabilities* (pp. 479–497). Baltimore, MD: Paul H. Brookes.

Finnie, N. R. (2001). *Handling the young child with cerebral palsy* (3rd ed.). Oxford, UK: Butterworth-Heinemann.

Freed, D. B. (2012). *Motor speech disorders: Diagnosis and treatment* (2nd ed.). Clifton Park, NY: Delmar.

Hardy, J. (1964). Lung function of athetoid and spastic quadriplegic children. *Developmental Medicine and Child Neurology, 6*, 378–388.

Healy, A. (1983). Cerebral palsy. In J. Blackman (Ed.), *Medical aspects of developmental disabilities in children birth to three.* Iowa City, IA: University of Iowa Press.

Hixon, T. J., & Hoit, J. D. (1999). Examination of the abdominal wall by the speech-language pathologist. *American Journal of Speech-Language Pathology, 8*, 335–346.

Hixon, T. J., & Hoit, J. D. (2000). Examination of the rib cage wall by the speech-language pathologist. *American Journal of Speech-Language Pathology, 9*, 179–196.

Hoit, J. D. (1995). Influence of body position on breathing and its implication for evaluation and treatment of speech and voice disorders. *Journal of Voice, 9*, 341–347.

Huckabee, M. (2009). The development of swallowing respiratory coordination. *Perspectives in Swallowing and Swallowing Disorders, 18*, 19–24.

Kelly, B. N., Huckabee, M., Jones, R. D., & Frampton, C. M. A. (2007). The first year of life: Coordinating respiration and nutritive swallowing. *Dysphagia, 22*, 37–43.

Matsuo, K., Hiiemae, K. M., Gonzales-Fernandez, M., & Palmer, J. B. (2008). Respiration during feeding on solid food: Alterations in breathing during mastication, pharyngeal bolus aggregation, and swallowing. *Journal of Applied Physiology, 104*, 674–681.

McPherson, K. A., Kenny, D. J., Kohell, R., Bablich, K., Sochaniwskyl, A., & Milner, M. (1992). Ventilation and swallowing interaction of normal children and children with cerebral palsy. *Developmental Medicine and Child Neurology, 34*, 577–588.

Miller, C. K., & Willging, J. P. (2007). The implications of upper-airway obstruction on successful infant feeding. *Seminars in Speech and Language, 28*, 190–203.

Miller, M. J., & Kiatchoosakun, P. (2004). Relationship between respiratory control and feeding in the developing infant. *Seminars in Neonatology, 9*, 221–227.

Morris, S. E. (1985). Developmental implications for the management of feeding problems in neurologically impaired infants. *Seminars in Speech and Language, 6*, 293–316.

Morris, S. E. (1987). Therapy for the child with cerebral palsy: Interacting frameworks. *Seminars in Speech and Language, 8,* 71–86.

Mueller, H. (1972). Facilitating feeding and prespeech. In P. Pearson & C. E. Williams (Eds.), *Physical therapy services and developmental disabilities.* Springfield, IL: Charles C. Thomas.

Pinder, G. L., & Faherty, A. S. (1999). Issues in pediatric feeding and swallowing. In A. J. Caruso & E. A. Strand (Eds.), *Clinical management of motor speech disorders in children* (pp. 281–318). New York, NY: Thieme.

Redstone, F. (1991). Respiratory components of communication. In M. B. Langley & L. J. Lombardino (Eds.), *Neurodevelopmental strategies for managing communication disorders in children with severe motor dysfunction* (pp. 29–48). Austin, TX: Pro-Ed.

Redstone, F. (2012). Movement science for the SLP. In R. Golfarb (Ed.), *Translational speech-language pathology and audiology* (pp. 129–136). San Diego, CA: Plural.

Redstone, F., & West, J. (2004). The importance of postural control for feeding. *Pediatric Nursing, 30,* 97–100.

Seikel, J. A., King, D. W., & Drumright, D. G. (2005). *Anatomy and physiology for speech, language, and hearing* (2nd ed.). San Diego, CA: Singular.

Solomon, N. P., & Charron, S. (1998). Speech breathing in able-bodied children and children with cerebral palsy: A review of the literature and implications for clinical intervention. *American Journal of Speech-Language Pathology, 7,* 61–78.

Wolf, L. S., & Glass, R. P. (1992). *Feeding and swallowing disorders in infancy: Assessment and management.* Tucson, AZ: Therapy Skill Builders.

Workinger, M. S. (2005). *Cerebral palsy resource guide for speech-language pathologists.* Clifton Park, NY: Thomson Delmar.

Zemlin, W. R. (1998). *Speech and hearing science: Anatomy and physiology* (3rd ed.). Boston, MA: Allyn & Bacon.

CHAPTER 7

NDT and Speech Sound Production

Leslie Faye Davis and Fran Redstone

Introduction: The Speech Production System

Speech is the acoustic output of the coordination of the subsystems of the speech production system. Typically, we think of phonation as the output from the linkage of the respiratory and laryngeal subsystems. And then there is articulation, occurring in the oral cavity. But speech is so much more.

Some terms used to describe the skill of speaking are: "complex," "rapid," "precise," and "skilled" (Simonyan & Horwitz, 2011; Smith, Goffman, & Stark, 1995). The diversity of these adjectives stems from the fact that speech requires the coordination of respiration, phonation, resonance, and articulation (Mysak, 1976), all at the same time. Moreover, this speech system is but one part of a young child's development, which is changing constantly. The goal of this system is to convey linguistic meaning. Therefore, in this context, the word "complex" is a gross understatement.

A chapter on speech sound production and the child with cerebral palsy sounds like it should be a chapter on the larynx or the mouth. However, the production of speech, especially for the child with cerebral palsy, involves so much more than the vibration of the vocal folds and movements of the mouth. We, as speech-language pathologists (SLPs), need to address the whole speech system with its four major component parts. It is essential to think about it as one interrelated system. Whatever occurs in one segment of the system directly influences the functioning of the others.

The development of the integration of the system takes time in the typical child and is based on the child's normal muscle tone, movements, and support from the environment. However, this task is exceptionally difficult for the child with a neuromotor impairment such as cerebral palsy due to the lack of the basic requirements of normal muscle tone, posture, and movements.

We used to say that speech was an overlaid function of breathing and eating, but now we know more. There are indications that our system developed phylogenically, specifically for communication. MacLarnon and Hewitt (1999) demonstrated that modern humans evolved expanded thoracic vertebra to support the breath control necessary for speech production compared to early hominids and nonhuman primates. Additionally, Simonyan and Horwitz (2011) hypothesized that the direct connections from the laryngeal motor cortex to the motorneurons in the brainstem seen in humans, and not apparent in nonhuman primates, represent an evolutionary development allowing voluntary speech. They discuss this recent evolutionary development as a prerequisite for human speech control.

Although researchers (Moore & Ruark, 1996; Steeve & Moore, 2009; Steeve, Moore, Green, Reilly, & McMurtrey, 2008) hypothesize that the underlying neurology for the speech system is different from that of nonspeech activities such as feeding, even they acknowledge that their research suggests that younger children demonstrate similarities between early sound production and chewing (Moore & Ruark, 1996). It appears that there is still "the possibility of shared neural control during early development" (Bahr, 2001, p. 4). In addition, it is acknowledged that speech is influenced by many factors including a developing linguistic system. And both feeding and speech skills are influenced by repetitive use.

Anatomy and Physiology

Hodge and Wellman (1999) describe the several muscle groups that generate and valve the air pressures producing speech. These muscles are part of the speech production system that includes the skeletal structures for respiration: the spinal column, rib cage, shoulder, and pelvic girdles. This respiratory framework supports the trunk or thorax, which encloses the lungs and the muscles of inhalation and exhalation. These muscles are responsible for controlled respiration for speech, but this same trunk musculature is required for movements like bending, sitting upright, turning, and the core stability for walking, as well as the primary function of gas exchange.

Respiratory control for speech is learned through use, during the process of meeting communication demands. Vegetative breathing rate is 12 to 18 breaths-per-minute (bpm) in the mature system (Seikel, King, & Drumright, 2005) while it is variable for speech. The time spent for inhalation during vegetative breathing is about 40% of the respiratory cycle. This makes our breathing fairly rhythmic. Our diaphragm contracts and increases the vertical dimension of the thorax. The lungs are attached to the chest wall through pleural linkage. As the chest wall expands due to muscle contractions, the lungs expand. Because the chest wall expands, negative pressure is created in the lungs, and air rushes in to equalize the pressure. This is inhalation. During vegetative breathing, exhalation occurs through relaxation. It is passive. This relaxation is the response to the pressures of gravity, elasticity, and torque. These natural forces compel the respiratory system to return to a resting state and are typically referred to as recoil forces.

No matter what position we are in, inhalation is an antigravity action that occurs in one or more dimensions. For speech, the external intercostal muscles contract to expand the chest cavity, and the force of gravity is challenged. As the diaphragm contracts, it lowers, creating greater volume and decreased pressure in the lungs, and pushes out the abdominal muscles. Hence, the constant of gravity as a force is something we can take advantage of when establishing intervention strategies. We can change the child's position to take advantage of the force of gravity.

The demands to maintain the energy source for speech production require the ability to adjust the pressures of recoil. During speech breathing, exhalation is extended from the 50 to 60% for vegetative breathing to 80 or 90% of the respiratory cycle. To accomplish this, both passive and active forces are required, depending on the length of utterance. Holding off the forces of exhalation is called checking action (Seikel et al., 2005). The muscles of inspiration remain active longer so that the thorax is prevented from returning to resting level.

Checking action and laryngeal grading help to extend exhalation, and are sufficient for conversational speech. However, when we speak longer utterances, we may need a continued energy source. The muscles of exhalation become active to push air out of the lungs. Our intercostals can slowly pull our rib cage down and our abdominals can push the diaphragm farther up. This allows the prolongation of exhalation and provides an increased energy source for speech.

The respiratory framework has muscle attachments that span the entire speech production system. This highlights the anatomical relationships between the larynx, mouth, and respiratory framework. For example, the hyoid bone, which is closely associated with laryngeal structures and is considered part of the phonatory system, has muscle attachments to the respiratory framework (sternohyoid and omohyoid) (Jones-Owens, 1991; Wolf & Glass, 1992). This rather small bone is unique in that it has no direct attachments to any other bone, yet there are nine muscles attached to it. The supralaryngeal extrinsic muscles of the larynx (mylohyoid, geniohyoid, and digastric) attach to part of the articulatory framework: the mandible. Similarly, while the genioglossus is considered a tongue muscle for articulation, it also elevates the larynx, playing an essential role in pitch and resonance. The interaction of these muscles, which span the entire skeletal framework for speech, provides the stability for control for phonation (Jones-Owens, 1991; Seikel et al., 2005). Moreover, the relationship among the subsystems exemplifies how dynamic the system is, and further demonstrates the dependence of the system on muscle tone, posture, and head/trunk alignment.

Coarticulation

Coarticulation is another example of the interrelationship among the subsystems. Although Van Riper's traditional approach to speech production is one that deals with sound segments, the *McDonald Deep Test of Articulation* (1964) notes that in fluent speech, there is no such thing as initial, medial, and final sounds. McDonald concludes that the basic unit of speech is the syllable, not a sound in isolation. In fact, we now use the terms intervocalic, pre-, and postvocalic to indicate the fluency within a word's production (Bauman-Waengler, 2012). Intelligible speech requires more than saying one sound after another. It results from the ability to form syllables into words and phrases (Bernthal & Bankson, 2004). Recent nonlinear phonologies note the need to incorporate linguistic elements into our analyses of a child's speech production. The features of one segment influence adjacent segments (Bernhardt, 2003).

Our system must be anticipatory to be able to accomplish this fluently. This means that the structures are constantly being modified by the anticipation of the coming sound and the previous sound. Most SLPs are familiar with the concept of coarticulation. This preparatory preforming of speech sounds requires a great deal of coordination of the entire system. To motorically anticipate a target sound, it is easier if one has a consistent motoric system from which to make judgments and predictions. Children with cerebral palsy, especially the athetoid type, are rarely consistent in their movements. Therefore, making consistent articulatory judgments for sound production is an even greater challenge, and timing for voice onset and termination is typically distorted.

Sussman, Duder, Dalston, and Cacciatore (1999) studied the development of coarticulation for stop sounds in one child from 7 to 40 months, at which time their subject attained coarticulatory patterns typical of adults. They sought to determine how children develop the motor control for various consonant–vowel (CV) segments requiring coarticulation. They began with the child during babbling that they describe as the "primordial CV" (p. 1081). At this stage the child experiments with a range of articulatory movements. Interestingly, these researchers found that each stop consonant followed a different pattern of development.

Coarticulation for labials plus a vowel appears to be easier to develop because labials require less control over fewer structures. When the jaw and lips are closed, the tongue is free to adopt any tongue position. Sussman et al. (1999) describe the difficulty in learning differential tongue control for coarticulation of alveolar stops plus vowels, as the child needs greater stability and dissociation of the tongue musculature for tongue tip movement. Similarly, Hayden and Square (1994) suggest that early CV sound combinations, that is, [na, da], which occur in Stage III of the PROMPT hierarchy, are accomplished by jaw movement with the tongue flat on the floor of the mouth. In Hayden and Square's Hierarchy of Movement (1994), the vertical plane is the first dominant oral movement that is accompanied by the wide, ungraded excursion of the jaw (Figure 7–1).

As noted, the larynx also participates in coarticulation. Our system anticipates words that include sounds with varying voice onsets. Laryngeal muscles are constantly changing the position of the glottis, as well as the mass of the vocal folds, for various frequencies of the sounds being produced. Our system is enabled by the coordinated movements of the muscles that stabilize the laryngeal system to allow dissociated mobility of its parts. This stability comes from the overlapping muscular connections among the subsystems of the speech production system. For example, the dissociation between the head and shoulder girdle allows for the elongation of the neck, which contributes to the increase of pharyngeal space. This leads to a decrease of hypernasality in the developing child. Furthermore, without this basic structural alignment, the jaw and, in turn, the lips and tongue, will not develop adequate dissociation, which is critical in the emergence of varied sound play.

Simply put, we don't talk by synthesizing one sound after another. We are anticipating sounds that are four or five phonemes ahead of what we are producing at any given millisecond. The subtle nature of these rapid movements depends on the stability discussed above. We learn a preset of muscle movements and store this information centrally in order to appropriately anticipate articulatory demands. This concept of feedforward is consistent with other forms of movement. For example, in the gross motor area, when you walk down a staircase expecting 10 stairs and there are only nine, you get to the bottom and feel like a fool! So, where is the other stair? You have preset your muscles in anticipation of a certain motor demand. A similar preset musculature anticipation happens when you lift up a pitcher and expect that it is full but it is not. The same phenomenon

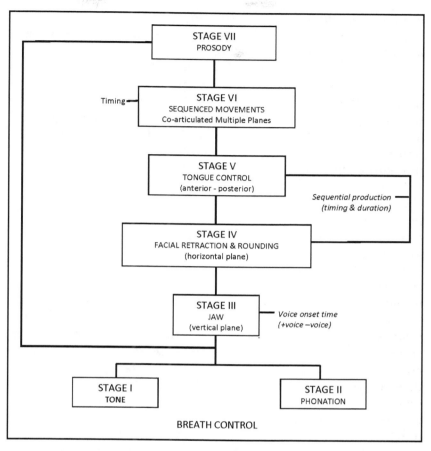

Figure 7–1. The PROMPT Hierarchy of Movement demonstrating the stages of movement complexity for speech. (This article was published in *Clinics in Communication Disorders, 4,* Hayden, D. A., & Square, P. A., Motor speech treatment hierarchy: A systems approach, 162–174, Copyright Elsevier [1994]. Reproduced with permission.)

occurs in the speech arena. If you are saying a word like "Mississippi," your system feeds you information to anticipate this four-syllable string of voiced and voiceless phonemes. Motor demands are placed on the articulatory system and also produce on–off demands in the laryngeal valving mechanism. While producing the /p/ in this word, there is a hold on exhaled air or delayed voice onset time. This intricate balancing of systems is indeed dependent on muscle tone and postural alignment or stability. The concept of feedforward is dependent on consistency in movements as a child develops.

As clinicians working with young children, we need to realize that it is a mistake to teach sound production as a string of unrelated segments. This is discussed in the section on therapy where, hopefully, it will become clear that a major goal for the SLP should be to help the child with cerebral palsy establish a predictable base of support from which respiratory, phonatory, and coarticulatory movements can develop.

Development

The timing and grading of the muscles within and among the systems is complex and develops over time in the typically developing child (MacLarnon & Hewitt, 1999; Solomon & Charron, 1998). Mueller (2001) reminds us that the typical child takes at least 5 years to develop fluent speech. Others suggest that the system continues to change until the child reaches adolescence. For speech to develop, voluntary control over each system is needed (Hayden & Square, 1994) for the integration of the systems to occur.

The oral structures of the neonate influence the primary function, feeding. Over the next 2 years these structures change significantly, providing increased ability to produce phonemic distinctions. Increased motor control, as a function of dissociated movement, will improve along with the underlying neurology, reflecting the increased importance of linguistic functions. Currently, there is much discussion in our field regarding the relationship between the development of feeding and speech skills. There are those who believe the relationship between these functions is irrelevant (Lof, 2003). However, we would like to point to the significance of the development of dissociated oral movements over time. Initially, an infant uses the oral structures as a total unit. The jaw, cheeks, tongue, lips, and soft palate work together during reflexive suck/swallow. As children learn to manipulate various food textures, they begin to move the oral structures in a variety of ways. The jaw starts to grade opening; the tongue lateralizes, extends, and bunches; and the lips move independently from the jaw (unlike the suck/swallow). The ability to isolate and combine movements increases the repertoire of movements that can be incorporated into speech and coarticulation. This is not to say that feeding is the only way in which the child learns this dissociation. However, this may be one helpful tool to treat children with motor deficits. Let's look at some specifics to demonstrate the constant state of change of the speech production system for the youngster in the first few years.

Birth to 3 Months

Bleile (1995) notes that infants practice using their vocal mechanism, which will be the basis of later speech. The sounds that are made during early infancy are influenced by the child's position and movements that are typically unstable. Davis (1987) describes these young infants as "belly breathing" (p. 101) and "barrel chested" (p. 102). The diaphragm contracts and pushes the abdomen. There is no involvement of the thorax, no dissociation, and no stability. The very early nonreflexive sounds heard include nasals. This is due to the tongue taking up much of the oral space as well as passive physiological flexion, which lowers the velum. By 3 months of age, there may be vowels (cooing) and CV-VC syllables because of the development of extension and movement.

The development of active flexion in the upper trunk, used for prone propping (Redstone, 1991), occurs slightly later than active extension, producing the desired balance between extension and flexion. This is rarely seen in children with cerebral palsy. At 3 months for typical children, this balance produces cervical elongation and an ability to flex the neck. This is called capital flexion and allows for the chin-tuck position. This alignment is further reinforced by the muscles used in the child's strong suck (Redstone, 1991). Here we see another interaction between systems.

Three to 5 Months

According to several authors (Alexander, Boehme, & Cupps, 1993; Kent, 1999), the increased variety in sounds produced in the 3- to 5-month period reflects an increase in oral activity, which, in turn, reflcts the child's increased general movement activities. Kent (1999) notes that by the end of this period the infant has developed the distinctive right-angled orientation of the human "craniovertebral relationship" (p. 51). The child is developing extension against gravity in the head, neck, and thoracic spine (Alexander et al., 1993; Bahr, 2001) that produces good head control and allows the infant to hold himself up against gravity. This upright position indicates good stabilization of the pharyngeal area necessary for the resonation of vowels (Bauman-Waengler, 2012).

In supine we see greater variety of movements, suggesting the fact that the child is no longer influenced only by the physiological flexion. There is now a balance between extension and flexion. The infant is reaching out, hips may flex with feet in the air, hands to feet, hands to midline, or lateral flexion. The mouth may be open but the child can attain a chin tuck due to elongation of the neck extensors along with the development of active neck flexion. We hear back sounds /g, ŋ / due to gravity influencing the posterior position of the tongue, but more forward, open, "happy" sounds (Mueller, 2001) are also heard secondary to the increased extension.

We see greater dissociation of the head and shoulder, and the infant is able to play in prone during this period. Stability allows for forearm support and the ability to weight shift. This strengthens the thorax (Davis, 1987). The child may reach and bring things to the mouth for exploration. Increased lip movements are seen in prone and greater bilabial sounds produced. With greater extension and head control allowing for increased pharyngeal space during this period, vocalizations become less nasal and more varied. Additionally, the tongue no longer fills the majority of the oral cavity, which allows greater pharyngeal and oral resonance. When supported in sitting, the child's balance is poor, but attempts to stabilize are evident. At this time, we hear more alveolar sounds as a result of greater jaw grading and closure.

The new postures and movement experiences during this period produce muscular activity that will be used functionally in future sound productions (Alexander et al., 1993). The majority of consonants heard during the first half of the infant's first year are glottals and velars whereas the second half of the first year produces labials and alveolars (Kent, 1999). This is reflected in Hayden and Square's (1994) Stage IV (rounding) and V (tongue control) of their hierarchy.

Six Months to 1 Year

During the second part of the first year, the pelvis becomes the child's center of gravity as observed in Figure 7–2. We see

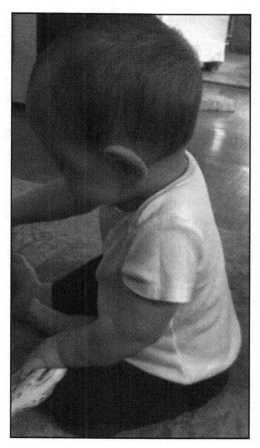

Figure 7–2. Trunk elongation in early stable floor sitting of a typically developing child.

controlled balance of flexion and extension, which allows independent sitting, reciprocal crawling, and rotation. The same musculature is used for respiratory control (Redstone, 1991). Structurally, the rib cage moves downward (Davis, 1987) due to the influence of antigravity positioning and muscle activations of the abdominals during weight shifting and rotation. Although the diaphragm will always be the primary mover for respiration, the thorax is now observed to move during inspiration, especially under maximal effort such as crying or loud vocal play.

Connaghan, Moore, and Higashakawa (2004) note that the structural changes in this period reduce the need for abdominal activity and increase rib cage contribution. The rotation seen at this time requires elongation of the obliques and intercostals. As a result, thoracic movements are seen during respiration (Redstone, 1991), and by 1 year trunk control has increased to allow for independent thoracic and abdominal movements for respiratory control for phonation and speech (Connaghan et al., 2004; Davis, 1987). By 1 year the child's respiratory pattern is approaching that of the adult. The respiratory rate for cry is 23 bpm (Langlois, Baken, & Wilder, 1980).

There is greater variation in the prosody of babbling and jargon and phonations are longer. This allows for the mimicking of the language produced in the environment (Davis, 1987). The infant is on the way to communicating through speech, and this pitch variation is the foundation for the emergence of pragmatics (i.e., raising pitch for question form). It is interesting to note that the prosody typical to the culture of children can be detected in their vocal play even without specific words.

One Year +

Hemispheric localization indicated by dendritic branching in Broca's area occurs between 1 and 2 years (Bahr, 2001). The influence of linguistics impacts the subsystems of speech production of the 1-year-old. But speech requires a continuous refinement of the underlying systems. Again, the infant needs to use the two major parts of the chest wall, the rib cage and abdomen, independently (Connaghan et al., 2004). The strategies for this control develop over time (Connaghan et al., 2004; Redstone, 2004).

This control is reflected in the child's ability to put words together for communication between 1 and 2 years of age. Once again, it requires the coordination between the subsystems of the speech production system. However, Kent (1999) notes that the connection between respiration and language patterns develops after the child begins to put words together, between 2 and 3 years. The child continues to practice the ability to match respiratory control with intended communication until about age 7. Until that time the effort required by the child is greater than the adult's (Kent, 1999).

The production of a constant air pressure through adducted vocal folds requires the coordination of the muscles of the chest wall, described previously as checking action, and the muscles of the laryngeal area (Davis, 1987; Redstone, 1991). The child practices this coordination for quite some time in order to produce appropriate loudness. Solomon and Charron (1998) report that oral pressures for children are typically higher than adults. How often is a child told to "use your indoor voice"? This suggests a difficulty in laryngeal grading as well as the coordination of thoracic muscle activity.

Familiarity with normal development permits us to better recognize when a behavior is not emerging or when it is emerging abnormally. This knowledge also allows the therapist to facilitate the motoric prerequisites that aid in the emergence of a target behavior or skill. In this way both our assessment and intervention abilities are enhanced.

Assessment

Many clinicians and researchers acknowledge the strong interrelationship between the subsystems of speech production. We noted this in relation to normal development but it also impacts abnormal development. Mysak (1976) and Pennington, Smallman, and Farrier (2006) note the dysfunctions of the subsystems of speech production in children with cerebral palsy leading to dysarthric speech. In addition, while discussing the respiration of children with cerebral palsy, Solomon and Charron (1998) note that the air flow abnormalities found during speech are not attributable solely to the respiratory musculature but also to the laryngeal, velopharyngeal, and articulatory muscles as well.

Although the expiratory muscles of a child with cerebral palsy may be weak (Hardy, 1964; Solomon & Charron, 1998) or the chest wall too rigid due to hypertonicity, if the child has enough respiratory capacity for vegetative purposes, there are also sufficient resources for speech (Rosenbek & Lapointe, 1978). An observation by Hull (1940) notes that respiration in children with cerebral palsy deviates from normal and this deviation increases with speech.

Davis reports that she once observed the TV interview of a woman with polio-induced quadriplegia who was highly motivated to function independently. During the interview the woman noted that she had 12% of typical lung capacity. But despite this limitation, she was totally intelligible and demonstrated normal phrase length, employing five to ten word utterances, depending on the linguistic content. Typically, air is graded by the use of both laryngeal and chest wall musculature, but she did this by primarily using laryngeal musculature. SLPs need to remember that it is not sufficient to activate the thorax alone. The entire system must work together in a coordinated, graded manner. It is apparent from the observation of this woman that it is not how much air is in the lungs, but how it is graded.

Gross Motor Influences on Respiration

When assessing respiration for phonation and speech, it is important to observe the movements of regions of the thorax. In research studies this is often accomplished using instrumentation. However, the clinician at a school or in a child's home will need to use a perceptual approach, which includes listening and observing. When assessing a child with cerebral palsy, it is also important to recognize and evaluate certain gross motor skills as well. The trunk musculature is responsible for the actions of the chest wall for respiration but also influences the child's ability to sit up and move.

Abnormal muscle tone of the trunk may be the reason for some structural abnormalities. The child with cerebral palsy who exhibits hypotonia may fix, or attempt to stabilize, by elevating, retracting, or internally rotating the shoulders. The result is the inability of the rib cage to expand for inspiration or to descend for exhalation for speech. In addition, the arms may remain adducted against the body due to lack of dissociation of the scapula with the upper arm. This may flatten the rib cage. Flared ribs may also be evident due to inactive abdominals and lack of stability of the upper thorax against the contraction of the diaphragm (Davis, 1987). Occasionally, there is a depression of the sternum. This looks as if the child is breathing in a paradoxical manner, and is often present in children with histories of respiratory distress at birth. The sternum is being drawn in as the diaphragm descends due to a lack of musculature support and shoulder stability (Redstone, 1991).

Compensations

What is the typical rate of respiration, and can the child adapt this for speech? Is speech interrupted with need for inhalations? Youngsters with cerebral palsy often have a rapid, shallow rate of respiration (Mueller, 1972) due to hypertonicity. Agonists and antagonists are working at the same time. In general, too many muscles are working at once leading to a limited range of movement. The system compensates by increasing respiratory rate.

What is most important is the ability of the child to change the I-fraction for speech. This is done by grading at the larynx and use of the trunk musculature. As noted previously, respiration for sound production is active. The chest wall expands for inspiration in three directions: vertical, anterior–posterior, and lateral. This movement was described by Zemlin (1998) as the lifting of the "handle of a water bucket" (p. 52). For this expansion to occur, muscle activity and a point of stability are needed. The stability is provided by the vertebral column, which is the point of attachment for the ribs.

Interactive Experience

Become kyphotic by hunching over and sitting on your coccyx (posterior pelvic tilt). Take a deep breath. Can you?

Go into hyperextension. Take a deep breath. How does this feel?

Now sit up. Take a deep breath. What moved?

When you were in hyperextension in the above experience, or when our children hyperextend, the vertebral column is compressed externally making the system too stable. Limited mobility of the rib cage will occur. When the thorax is hyperflexed due to sitting with posterior pelvic tilt, the vertebral column is also compressed, but this time it is internally compressed. Again, decreased mobility is the result.

If the thorax cannot stabilize and align on the vertebral column, then it cannot be active in the inspiratory phase of a cycle, leaving the individual with primitive diaphragmatic (belly) breathing. If the thorax is not active during inspiration, how can it remain active during expiration or hold against recoil forces? It cannot. Therefore, the ability to produce extended, graded exhalation for speech production is inhibited. While attempting to speak, it is most common for children with cerebral palsy to use hyperfunction to grade airflow. The child might use trunk flexion to push out air or strain at the vocal folds to grade airflow. Some children even use both strategies simultaneously. This pathological pattern is learned, centrally stored, and becomes more and more dysfunctional over time.

One of the typical postures we see in a child with cerebral palsy is head hyperextension. This leads to abduction of the vocal folds and an open glottis. This is what we utilize for CPR: an open airway but not for phonation! What we frequently hear is a breathy, low volume voice and short utterances or bursts of sound. The air is released rapidly without laryngeal grading.

Children with cerebral palsy who are motivated to communicate often attempt to initiate phonation by throwing their heads forward (flexion), and biomechanically closing the glottis. However, that adducts the glottis totally and shuts off sound production.

On the other hand, some children demonstrate the opposite. They are in hyperflexion, which strongly adducts the vocal folds. In an attempt to phonate, they throw their heads backward into hyperextension, thereby widely abducting the vocal folds. This is more typically seen in children with athetoid movements. In both cases, what is required are graded movements that will be possible with a more neutral head position. We would like to emphasize the importance of assessing the ability to phonate at will. It is critical for the SLP to recognize the compensatory patterns above as well as collecting and analyzing the child's phonetic/ phonemic inventory and doing an oral examination. However, the coordination of the systems as indicated by voluntary phonation during communication is an important component for the child with cerebral palsy. It is often overlooked because assessment protocols for physically typical children do not include this. Typical children rarely have difficulty in this area.

Sounds as Clues

The types of sounds that a child makes will give us direction for treatment. If we listen carefully, we will get clues as to which structures are active in the oral area. We are used to noting labial versus alveolar, palatal, or glottal sounds. It is imperative that the SLP also note these sounds in relation to the rest of the child's body. For example, a predominance of open vowels and glottal sounds tells us that the sounds being produced are from an open mouth with the tongue back. This is usually related to head extension. Similarly, a breathy quality tells us the glottis is wide, which is generally also associated with head extension. Harshstrained sounds that are produced by squeezing air through vocal folds that are too tense and constricted are due to spasticity at the level of the larynx. However, this spasticity is not localized to the larynx. Frequently, spasticity in the shoulders, arms, head, and neck are also present. Nasal quality often indicates a retracted tongue from the influence of gravity on the tongue in a hyperextended head, or a lack of mobility of the velum from the head, if the head is hyperflexed. Then, too, nasality is typical when the child's shoulders are elevated and there is limited pharyngeal space due to lack of dissociation between the head and the shoulders. The therapist must observe the relationship between sound production and posture.

The patterns noted may become habituated through use, leading to muscle changes, such as shortening of the capital extensors, which further limits movement possibilities. It is important for the SLP to note these abnormal postures because they impact the child's ability to produce and maintain the air pressures necessary and then shape the oral pharyngeal structures to resonate the air for speech. This should direct our treatment planning. Too often, SLPs do not observe the trunk control or head posture, because they feel the physical therapist should deal with these issues. This is an area where the SLP and the physical therapist should work together, because trunk stability and head control will lead to improved graded movements for respiration, phonation, and speech. Additionally, the SLP must become comfortable learning and using therapeutic handling as a way to facilitate improved speech. After all, team members are not always available.

Treatment

Alignment for Respiration/Phonation

NDT speech sound facilitation techniques have been developed by Mueller and are employed after normal tone and alignment have been attained through handling, movement, and/or positioning. Normal tone and alignment of the proximal muscles and structures provide the basis for developing a functional skill and are typically the first steps in developing a treatment program for a child with cerebral palsy. This allows more accurate, well-graded movements of distal structures such as oral structures for articulation as well as the coordination of respiratory muscles with laryngeal muscles for phonation. Mueller (2001) reminds us that this increases the possibility of making sounds without effort. Effortful sound production is so often seen in children with cerebral palsy.

If the child has head and trunk alignment, is stimulated appropriately, and is motivated, then sound production often develops, or improves, spontaneously. The authors of this chapter used to work directly on thoracic muscles but realized that getting greater central control with stability is more effective and efficient, and leads to greater carryover of function.

Handling

The NDT therapist handles in order to inhibit abnormal postures. This increases the possibility of a more normal response. When tone and posture are optimized, a more typical sensory experience can be introduced and the therapist can facilitate a more normal movement response. This sensory-motor pattern should be reinforced, repeated, and practiced in different contexts so that it can be "mapped" centrally. For example, one may observe that the improved posture leads to spontaneous bilabial closure during feeding. If so, this is the opportunity to incorporate the lip closure into another functional context, sound production.

All children with speech production problems will benefit from sitting with stability, alignment, and symmetry during speech sound production activities. Stable sitting is defined by the position of the pelvis. It is from pelvic stability that trunk elongation can occur (Figure 7–3).

SLPs working with children with cerebral palsy need to remember that "speech therapy begins at the hips and goes to the lips" (Anonymous, as cited in Zemlin, 1998, p. 52); or as Davis states, "What you want at the lips, you mediate at the hips" (Bahr, 2001, p. 45). In fact, both statements should be credited to Davis.

The child with hypertonicity may benefit from slow movement and attainment of symmetry. The child with low tone would benefit from joint compression resulting from gentle bouncing to improve tone in the trunk, whereas smaller areas would benefit from facilitatory techniques such as tapping. It is worthwhile to note here that massage for children with low muscle tone is NOT appropriate, because the goal of massage is to lower tone.

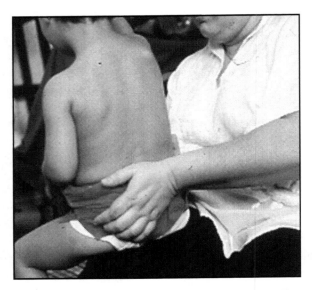

Figure 7–3. Attaining pelvic stability through handling during speech therapy.

Those who have received massages or facials should try now to recall those experiences. Do you remember that massage relaxes your body? However, tapping on the face during a facial is used to increase muscle tone.

Children with hypertonicity may benefit from massage, but those with low tone will not. Children with low tone require techniques to increase muscle tone such as joint compression or tapping.

NDT Handling for Respiration

The principle of postural control through therapeutic handling and positioning is the basis of NDT intervention for improved respiratory, phonatory, and articulatory functioning. A supportive environment is created through handling and maintained by proper positioning. Each subsystem can be addressed as needed following a thorough assessment of the primary and secondary impairments relevant to speech production.

An Example of Therapeutic Handling for Inspiration

In an effort to increase thoracic participation in inspiration, we can use the force of gravity to our advantage. By placing a child over a ball in a supine position while keeping the head in neutral flexion, the therapist can tilt the child, gently and slowly, upside down—but not too far. In this way, the external intercostals have less work to do as they are in a more progravity position. In this position the child has an opportunity to experience the expansion of the chest. Stimulating for sound production while the child is in a slightly backward position helps to inhibit the use of compensatory hyperflexion as a strategy to extend sound production.

Many NDT authors (Alexander, 1987; Davis, 1987; Mueller, 2001; Redstone, 1991) address the speech breathing needs of children with cerebral palsy by incorporating NDT respiratory techniques into phonation activities. For young children, respiratory/phonatory coordination is encouraged during early sound play, which is often the first step in the process. Sound play does not have the linguistic content often associated with effort. Sound play may begin with undifferentiated phonation or may be babbling. Early sound production and babbling in the typically developing child is closely associated with gross motor movements. The therapist can provide movement that will increase the likelihood of the child making vocal attempts. Gentle bouncing or rocking may facilitate sound production as well. Some early goals are listed below.

Early Respiratory/Phonatory Goals

Increase the frequency of vocal attempts.

Increase the length of vocal attempts.

Increase the number of syllables per exhalation.

Increase the variety of vocal attempts. This includes a change in the type of sound and position of the sound within a word.

The frequency, number, length, and type of vocalization expected for each child will vary depending on the child's functioning baseline. This is initially determined during assessment. However, good treatment requires an ongoing assessment. In addition, the goals noted above are not mutually exclusive. Several can be addressed at one time. Some traditional techniques to use may be modeling, imitation of the child's vocalization, and visual cueing. The NDT techniques of handling and movement should be employed if the traditional therapies did not produce an appropriate response. The addition of these NDT techniques can increase the likelihood of a well-graded response without the use of effort, compensations, or pathology.

NDT techniques that target respiration/phonation involve the activation of the intercostals and abdominal muscles. Initially, trunk elongation should be targeted. This allows greater intake of air on inhalation and can be accomplished through presentation of stimuli at appropriate levels after a stable base of support has been provided. However, a flexor component is necessary so that total extension does not occur. This treatment scenario can be accomplished through good capital flexion and the presentation of stimuli at, or below, eye level. A midline component in the upper trunk is also desirable and easily attained by encouraging reaching and holding a two-handed object/toy in front of the child as is seen in Figure 7–4.

It is during simple tasks like these that modeling of target phonation should be provided. These activities can be provided during the speech session or during play at home or in school settings. During speech sessions equipment such as rolls and balls can also be used to facilitate elongation of the trunk as seen in Figure 7–5. Note how the equipment can be used to facilitate play, language stimulation, and movement to enhance phonation. Remember, it is important for the activity to be salient to the child. This means that it is both motivating and appropriate for the child's functioning level. Providing elongation of the trunk within an age-appropriate activity demands creativity on the part of the clinician.

Another movement easily incorporated to develop respiratory musculature and coordination for phonation includes rotation. This allows the respiratory musculature to be used in a dissociated manner, which then needs to be incorporated

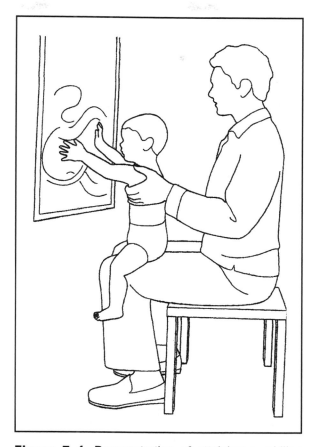

Figure 7–4. Demonstration of attaining a midline component with a child during therapeutic play. Note elongation of trunk, head and trunk alignment, and symmetry. (Reprinted from Bower, E. [2009]. Play. In E. Bower [Ed.], *Finnie's handling the young child with cerebral palsy at home* [4th ed.]. Copyright [2009], with permission from Elsevier.)

into a speech event. Rotation without a phonatory or speech component will not automatically improve speech production according to the principle of specificity. If speech is the desired outcome, then speech needs to be incorporated into the session. Figure 7–6 demonstrates the incorporation of rotation into a speech-related activity.

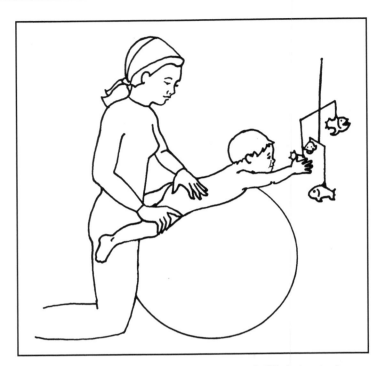

Figure 7–5. The use of a ball in therapy to facilitate trunk elongation and head/trunk alignment while incorporating a play component. (From illustration by Barbro Salek in Connor, F., Williamson, G. G., & Siepp, J. M. [1978]. *The program guide for infants and toddlers with neuromotor and other developmental disabilities.* New York, NY: Teachers College Press. Public domain.)

Coordination of respiratory activity within a movement becomes greater as the movement is repeated and learned (Alexander et al., 1993). Activities that encourage rotation are also used to prepare the external intercostals and obliques for active participation during respiration. This is an excellent time for PTs and SLPs to cotreat. Through modeling, the SLP can facilitate inspiration as the PT is elongating and facilitating lateral twisting.

When therapists work alone, therapeutic handling becomes their responsibility. This is true for SLPs as well as PTs or OTs. For example, while maintaining the child in supported sitting with a stable pelvis, the SLP may move an object to be reached so that the child will need to stretch across midline, thereby elon-

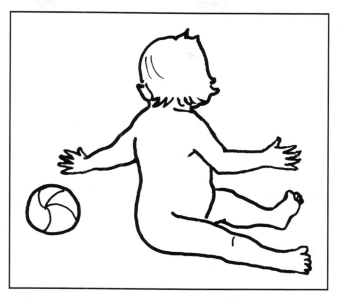

Figure 7–6. Rotation is being facilitated during play. (From illustration by Barbro Salek in Connor, F., Williamson, G. G., & Siepp, J. M. [1978]. *The program guide for infants and toddlers with neuromotor and other developmental disabilities.* New York, NY: Teachers College Press. Public domain.)

gating the intercostal and oblique trunk muscles. Of course, this needs to be done on both sides to stimulate the trunk muscles symmetrically. Sound production should be encouraged as the child is brought back to symmetry. Phonation can be prolonged as handling prevents a collapse into hyperflexion, which is a typical strategy utilized by children with cerebral palsy while attempting to phonate. Unfortunately, cotreatment is often a luxury and therefore the SLP should know how to facilitate elongation and rotation.

When targeting more complex linguistic material during language therapy, these same principles apply. However, for some of the therapy time, chair positioning may be appropriate. Sitting with pelvic stability, trunk elongation, and shoulder stability can also foster improved respiratory functioning for speech. Figure 7–7 illustrates appropriate chair sitting. This is more likely to produce a noneffortful, verbal response from the child.

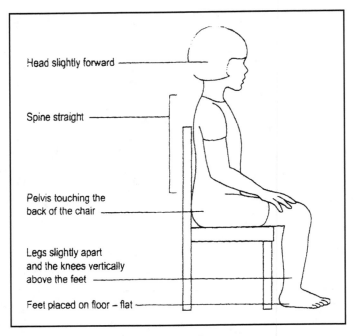

Head slightly forward

Spine straight

Pelvis touching the
back of the chair

Legs slightly apart
and the knees vertically
above the feet

Feet placed on floor – flat

Figure 7–7. Chair sitting with foot support, pelvic stability, shoulder stability, and symmetry. This starting position is more likely to result in voice output that is effortless. (Reprinted from Bower, E. [2009]. Chairs, pushchairs, and car seats. In E. Bower [Ed.], *Finnie's handling the young child with cerebral palsy at home* [4th ed.]. Copyright [2009], with permission from Elsevier.)

Another valuable NDT respiratory technique, besides positioning and movement, is called vibration and is often incorporated into handling during movement. It is typically taught in NDT courses, practiced, and then used with children during supervised practicums. Vibration is primarily intended for children with high muscle tone. Mueller (1972) describes it as "intense movement" (p. 306). It actually is low-amplitude, low-frequency vibration provided by the clinician's hands. According to Cherry (1980), this type of vibration reduces spasticity and allows more normal movement to occur. The clinician's hands remain in contact with the child's body, without pushing or pressure, to avoid extra stimulation. Light pressure with vibration can be applied by the therapist's hands to the upper trunk when the child spontaneously exhales, and is stopped just before the next inhalation occurs. Also, the therapist can gently elevate the upper trunk if the child is attempting to use hyperflexion as a strategy to "push" air during phonation. Vibration can be used anywhere the hands are placed on the child's body. However, to affect respiration for phonation, the upper rib cage or back is best. If done correctly, it will produce greater movement in the thorax and a longer vocalization with improved quality within the session. If increased thoracic movement and improved quality does not occur, the technique should be discontinued. Clearly, this is true of any strategy, for any child, with any disorder. In the case at hand, thought should be given to going back to basics and making sure that alignment and tone were adequate.

Whereas vibration is used for children with hypertonicity affecting respiratory musculature, joint compression is a technique that may be used for children with hypotonia. This can be done with the child sitting securely on the therapist's lap in an upright position with good alignment. Now, with the therapist's toes on the floor, heels could be raised an inch and then put down, providing a gentle input to the child's trunk. This should only be done a few times and then stopped to wait for the child's reaction. Typically, the child indicates a desire for more by moving the body up and vocalizing. Again, appropriate phonation should be modeled, and then the therapist should wait expectantly for the child's reaction, an important part of any therapy. This activity can be done with the child facing the therapist, if the child is more stable independently. In addition, this same type of input can be provided on a ball. The key is graded input with good alignment and constant monitoring by the handler. Otherwise, poor posture will be reinforced.

It is important to note that an NDT approach is not employed in lieu of other speech techniques—but in addition to them. The quality of the therapy depends on the ability of the clinician to individualize the treatment program for each child, to incorporate appropriate techniques, and to make the activity enjoyable so that the child actively participates. As in all therapeutic handling, the therapist's hands guide the child. The purpose of handling for improved respiratory control is to facilitate both greater inspiration and the subsequent checking action of the chest wall during vocalization. The objective is for the child to get more appropriate proprioceptive and auditory feedback while actively participating. The stimulus for sound production may be a model, an auditory closure task, a response to a picture, or even a song.

NDT-Speech Sound Production

As SLPs we know a great deal about the production of speech sounds. For example, we know that central vowels are ones in which the tongue does not move a great deal, /i/ is produced with the tongue high and forward, and /u/ is produced with the tongue still high but more posteriorly positioned. Some vowels are produced with the tongue low, which often accompanies more open mouth posture. Figure 7–8 is the vowel quadrangle, which demonstrates the position of the tongue for English vowels. It is important to remember that the child's tongue position is related to head position. A hyperextended head will lead to a posteriorly positioned tongue. In addition, a back, low vowel is more likely to produce hyperextension of the jaw. We can use this information to determine the sound environments of words chosen in therapy that will be most likely to produce an effortless, successful sound production. The sound one chooses for the child to produce is critical. For example, having a child phonate an open vowel such as /ɑ/ will encourage head and jaw extension. Therefore, using the more closed sound /u/ helps maintain head flexion, which helps with the adduction of the vocal folds and prolongation of the sound. Furthermore, the more graded jaw and lip closure facilitates preparation for movement to the next sound.

Using the Vowel Quadrangle in Figure 7–8 produce the front vowels.

Do the same for the back vowels.

Do you notice how your tongue goes from high to low?

Also notice how your jaw extends to produce low vowels.

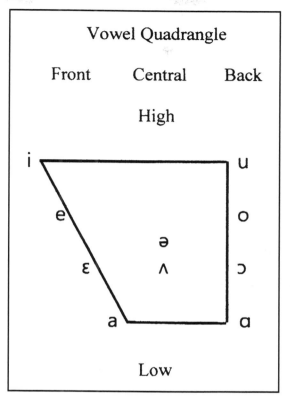

Figure 7–8. The vowel quadrangle indicating the position of the tongue during vowel production. The tongue position will influence the jaw position. This information helps SLPs make decisions regarding words to target in therapy.

Consonants are produced with greater constrictions than vowels. For example, to make the /b/ sound, the lips close, and voice onset begins. However, when we produce a /z/, the closure is not complete and the constriction is made with the tongue. The /g/ is also made with the tongue, but closure is complete and is made in the back of the mouth (velar). The jaw is also slightly open to a greater extent to produce the /g/ than it is for the /b/ or /z/. The ability to change the shape of our vocal tract by moving our jaw, tongue, or lips, allows us to produce the great range of sounds we use for communication (Ferrand, 2001). Children with cerebral palsy have difficulty making the subtle jaw, lingual, and labial movements required for speech production. Often the child's oral area is dominated by jaw extension secondary to head extension. This jaw position limits the type of sounds that are likely to be produced.

While sitting in your chair, produce a /b/ sound.

Now hyperextend your head and attempt it again.

Your jaw has to move a greater distance against gravity to produce the bilabial closure when your head is extended.

Do the same exercise for the /z/ or /d/ or any other alveolar sound.

Again, with the jaw extended, it is more difficult to produce a sound that requires closure of the lips or the anterior tongue. We typically produce these sounds with nearly closed jaws.

Now, with your head hyperextended, is it easier to make a /g/ or a /d/?

Gravity makes it easier to produce the /g/.

Moto-Kinaesthetic Methods

The Moto-kinaesthetic method was described nicely by Travis (1940) as a method in which the "teacher actually guides by manual manipulation the parts of the speech apparatus into the necessary movements for the production of correct sound sequences" (p. 283). Travis is describing the method developed by Hill-Young and used in a school in Los Angeles. The method was used with children who were deaf/blind and who had cerebral palsy. Hill-Young emphasized errorless learning and helping the child go through the actual motions to get the experience of sound sequencing. This approach was first described in detail by Stinchfield-Hawk (1937) and notes the importance of functional speech, early training, and practice. These are all concepts that are respected today.

Mueller devised speech sound facilitation techniques for children with cerebral palsy. This entails an analysis of the sounds the child makes along with the muscle tone and postures the child uses. Clinicians use their hands to facilitate the movement of the child's articulators along with appropriate movement or positioning to influence airflow and valving of the vocal folds. This is performed within an activity, along with appropriate speech stimulation, typically modeling, to prompt a response from the child. Again, this would not be attempted until tone and alignment had been addressed. In addition, it is performed while also addressing exhalation through movement, vibration, or compression.

Speech sounds are never introduced in isolation and usually are encouraged in an intervocalic or medial position. This produces a better production of consonants. If the constriction occurs in the initial position, there is a tendency to halt phonation. The medial position allows for "soft voice initiation" (Mueller, 1972, p. 307). The therapist may use one hand to begin vibration, if needed. Then, the child would make a central vowel and the clinician would facilitate momentary mouth closure and opening with the other hand. This is done passively so that the child experiences effortless voice production. The facilitation of oral closure should be done without interrupting the child's phonation so that the child experiences a multisyllable vocalization. The goal is for the child to experience this, repeat it, and practice it, so that neural pathways are enhanced, synergies developed, and programs stored centrally (see Chapter 2) for later use.

When we describe the typical speech pattern of individuals with cerebral palsy, several phrases come to mind: slow and labored, poor voice quality, short bursts of sounds or words, and articulatory errors. All of these descriptors have a common foundation—errors in timing. In other words, as we have been saying throughout this chapter, motor coordination is the root of the problem. Treatment goals, therefore, need to address the child's ability to make varied contacts and initiate or terminate voice more quickly.

It is easier for the SLP to work on sounds that can be facilitated externally. These involve jaw and labial musculature. However, /l/ can be introduced fairly easily by raising the tongue with a tool, such as a tongue depressor, or the clinician's gloved finger. Tongue tip /d/ can also be easily facilitated.

Timing and Phonemic Value

An example of the importance of timing from the first author's clinical practice is the extreme frustration of a young client who was attempting to describe his activity the previous day. This clinician heard the client say, "I go poat." It took many trials to realize the client was telling her that he went on a BOAT

Analysis tells us this client's underlying problem was his inability to release his bilabial closure and initiate voicing simultaneously to make the sound that we hear as /b/. Rather, his release time was delayed and voicing was delayed, giving the listener the perception of /p/.

Having this client practice minimal pairs of /b-p/ in isolation or in words would be foolish and frustrating. He needed the therapist to help him produce a quicker release with voice onset. Postural alignment was the start, but adding a tactile cue to break lip contact while providing vibration to the upper chest to help initiate voice was the method that enabled him to communicate his intent. After establishing the sequence, practice and repetition would be worthwhile.

Hayden and Square (1994) suggest that the pattern of sound development follows a motor hierarchy. They note that the infant must establish stability and then learn to move the jaw in a vertical plane allowing for graded jaw opening. This then leads to velar and alveolar sounds. Later, the child learns facial retraction and lip rounding that is followed by variation in vowels and bilabial sounds. Hayden and Square developed this hierarchy primarily for children with apraxia of speech. However, the concepts are generalizable.

An Eclectic Approach

SLPs learn a great deal about therapy for speech sound disorders in physically typical children. The child with cerebral palsy, like a child with CAS or a phonological disorder, may have a small phonetic inventory (PI). Similar strategies for all of these children can be used to increase the child's expressive vocabulary. One strategy is to teach new words that include the sounds already in the child's PI (Bleile, 1995). While the SLP works on increasing the PI, the family, along with other members of the team, can put together a core vocabulary of new functional words that can be used throughout the day. An NDT speech clinician can alert the team to sounds that lead to either hyperextension or hyperflexion in the child with cerebral palsy. These would be done after the assessment and analysis of the child's speech production system. For example, although the child may have /h/, encouraging "hi" is likely to lead to an extensor pattern due to the jaw hyperextension for the vowel. However, a social greeting is definitely worthwhile, and, therefore, "hello" might be placed on the word list. Although a child may have the /g/ sound in the PI due to posterior tongue position, it can be placed within a sound environment that encourages forward movement such as in the phrase /ʌ gem/ that facilitates forward movement with the lips, along with a front vowel.

Another strategy to increase an expressive vocabulary is to increase the phonetic inventory (Bauman-Waengler, 2012). When deciding what sounds to target in therapy, an NDT approach would incorporate typical selection strategies along with the knowledge that some sounds in some positions are more likely to lead to blocking or use of pathology in the child with cerebral palsy. As previously noted, voiced consonants in an intervocalic or medial position are more likely to be successfully produced without effort. This may avoid the voice onset timing issues noted above.

Conclusions

As NDT speech clinicians for many years, the authors of this chapter have found that using the knowledge of development, components of movements, handling, and problem-solving skills learned during our NDT courses have helped us treat children with cerebral palsy. NDT gives us the specific information about cerebral palsy that can be used in therapy for children with neuromotor issues. However, into this specific information we need to incorporate our knowledge of speech and language learned in graduate programs, continuing education courses, presentations at conventions, journals, and books. NDT, along with all the other techniques and information acquired, can lead to a powerful arsenal of therapeutic tools to benefit children with cerebral palsy.

It is essential for the SLP to understand the importance of therapy techniques that utilize motor facilitation, touching, and cueing for improvement in overall speech production. These are not new concepts. Movement and cueing methodologies have been discussed in our field as early as the 1930s. Cerebral palsy is by definition a motor disorder and, therefore, attempting to improve the child's speech by only using auditory and visual stimuli will not address the primary dysfunction. Helping the child to normalize general muscle tone and posture and to feel the subtle movements used for articulation is essential to the therapy process. Input that provides tactile, kinesthetic, and proprioceptive experiences helps the child to feel the desired sound production goals.

Therapeutic methodologies, which are multisensory (auditory, visual, tactile–kinesthetic) provide greater potential for achieving the child's goals. The authors of this chapter strongly suggest that the SLP interested in working with children with cerebral palsy enroll in a multitude of continuing education courses that emphasize the nature and needs of those with motor impairment. This would include, but not be restricted to, information related to sensory-motor approaches and multidisciplinary team approaches such as NDT.

Ten Items to Remember to Improve Intervention

1. All the subsystems of the speech production system are interrelated.
2. Cerebral palsy affects the motor components of all the subsystems of speech production.
3. It is important to assess and treat the ability to initiate voice at will.
4. During assessment and treatment, watch for compensations such as the use of extension/flexion to initiate voice.

5. Analyze sounds produced by the child in relation to postures and movements.
6. Treatment begins with stability, alignment of head/trunk, and symmetry.
7. Sitting during speech therapy should provide upright positioning and stability, which targets the pelvis for good trunk support.
8. Treatment includes handling. Do not hesitate to use your hands to move and facilitate gross and oral movements.
9. Help the child produce sounds with facilitation. Encourage the child to repeat and practice sounds. Then change the contexts of the sounds for generalization.
10. Choose sounds for intervention that are functional and developmentally appropriate, but do not trigger compensations or pathology.

Think Critically for Self-Study or Classroom Discussion

1. Put "what you want at the lips, you mediate through the hips" in your own words.
2. Why is head alignment so important to sound production?
3. What sounds will a child with neck hyperextension have difficulty producing?
4. What strategy is often used by a child with cerebral palsy to initiate voice?
5. With what strategy would you begin treatment in order to attain mouth closure for speech production?

References

Alexander, R. (1987). Oral-motor treatment for infants and young children with cerebral palsy. *Seminars in Speech and Language, 8,* 87–100.

Alexander, R., Boehme, R., & Cupps, B. (1993). *Normal development of functional motor skills.* San Antonio, TX: Therapy Skill Builders.

Bahr, D. C. (2001). *Oral motor assessment and treatment: Ages and stages.* Boston, MA: Allyn & Bacon.

Bauman-Waengler, J. (2012). *Articulation and phonological impairments: A clinical focus* (4th ed.). Boston, MA: Allyn & Bacon.

Bernhardt, B. H. (2003). Nonlinear phonology: Application and outcomes evaluation. *Perspectives in Language Learning and Education, 10,* 26–30.

Bernthal, J. E., & Bankson, N. W. (2004). *Articulation and phonological disorders* (5th ed.). Boston, MA: Pearson.

Bleile, K. M. (1995). *Manual of articulation and phonological disorders.* San Diego, CA: Singular.

Bower, E. (2009). Play. In E. Bower (Ed.), *Finnie's handling the young child with cerebral palsy at home* (4th ed., pp. 309–330). Oxford, UK: Butterworth-Heinemann.

Cherry, D. B. (1980). Review of physical therapy alternatives for reducing muscle contractures. *Physical Therapy, 60,* 877–881.

Connaghan, K. P., Moore, C. A., & Higashakawa, M. (2004). Respiratory kinematics during vocalization and nonspeech respiration in children from 9 to 48 months. *Journal of Speech, Language, and Hearing Research, 47,* 70–84.

Davis, L. F. (1987). Respiration and phonation in cerebral palsy: A developmental model. *Seminars in Speech and Language, 8,* 101–106.

Ferrand, C. T. (2001). *Speech science: An integrated approach to theory and clinical practice.* Boston, MA: Allyn & Bacon.

Hardy, J. (1964). Lung function of athetoid and spastic quadriplegic children. *Developmental Medicine & Child Neurology, 6,* 378–388.

Hayden, D. A., & Square, P. A. (1994). Motor speech treatment hierarchy: A systems approach. *Clinics in Communication Disorders, 4,* 162–174.

Hodge, M. M., & Wellman, L. (1999). Management of children with dysarthria. In A. J. Caruso & E. A. Strand, (Eds.), *Clinical management of motor speech disorders in children* (pp. 209–280). New York, NY: Thieme.

Hull, H. (1940). A study of the respiration of fourteen spastic paralysis cases during silence and speech. *Journal of Speech Disorders, 5,* 275–276.

Jones-Owens, L. (1991). Prespeech assessment and treatment. In M. B. Langley & L. J. Lombardino (Eds.), *Neurodevelopmental strategies for managing communication disorders in children with severe motor dysfunction* (pp. 49–80). Austin, TX: Pro-Ed.

Kent, R. D. (1999). Motor control: Neurophysiology and functional development. In A. J. Caruso & E. A. Strand (Eds.), *Clinical management of motor speech disorders in children* (pp. 29–72). New York, NY: Thieme.

Langlois, A., Baken, R., & Wilder, C. (1980). Prespeech respiratory behavior during the first year of life. In T. Murray & J. Murray (Eds.), *Infant communication cry and early speech*. San Diego, CA: College-Hill.

Lof, G. (2003). Oral motor exercises and treatment outcomes. *Perspectives on Language Learning and Education, 10*, 7–11.

MacLarnon, A. M., & Hewitt, G. P. (1999). The evolution of human speech: The role of enhanced breathing control. *American Journal of Physical Anthropology, 109*, 341–363.

McDonald, E. T. (1964). *McDonald deep test of articulation*. Pittsburgh, PA: Stanwix House.

Moore, C. A., & Ruark, J. L. (1996). Does speech emerge from earlier appearing oral motor behaviors? *Journal of Speech and Hearing Research, 39*, 1034–1047.

Mueller, H. (1972). Facilitating feeding and prespeech. In P. Pearson & C. Williams (Eds.), *Physical therapy services in the developmental disabilities*. Springfield, IL: Thomas.

Mueller, H. (2001). Feeding. In N. R. Finnie (Ed.), *Handling the young child with cerebral palsy at home* (3rd ed., pp. 209–221). Boston, MA: Butterworth-Heinemann.

Mysak, E. D. (1976). *Pathologies of speech systems*. Baltimore, MD: Williams & Wilkins.

Pennington, L., Smallman, C., & Farrier, F. (2006). Intensive dysarthria treatment for older children with cerebral palsy: Findings from six cases. *Child Language Teaching and Therapy, 22*, 255–273.

Redstone, F. (1991). Respiratory components of communication. In M. B. Langley & L. J. Lombardino (Eds.), *Neurodevelopmental strategies for managing communication disorders in children with severe motor dysfunction*. Austin, TX: Pro-Ed.

Redstone, F. (2004). The effects of seating position on the respiratory patterns of preschoolers with cerebral palsy. *International Journal of Rehabilitation Research, 27*, 283–288.

Rosenbek, J., & LaPointe, L. (1978). In D. Johns (Ed.), *Clinical management of neurogeniccommunication disorders*. Boston, MA: Little Brown.

Seikel, J. A., King, D. W., & Drumwright, D. G. (2005). *Anatomy and physiology for speech, language, and hearing* (4th ed.). Clifton Park, NY: Delmar, Cengage.

Simonyan, K., & Horwitz, B. (2011). Laryngeal motor cortex and control of speech in humans. *Neuroscientist*. Retrieved from http://nro .sagepub.com/content/early/2011/02/27/1073858410386727

Smith, A., Goffman, L., & Stark, R. (1995). Speech motor control. *Seminars in Speech and Language, 16*, 87–98.

Solomon, N. P., & Charron, S. (1998). Speech breathing in able-bodied children and children with cerebral palsy: A review of the literature and implications for clinical intervention. *American Journal of Speech-Language Pathology, 7*, 61–78.

Steeve, R. W., & Moore, C. A. (2009). Mandibular motor control during the early development of speech and nonspeech behaviors. *Journal of Speech, Language, and Hearing Research, 52*, 1530–1554.

Steeve, R. W., Moore, C. A., Green, J. R., Reilly, K. J., & McMurtrey, J. R. (2008). Babbling, chewing, and sucking: Oromandibular coordination at 9 months. *Journal of Speech, Language, and Hearing Research, 51*, 1390–1404.

Stinchfield-Hawk, S. (1937). Moto-kinaesthetic speech training for children. *Journal of Speech Disorders, 2*, 231–238.

Sussman, H. M., Duder, C., Dalston, E., & Cacciatore, A. (1999). An acoustic analysis of the development of CV coarticulation: A case study. *Journal of Speech, Language, and Hearing Research, 42*, 1080–1096.

Travis, L. E. (1940). The pedagogical significance of the moto-kinaesthetic approach in speech therapy. *Journal of Speech Disorders, 5*, 281–284.

Wolf, L. S., & Glass, R. P. (1992). *Feeding and swallowing disorders in infancy: Assessment and management.* Tucson, AZ: Therapy Skill Builders.

Zemlin, W. R. (1998). *Speech and hearing science: Anatomy and physiology* (4th ed.). Boston, MA: Allyn & Bacon.

CHAPTER 8

Saliva Control and Drooling in Children with Cerebral Palsy

Fran Redstone

Introduction

Saliva is the watery substance that protects our teeth, provides lubrication for swallowing, aids in digestion, and leads to oral comfort (Blasco & Allaire, 1992). Although two to six cups (Bakke, Bardow, & Moller, 2012) are produced daily by the six salivary glands (Arvedson & Brodsky, 2002), we are typically unaware of its existence because we automatically control it through swallowing. We swallow at least 600 times a day (Arvedson & Brodsky, 2002), less frequently at night, and more when eating and speaking.

Drooling, or sialorrhoea, is the loss of saliva control. It is the unintentional spilling of saliva from the mouth, and it has both health and social consequences (Walshe, Smith, & Pennington, 2012). The most common type of drooling is anterior drooling, which is what we observe when saliva spills from the mouth.

However, posterior drooling may lead to pooling of saliva in the hypopharynx. If not swallowed this may cause coughing, gagging, or even possible aspiration (Bakke et al., 2012; Blasco & Allaire, 1992).

Although all children lose saliva control at times throughout childhood, drooling is often persistent and severe in children with cerebral palsy (Acs, Ng, Helpin, Rosenberg, & Canion, 2007). This affects social integration as well as the child's development of self-esteem (Reid, Johnson, & Reddihough, 2009), and may impact the decision for educational inclusion. In addition, although parents may be very accepting, other caregivers may be less "hands on" due to the child's drooling and need for constant face wiping and changing of clothes (Acs et al., 2007, p. 499; Arvedson & Brodsky, 2002; Bakke et al., 2012). Drooling may also be socially stigmatizing (Love, 2000). In fact, social avoidance is the typical reaction to someone who drools (Blasco & Allaire, 1992). Moreover, drooling impacts the quality of life for both the child and the child's caregiver (Reid et al., 2009).

Drooling is a topic of interest in many disciplines. Because of its social consequences, much drooling related material has been published by educators and psychologists. In addition, the medical and dental professions have provided a great deal of research. However, it is acknowledged that the speech pathologist (SLP) treating the child with cerebral palsy may be one of the first professionals to see this child and possibly prevent the development of severe drooling through a program that addresses both postural and oral-motor needs. In fact, these are most often included in a comprehensive feeding program.

Development of Saliva Control

Control of saliva requires normalized oral sensation and oral-motor control. The oral control can be facilitated by the development of proximal stability, especially of the head, neck, and shoulder areas. During the first year of life, infants have periods of intense drooling. This is associated with jaw instability and the stimulation caused by teething. These are two causations that we should keep in mind when considering treatment planning.

An increase in saliva occurs with the maturation of the salivary glands, which is related to the infant's change in diet and the increased need of saliva for digestion. The infant must also learn to control the increased saliva production at nonfeeding times. In many ways saliva control parallels the control for feeding. This is not unexpected because the oral requirements for both are similar. Alexander, Boehme, and Cupps (1993) note that drooling is evident in 2-month-olds, due to large jaw excursions from an unstable mandible. Drooling decreases at about 5 months of age in positions that give the infant postural stability. At 6 months the infant may again begin to drool because of teething. But by about 9 months drooling is rare. This is the period when the child may be sucking from a bottle, actively taking food from a spoon, lateralizing food, as well as beginning to chew and cup-drink. In fact, saliva control is typically mature by 2 years of age when the child has attained internal jaw stability and is self-feeding with utensils. Drooling is rarely seen at age 4 and is considered atypical at 5 (Bakke et al., 2012).

Drooling and Cerebral Palsy

The reports of the prevalence of drooling in children with cerebral palsy range from 10% to 58% (Bakke et al., 2012; Chavez, Grollmus, & Donat, 2008). The salivary glands of children with cerebral palsy do NOT produce more than physically typical children (Erasmus et al., 2009; Senner, Logemann, Zecker, & Gaebler-Spira, 2004; Tahmassebi & Curzon, 2003). This was initially considered to be the cause of the drooling. Instead, the problem results from the fact that children with cerebral palsy who drool cannot *control* their saliva. These children do have a reflexive swallow (Chavez et al., 2008; Iammatteo, Trombly, & Luecke, 1990), but they swallow less frequently (Domaracki & Sisson, 1990). This is caused by a lack of oral-motor control, which leads to an incoordination of the swallow.

Most of the saliva pools anteriorly, which is the most vulnerable area for children with cerebral palsy (Harris & Dignam, 1980). Drooling often results from poor proximal stability, causing poor head control and an open mouth posture. In addition, lack of oral stability leads to a poor oral seal with an inability to move saliva posteriorly.

It is important to consider that children with cerebral palsy have sensory deficits, which, according to Blasco and Allaire (1992), may be the primary cause of drooling. Pinder and Faherty (1999) discuss drooling in children who demonstrate hyposensitivity. These children are unaware of the accumulation of saliva or their wet chins. Some children stuff their mouths, pocket food, or chew inadequately due to the lack of sensory input. Children with sensory aversion and hypersensitivity may posture their head and retract their tongue to avoid any oral sensations. This fixing leads to drooling because no movement of the saliva occurs.

Additional problems noted in this population may also lead to drooling. Seizure medications may actually increase saliva production as well as dental disease. Reflux, too, has also been implicated as a confounding factor. The loss of saliva may exacerbate reflux symptoms (Senner et al., 2004). Others feel that reflux may intensify drooling.

Assessment for Drooling

Because drooling is typically considered a disturbance of oral-motor control (Blasco & Allaire, 1992; Rodwell, Edwards, Ware, & Boyd, 2012), evaluation of saliva control needs to be part of a comprehensive speech/feeding assessment of the oral structures and functions. Blasco and Allaire (1992) note that severe drooling without a speech disorder does not occur. If children have speech, drooling is typically mild. Sittig (1947) also notes the relationship between speech and drooling. Although we typically consider treating severe drooling, we need to remember that mild to moderate drooling may be more devastating to the child who is less impaired and cognitively intact, because this child is more likely to be affected by the resulting social isolation.

One component of the assessment is gathering information from a medical report or parent interview. This may indicate gastrointestinal issues such as reflux or medications that can contribute to the child's drooling. Although reflux may increase the production of saliva as a defense against acid irritation (Senner et al., 2004), Heine, Catto-Smith, and Reddihough (1996) found no difference in drooling between their treatment and placebo groups following the administration of standard doses of anti-reflux medication. Therefore, we are uncertain about the relationship between reflux and saliva production. However, this information should still be collected.

Because swallows increase during feeding, drooling is most likely to occur during nonfeeding times. Therefore, examination and observations need to be conducted during play. Both objective and subjective measures of drooling are recommended. The Drooling Quotient is an objective measure of drooling frequency. It was developed by Rapp (1980) and entailed the use of an electronic device that made 40 random beeps over a 10-minute period. This reminded teachers to record a drooling event or its absence. The drool was defined as anterior loss of saliva. The Drooling Quotient procedure was revised by Van Hulst, Lindeboom, Van der Burg, and Jongerius (2012), who determined that a 5-minute quotient (DQ5) was more efficient and equally valid. These researchers used a score of 18 to serve as a "'rule of thumb" for clinical decision making in drooling treatment" (p. 1125). Another objective measure used in research studies has been the weighing of saliva on a bib after specified time periods (Harris & Dignam, 1980).

Subjective measures have been used, which include a rating scale. Typically, a score of one indicates a child who seldom drools, whereas a four indicates profuse drooling. Another measure is the Drooling Impact Scale (Reid et al., 2009), which was developed to measure drooling, based on its impact on families. In addition, research has concluded that this scale is sensitive enough to demonstrate effectiveness of intervention. Items include questions of frequency, severity, need to change clothes and wipe furniture, as well as the caregiver's perception of how drooling affects family life and the child's life.

These instruments are, however, more often used in research. Generally, an SLP performing an evaluation will observe, question the parents regarding medications, and subsequently make a determination concerning the presence and severity of drooling. If assessment determines that drooling is present to a degree that requires intervention, it is imperative to determine the cause. Intervention will be based on the underlying cause (Arvedson

& Health, 2001). The items typically observed during a drooling evaluation are those made during the feeding assessment as presented in Chapter 4.

It is likely that this comprehensive assessment and subsequent intervention will be multifaceted with several disciplines involved. The posture and muscle tone of the child should be noted, especially in relation to its influence on oral structures and movements. Postural stability for head control, head posture in various positions, jaw stability, and tongue placement will all have an effect on the child's ability to swallow and control saliva. If the child's muscle tone is low and the head lies on the chest, saliva will fall from the mouth due to gravity, unless there is strong lip closure—which is unlikely if the child has hypotonia! On the other hand, if the child's mouth is open due to an extended head posture, lip closure to retain saliva and initiate a swallow will be difficult.

In addition to observation, direct assessment through handling should be made of oral structures and sensitivity. How mobile is the tongue? Does it push saliva forward with forward tongue movement? In addition, it is important to keep all treatment options open. An assessment of receptive language and the cognitive level will facilitate treatment planning because some therapies require comprehension and memory. Another item to assess involves the family and its ability to participate in intervention by providing carryover activities between sessions. Once these items are evaluated and carefully analyzed, a comprehensive plan for saliva control can begin.

Intervention

Like many clinical interventions for children with cerebral palsy, the evidence indicating effective drooling treatments is scarce. Walshe et al. (2012) performed a systematic review of randomized control trials (RCT) and controlled clinical trials (CCT) of interventions for drooling in children with cerebral palsy. CCTs are trials with no randomization. They found only six studies to include in their review. None of these studies addressed physical, behavioral, or oral-motor approaches. The six studies included Botox and other pharmacological treatments only.

Arvedson and Brodsky (2002) present a flowchart for treating drooling, which indicates the initial step as the elimination of contributing factors, one of which is posture. An NDT approach advocates this as well. However, for children with complex needs such as those with cerebral palsy, this may just be preliminary. Mueller (2001) indicates that a program to improve drooling should include a sensory and behavioral approach as well as a feeding program that establishes correct swallowing. Of course, as clinicians we appreciate the need for regular re-evaluation of any nonmedical technique we initiate in order to determine if the selected protocol is working or if changes need to be made (Arvedson & Brodsky, 2002).

Postural Control

Most clinicians who treat children with cerebral palsy initially address saliva control through postural control, leading to better head and trunk alignment, resulting in improved oral functioning. Pinder and Faherty (1999) note that the SLP should target the development of gross motor skills to provide the foundation for oral functioning. Arvedson and Brodsky (2002) also note that oral-motor programs for drooling include head control and positioning.

The goal of postural control for the child who drools is to provide the trunk stability for head control. Without this, jaw stability will not be attained, and it is required for efficient tongue and lip movements needed for effective saliva control. This concept was proposed by Mueller in 1972. It is the basis of neurodevelopmental treatment (NDT) and has been discussed at length by such NDT SLPs as Morris (1977), Pinder (Pinder & Faherty, 1999), and Redstone (Redstone & West, 2004). It is interesting to note that these principles have been incorporated into common practice.

Sensorimotor programs for saliva control, which target the jaw, lips, and tongue, all begin with the provision of positioning to provide postural stability along with head alignment. Specific sensorimotor treatment techniques to improve drooling include procedures such as oral control and normalization of oral sensitivity through graded stimulation.

Sensorimotor Programs

It is important for all SLPs to be aware that any program that provides oral stimulation increases saliva production. This, in turn, may lead to increased drooling. Therefore, clinicians need to be sure that all saliva has been swallowed before transitioning to another activity.

These "oral-motor programs" include most of the non-medical approaches used by SLPs as part of a feeding program (Arvedson & Brodsky, 2002). It is appropriate to review many oral-motor programs and choose, or combine techniques, that best meet the needs of the children with cerebral palsy whom we work with. In fact, most clinicians do combine approaches (DeGangi & Royeen, 1994).

Ray, Bundy, and Nelson (1983) used procedures described by Mueller (1972) and Morris (1977) to facilitate mouth closure to reduce drooling in a single subject case study of an 11-year-old. This program began with stable positioning, provided oral stimulation, and gave the child oral control. The authors noted that oral control was provided immediately prior to stimulation in order to prevent head and jaw extension. Then oral control was faded as jaw closure became automatic. Results of this study indicated that mouth closure resulted in decreased drooling. In addition, an informal observation made during the course of the intervention was that vocalizations increased.

Samelstad (1988) used similar procedures as Ray et al. (1983) on two subjects with cerebral palsy who were 14 and 21 years of age. Samelstad began with positioning, used Mueller's oral control techniques, and provided stimulation through stroking various areas of the face and neck. This protocol used oral control while the subjects sucked on a popsicle and then continued while more stroking stimulation was applied. The researcher noted the importance of pausing regularly when applying stimulation to allow the subject time to swallow. The increase in salivation aided in triggering a swallow. Both subjects decreased drooling during the 2- to 4-week treatment phase.

Iammatteo et al. (1990) also replicated Ray et al.'s study with two subjects with cerebral palsy under the age of 3 who drooled severely. They investigated upright, symmetrical, stable positioning along with oral control during feeding. The program also included a tactile sensory component in order to prepare the participants for oral control. This is often needed with children with cerebral palsy who have sensory issues. The researchers used procedures described by the NDT practitioners Mueller and Morris. Results indicated that drooling was reduced by the techniques which enhanced mouth closure. Although some drooling may also be observed in typical children of this age, these children drooled severely. Additionally, the authors noted that a decrease in drooling was observed almost immediately, which they attributed to the young age of their subjects. This suggests that being proactive and treating early is appropriate and efficient.

Mueller (2001) states that if the child is constantly reminded to close the mouth, drooling will not disappear. She encourages parents to give a tactile prompt with firm pressure during the day while using oral control during feeding to "establish a proper swallowing pattern" (p. 120). In addition, Mueller (1972) presents a program for normalizing oral sensation, which is one major cause for drooling. This technique is taught and practiced in NDT courses and has been summarized in Chapter 4 as part of a comprehensive feeding program for children with sensory problems.

Another sensory program was studied by Domaracki and Sisson (1990) with two school-aged children with cerebral palsy. The researchers provided a sensory intervention using a NUK stimulator for 3 to 5 minutes at hourly intervals throughout the school day. The stimulator was chosen because of its size and ease of manipulation. The technique described by Mueller uses the clinician's gloved finger instead. This allows the clinician to receive tactile information regarding tone and movements. The positive aspects of sensory programs like these are the multiple presentations of graded stimuli to children daily and the emphasis on allowing the child time to swallow between exercises. Too often, sensory programs emphasize the stimulation, which increases saliva production. It is imperative that the child increase swallowing frequency, otherwise we may unintentionally exacerbate drooling.

Behavioral Programs

Although some authors have concluded that behavioral programs using praise, cues, and positive reinforcement have demonstrated success (Blasco & Allaire, 1992; Domaracki & Sisson, 1990), others have asserted that they are "laborious, time consuming, or inappropriate for toddlers" (Iammatteo et al., 1990). In addition, generalization to different settings has proven to be problematic (Blasco & Allaire, 1992). However, I would argue that most of the therapies described previously have also included a behavioral component. For example, if mouth closure is an initial objective, a clinician will typically use positive reinforcement, praising the child for employing closure for a predetermined time. In addition, it is not uncommon for children to associate mouth closure with specific activities (e.g., eating and drinking) or with certain people (SLPs and teachers). Behavioral techniques are based on the principles of conditioning and behavior modification. However, the child must first be able to physically attain closure independently. And that typically requires an oral-motor program for most children with cerebral palsy.

An example of a time-consuming behavioral program is Rapp's study (1980) that utilized an electronic device (described previously) to determine drooling frequency. It reminded teachers to gather baseline drooling information 40 times within two 10-minute periods from cognitively challenged adolescents with cerebral palsy. Rapp developed a behavioral modification device for the subjects in the study that provided an auditory signal to remind them to swallow. However, Rapp notes that the subjects learned to swallow *prior to* using the device. The electronic device was therefore used as a "link" (p. 449), allowing the children to implement the swallow behavior previously learned. Rapp concludes that this study demonstrates that swallowing can be shaped and conditioned. Recently, "apps" have been developed for use on smartphones (iPhones), and can be used with earphones or Bluetooth devices (Speech and Language Solutions Limited, 2012). This app signals clients to swallow at predetermined intervals.

Overcorrection is a behavioral approach developed by Foxx and Azrin (1973) to eliminate undesirable behaviors, aside from drooling, in populations other than cerebral palsy. These authors attempted to eliminate self-stimulatory behaviors in three cognitively challenged and one autistic child. Foxx and Azrin describe two components in this program: Restitution, when the individual corrects the effects of the behavior; and positive practice, when the new behavior is actually implemented.

Trott and Maechtlen (1986) used overcorrection to control drooling in two children when past attempts using verbal reminders and praise had not been effective. These children had severe cognitive challenges but no physical disabilities. The authors defined drooling as a drop of saliva on the lips. The children were required to clean the saliva from clothing and furniture. This was paired with negative verbal input and considered the restitution part of overcorrection. Then the children needed to press a tissue to their lips (positive practice). These authors conclude that overcorrection can reduce drooling. However, they warn that a program using this approach for children with motor deficits may also need to include "other measures to facilitate lip and mouth closure" (p. 704).

Goldfarb and Guglielmo (1976) used this approach with a 5-year-old with cerebral palsy. They defined drooling as a drop of saliva on the chin, which the child would not be able to self-correct. These authors felt that if the saliva was on the lower lip, the child could draw it back into the mouth. A verbal warning was given, and then the child was told to wash and dry her face. This would be considered Foxx's and Azrin's restitution phase. In addition, the child had to wash and dry her desk (positive practice). The number of drools recorded in a 45-minute session decreased over a 12-week period from nearly 100 to zero.

A similar approach was used to develop self-control of swallowing (Dunn, Cunningham, & Backman, 1987). This was trained in a motivated 16-year-old with cerebral palsy. He learned to monitor, evaluate, and reward himself. The authors, however, acknowledge that this subject probably had the oral-motor skills for controlling drooling and only needed "an effective management strategy" (p. 309).

Prosthetics

An intraoral appliance called the Innsbruck Sensorimotor Activator and Regulator (ISMAR) has been studied by Johnson et al. (2004) to determine its effectiveness in improving drooling and feeding skills. The main goal of the ISMAR is to provide jaw stability, position the tongue for improved swallow, and develop improved lip closure. The prosthesis was developed by a team that included a dentist and speech therapist. The study indicated that some drawbacks to the use of this device included its discomfort and possible damage to the oral area if the child disliked it. It was time-consuming for the parents to motivate the children while tolerance was being established. Only one third of the participants completed the study due to these problems. However, feeding and drooling improved significantly for the children who completed it. The best candidates for this intervention used wheelchairs, were not seizure prone, and were relatively intact cognitively. The authors also acknowledge that the frequency of drooling remained the same while the severity decreased.

An interestingly "reciprocal" (p. 227) influence between posture of the body and oral structure functioning was noted by Gisel, Schwartz, Petryk, Clarke, and Haberfellner (2000). Typically, we consider the influence of body position on the oral structures. This concept is the basis of much of the oral-motor intervention provided by therapists who are neurodevelopment treatment (NDT) trained and include a number of techniques described in this book. Gisel et al. studied the ISMAR described above in a group of children with cerebral palsy and found a positive interaction between oral structures and postural control for sitting and ambulation. In other words, good oral alignment led to improvement in gross motor skills.

Reciprocity of Gross-Motor and Oral-Motor

NDT therapists are deeply concerned with proper alignment in order to facilitate the best possible motoric functions for feeding and communication. Although I have never had the opportunity to study or use the ISMAR, there are children I've treated who demonstrate what Gisel et al. (2000) described. Through treatment, two children with athetoid cerebral palsy who were cognitively intact learned very quickly that they needed to adjust their bodies in order to communicate effectively and be independent feeders. As soon as they desired one of these functions, they sat upright spontaneously, became symmetrical, and provided their own stability, usually through weight bearing. The need for better oral functioning provided the motivation to improve their gross-motor skills.

Another prosthetic device used for saliva control is a chin-cup. It was originally developed by orthodontists to decrease jaw protrusion by putting pressure on the jaw. Harris and Dignam (1980) noted an increase in anterior seal or lip closure and modified the chin-cup using very light pressure. These researchers also included oral exercises to strengthen the lips and jaw and to increase automatic swallows. The results indicated that a combination of both oral exercises and the use of a chin-cup were optimal.

Surgery

The SLP is involved in the assessment and follow-up of clients who undergo surgery for drooling. The first surgical procedure developed to decrease drooling was performed in the 1960s. It rerouted the saliva ducts so that swallowing could be facilitated (Harris & Purdy, 1987). The rationale for this operation made sense because tongue movement to propel the saliva posteriorly is often poor in children with cerebral palsy. Another early procedure entailed the removal of the salivary glands. Now, surgery for drooling typically involves one of these surgical interventions or combination of them.

Postsurgical problems may occur and include loss of taste, swelling, and pain (Harris & Purdy, 1987). The most severe complication was reported by Stevenson, Allaire, and Blasco (1994) who presented a case study of a young man with athetosis who developed feeding difficulties and pneumonia leading to placement of a gastrostomy tube after surgery to improve drooling. Blasco (2002) notes another practical problem in that these surgical procedures occur infrequently. Therefore, finding an experienced surgeon may be difficult. In addition, he states that "no one procedure has emerged as the most effective" (p. 980). A reasonable "dual approach" has been prescribed by Harris and Purdy (1987) who suggest therapy for a trial period before a referral for surgery is made.

Botox and Other Medications

The most frequently studied drugs have been those that inhibit secretion by the salivary glands typically through the use of an anticholinergic agent that blocks the production of saliva. They may be administered orally or by injection. One of the injected agents is botulinum toxin (BoTN). This is widely referred to as Botox and is the brand most often used in studies. The Cochrane review of randomized control trials (RCT) by Walshe et al. (2012) found six studies using Botox or oral medications to decrease drooling. All studies demonstrated some effectiveness up to 1 month posttreatment. Another review by Rodwell et al. (2012) found 16 studies of Botox treatment for drooling. These authors also conclude that Botox is effective, but temporary.

A variation in outcomes is demonstrated in a study by Reid, Johnstone, Westbury, Rawicki, and Reddihough (2008). One group was treated with Botox while another group had no treatment. A significant difference was found between groups. However, while two-thirds of the treated group improved significantly, the other third demonstrated no change or only minor improvement.

Pharmacological interventions have been considered a "possibility" although no strong conclusions can be made regarding the average effect on drooling in children with cerebral palsy (Jongerius, van Tiel, van Limbeek, Gabreels, & Rotteveel, 2003). It has been suggested that after oral-motor and behavioral programs have been attempted and drooling persists, pharmacological interventions should be initiated. Success is variable and, unlike behavioral or oral-motor interventions, these may have side effects (Arvedson & Brodsky, 2002; Cockerill, 2009). In fact, Reid et al. (2008) note that one RCT was discontinued due to unexpected, serious events that included dysphagia and speech difficulties.

Conclusions

Although "no obvious treatment of choice has emerged" (Love, 2000, p. 148) for drooling, when treating children with cerebral palsy, the inclusion of an oral-motor component is imperative. This sentiment has been echoed by others (Blasco, 2010). If no motor deficits are apparent, behavioral approaches alone may be worthwhile (Garber, 1971). However, a combined program, or dual approach, after a comprehensive assessment is the most appropriate intervention. This is the approach NDT has advocated for drooling as well as for all other facets of speech therapy.

Children with cerebral palsy differ from physically typical children who drool. Blasco (2002) states that "hands-on oral-motor therapy techniques and proper positioning interventions remain the fundamental management modalities" (p. 780). We must always remember to address motor aspects when treating children with motor deficits. This is as true for feeding as it is for communication, speech, and saliva control. And it is this principle that has been stressed repeatedly throughout this book.

Ten Items to Improve Intervention

1. Drooling is intermittently seen in typically developing children up to age 4 years and is associated with teething or periods of intense concentration.
2. Children with cerebral palsy typically drool due to poor oral-motor control.
3. Drooling occurs less frequently during feeding because the frequency of swallowing increases during this activity.
4. A program of oral-motor control that includes postural support and positioning is considered the first choice for children with cerebral palsy.
5. Strict behavioral programs are worthwhile but time-consuming.
6. Combining a behavioral approach along with an oral-motor program should be considered.
7. The SLP should consult with dentists and doctors when surgery, medications, or appliances are being considered.
8. No one program has been developed that is the answer for all children with cerebral palsy who drool. A multi-modal, individualized approach is best.
9. Any program that is developed for a child with cerebral palsy needs to address the child's oral-motor control issues.
10. It is imperative to evaluate and treat the cause of the drooling.

Self-Study and Classroom Discussion

1. Why would a program of saliva control be included in a comprehensive feeding program for a child with cerebral palsy?
2. A behavioral program alone may not work for a child with cerebral palsy. Why?
3. List three reasons for drooling.
4. How are NDT oral control and the use of a chin-cup similar, and how do they differ?
5. Why is it likely that a child picked up for early intervention might not develop drooling?

References

Acs, G., Ng, M. W., Helpin, M. L., Rosenberg, H. M., & Canion, S. (2007). Dental care: Promoting health and preventing disease. In M. L. Batshaw, L. Pelligrino, & N. J. Roizen (Eds.), *Children with disabilities* (pp. 499–510). Baltimore, MD: Paul H. Brookes.

Alexander, R., Boehme, R., & Cupps, B. (1993). *Normal development of functional motor skills*. San Antonio, TX: Therapy Skill Builders.

Arvedson, J. C., & Brodsky, I. (2002). *Pediatric swallowing and feeding: Assessment and management* (2nd ed.). San Diego, CA: Singular.

Arvedson, J. C., & Health, K. (2001). Pediatric clinical feeding and swallowing evaluation. *Perspectives in Swallowing and Swallowing Disorders, 10*, 17–23.

Bakke, M., Bardow, A., & Moller, E. (2012). Severe drooling and treatment with botulinum toxin. *Perspectives in Swallowing and Swallowing Disorders, 21*, 15–21.

Blasco, P. A. (2002). Management of drooling: ten years after the consortium of drooling: 1990. *Developmental Medicine and Child Neurology, 44*, 778–781.

Blasco, P. A. (2010). The treatment of drooling. *Developmental Medicine and Child Neurology, 52*, 980.

Blasco, P. A., & Allaire, J. H. (1992). Drooling in the developmentally disabled: Management practices and recommendations. *Developmental Medicine and Child Neurology, 34*, 849–862.

Chavez, M. C. M., Grollmus, Z. C. N., & Donat, F. J. S. (2008). Clinical prevalence of drooling in infant cerebral palsy. *Medicina Oral, Patalogia Oral y Cirugia, Bucal, 13*, e22–e26.

Cockerill, H. (2009). Feeding. In E. Bower (Ed.), *Finnie's handling the young child with cerebral palsy at home* (4th ed., pp. 149–164). Edinburgh, UK: Butterworth-Heinemann.

DeGangi, G. A., & Royeen, C. B. (1994). Current practice among Neurodevelopmental Treatment Association members. *American Journal of Occupational Therapy, 48*, 803–809.

Domaracki, L. S., & Sisson, L. A. (1990). Decreasing drooling with oral motor stimulation in children with multiple disabilities. *American Journal of Occupational Therapy, 44*, 680–684.

Dunn, K. W., Cunningham, C. E., & Backman, J. E. (1987). Self-control and reinforcement in the management of a cerebral-palsied adolescent's drooling. *Developmental Medicine and Child Neurology, 29*, 305–310.

Erasmus, C. E., Van Hulst, K., Rotteveel, L. J. C., Jongerius, P. H., Van Den Hoogen, F. J. A., Roeleveld, N., & Rotteveel, J. J. (2009). Drooling in cerebral palsy: Hypersalivation or dysfunctional oral motor control? *Developmental Medicine and Child Neurology, 51*, 454–459.

Foxx, R. M., & Azrin, N. H. (1973). The elimination of autistic self-stimulatory behavior by overcorrection. *Journal of Applied Behavior Analysis, 6*, 1–14.

Garber, N. B. (1971). Operant procedures to eliminate drooling behavior in a cerebral palsied adolescent. *Developmental Medicine and Child Neurology, 13*, 641–644.

Gisel, E. G., Schwartz, S., Petryk, A., Clarke, D., & Haberfellner, H. (2000). Whole-body mobility after one year of intraoral appliance therapy in children with cerebral palsy and moderate eating impairment. *Dysphagia, 15*, 226–235.

Goldfarb, R., & Guglielmo, H. (1976, April). *The efficacy of an overcorrection procedure in the management of tongue thrust and drooling behavior.* Paper presented at the Annual International Convention of The Council for Exceptional Children, Chicago, IL.

Harris, M. M., & Dignam, P. F. (1980). A non-surgical method of reducing drooling in cerebral-palsied children. *Developmental Medicine and Child Neurology, 22*, 293–299.

Harris, S. R., & Purdy, A. H. (1987). Drooling and its management in cerebral palsy. *Developmental Medicine and Child Neurology, 29*, 805–814.

Heine, R. G., Catto-Smith, D. S., & Reddihough, A. G. (1996). Effect of antireflux medication on salivary drooling in children with cerebral palsy. *Developmental Medicine and Child Neurology, 38*, 1030–1036.

Iammatteo, P. A., Trombly, C., & Luecke, L. (1990). The effect of mouth closure on drooling and speech. *American Journal of Occupational Therapy, 44,* 686–691.

Johnson, H. M., Reid, S. M., Hazard, C. J., Lucas, J. O., Desai, M., & Reddihough, D. S. (2004). Effectiveness of the Innsbruck Sensorimotor Activator and Regulator (ISMAR) in improving saliva control in children with cerebral palsy. *Developmental Medicine and Child Neurology, 46,* 39–45.

Jongerius, P. H., van Tiel, P., van Limbeek, J., Gabreels, F. J. M., & Rotteveel, J. J. (2003). A systematic review for evidence of efficacy of anticholinergic drugs to treat drooling. *Archives of Disease in Childhood, 88,* 911–914.

Love, R. L. (2000). *Childhood motor speech disability.* Boston, MA: Allyn & Bacon.

Morris, S. E. (1977). *Program guidelines for children with feeding problems.* Mount Joy, PA: Childcraft Education Corporation.

Mueller, H. (1972). Facilitating feeding and prespeech. In P. H. Pearson & C. E. Williams (Eds.), *Physical therapy services in the developmental disabilities* (pp. 283–310). Springfield, IL: Thomas.

Mueller, H. (2001). Feeding. In N. R. Finnie (Ed.), *Handling the young child with cerebral palsy at home* (3rd ed., pp. 209–221). Boston, MA: Butterworth Heinemann.

Pinder, G. L., & Faherty, A. S. (1999). Issues in pediatric feeding and swallowing. In A. J. Caruso & E. A. Strand (Eds.), *Clinical management of motor speech disorders in children* (pp. 281–318). New York, NY: Thieme.

Rapp, D. (1980). Drool control: Long term follow-up. *Developmental Medicine and Child Neurology, 22,* 448–453.

Ray, S. A., Bundy, A. C., & Nelson, D. L. (1983). Decreasing drooling through techniques to facilitate mouth closure. *American Journal of Occupational Therapy, 37,* 749–753.

Redstone, F., & West, J. (2004). The importance of postural control for feeding. *Pediatric Nursing, 30,* 97–100.

Reid, S. M., Johnson, H. M., & Reddihough, D. S. (2009). The drooling impact scale: A measure of the impact of drooling in children with developmental disabilities. *Developmental Medicine and Child Neurology, 52,* e23–e28.

Reid, S. M., Johnstone, B. R., Westbury, C., Rawicki, B., & Reddihough, D. S. (2008). Randomized trial of botulinum toxin injections into the salivary glands to reduce drooling in children with neurological disorders. *Developmental Medicine and Child Neurology, 50,* 123–128.

Rodwell, K., Edwards, P., Ware, R. S., & Boyd, R. (2012). Salivary gland botulinum toxin injections for drooling in children with cerebral palsy and neurodevelopmental disability: A systematic review. *Developmental Medicine and Child Neurology, 54*, 977–987.

Samelstad, K. M. (1988). Treatment techniques to encourage lip closure and decrease drooling in persons with cerebral palsy. *The Occupational Therapy Journal of Research, 8*, 164–175.

Senner, J. E., Logemann, J., Zecker, S., & Gaebler-Spira, D. (2004). Drooling, saliva production, and swallowing in cerebral palsy. *Developmental Medicine and Child Neurology, 46*, e801–e806.

Sittig, E. (1947). The chewing method applied for excessive salivation and drooling in cerebral palsy. *Journal of Speech Disorders, 12*, 191–194.

Speech and Language Solutions. (2012). *Swallow now for iPhone, iPad, iPod*. Retrieved October, 20, 2013, from http://www.speechlanguage solutions.co.uk

Stevenson, R. D., Allaire, J. H., & Blasco, P. A. (1994). Deterioration of feeding behavior following surgical treatment of drooling. *Dysphagia, 9*, 22–25.

Tahmassebi, J. F., & Curzon, M. E. (2003). The cause of drooling in children with cerebral palsy—hypersalivation or swallowing defect? *International Journal of Paediatric Dentistry, 13*, 106–111.

Trott, M. C., & Maechtlen, A. D. (1986). The use of overcorrection as a means to control drooling. *American Journal of Occupational Therapy, 40*, 702–704.

Van Hulst, K., Lindeboom, R., Van der Burg, J., & Jongerius, P. (2012). Accurate assessment of drooling severity with the 5-minute drooling quotient in children with developmental disabilities. *Developmental Medicine and Child Neurology, 54*, 1121–1126.

Walshe, M., Smith, M., & Pennington, L. (2012). Interventions for drooling in children with cerebral palsy. *Cochrane Database of Systematic Reviews, 2*. doi:10.1002/14651858.CD008624.pub3. Retrieved August 15, 2013, from http://www.ncbi.nlm.nih.gov/pubmed/23152263

CHAPTER 9

Early Language Intervention and Interaction

Fran Redstone

Introduction

When we hear the term "language" we typically think "speech." However, we need to remember that speech is just one form of *expressive* language. Other examples of expressive language include writing, gesture, sign language, and AAC. To begin with we should agree on some basic terminology. I'm sure you are all familiar with how linguists label the components of language: semantics, syntax, morphology, phonology, and pragmatics. In addition, we should all be aware that these terms have been classified in different ways. For example, Bloom and Lahey (1978) talk about content, which includes semantics; form, which is a big category and includes syntax, morphology, and phonology; and use, which comprises pragmatics. Some researchers emphasize the stages of prelinguistic communication, whereas others discuss the functions of language. The theories of language development attempt to incorporate each of these components.

Although the terminology differs, and it seems that each researcher has a different emphasis, there is much overlap. All agree that the basis of language development is started in infancy (Billeaud, 1998; Mueller, 2001).

Theories of Language Development

Language acquisition is a major accomplishment that is achieved rapidly and automatically (Drominey & Dodane, 2004). There are many theories of language development. Most agree with the premise that language is a form of social behavior. Its function is communication and it is learned and practiced through interactions with people in the child's environment. Most theories assume the importance of mental processing of environmental stimuli (Accardo, Accardo, & Capute, 2008) as well as some degree of reinforcement of behavior. In this clinician's view, there are parts of many theories that make sense. For example, it is likely that human infants are hard-wired for language acquisition (Nativist Theory), and that verbal behaviors can be increased through positive reinforcement (Behaviorist Theory). In addition, cognitive skills such as memory and attention are important (Cognitive Theory), and a major function of language is social communication (Social Interaction Theory). We need to keep in mind that anything interfering with the child's ability to interact with his environment is a possible cause for a communication delay (Rossetti, 2001). Based on Rossetti's assertion, the child with cerebral palsy is certainly at risk for a language and communication delay.

Bell (1971) proposed that the mother in a mother–child interaction has certain expectations. If those expectations are not met, she will provide more prompts and directives to elicit a response. Parents of typical children automatically change the rate of their speech and the complexity of their language as they perceive children's comprehension, based on their responses. The child with cerebral palsy is less spontaneous and takes longer to learn (Finnie, 2001). Research indicates that mothers of children with physical disabilities are more directive and ask more questions, whereas the children generally remain passive in the interactions (Hanzlik & Stevenson, 1986; Pennington &

McConachie, 1999). This process may reflect the parents' natural attempt to elicit more activity from their children.

Let's consider how typical children learn language and how integral this development is to early interpersonal interactions. I think you will recognize how important early motor skills are to this development.

Prelinguistic Development

Intentionality is developed throughout the child's first year. It begins when the young infant visually attends to the mother's face (Rossetti, 2001) as seen in Figure 9–1. This early eye contact, along with touch, has been found to be important for the

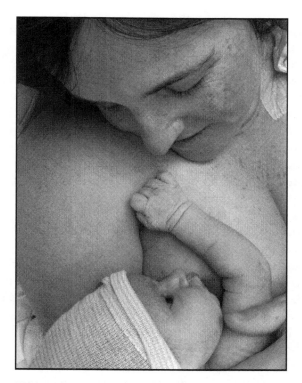

Figure 9–1. Early mother–child eye contact is the beginning of communicative interaction. It has been considered to have a turn-taking quality.

establishment of bonding and often has the quality of early turn-taking (Sachs, 2001). It also has been considered the basis for later interaction (Rosetti, 2001).

The infant's vocalizations and movements may be considered to be communication, but it is communication without intent. However, the adults in the child's environment act as if the child had demonstrated intention (Paul, 2007). This stage is called perlocutionary (Bates, 1976). Subsequently, the child enters the illocutionary stage (Bates, 1976), which is now intentional but not symbolic, and unconventional language is used. Intentional communication emerges around 9 months of age (Berko-Gleason, 2001). Now, the child depends greatly on the interactional quality of language in order to learn what works (Paul, 2007). The communication is still prelinguistic and not conventional. When children begin to use words more accurately they have entered the locutionary stage. In general, it appears that early communication acts are important in the ultimate development of language (Sigafoos et al., 2000A)

We should also be aware of the relationship between joint attention and language learning. Mundy and Newell (2007) note that caregivers often refer to new objects in unstructured activities by using eye gaze. Drominey and Dodane (2004) note that learning language is difficult due to all the possibilities of a word's meaning. However, the caregiver can aid in the mapping of important elements a word might mean. The caregiver does this through eye gaze as well as the acoustic elements of the verbal signal, which we refer to as motherese. This type of speech occurs at a higher pitch with greater pitch excursions. Drominey and Dodane (2004) note that these elements reduce "referential uncertainty" (p. 132).

Eye gaze also increases the child's ability to control the environment. It encourages the caregiver to look at the item the infant is looking at. The child is directing the adult's attention. In turn, the adult will usually label the item and may hand the child that item. Again, intention begins with very young infants' visual attention to faces as seen in Figure 9–2.

When a child begins to gaze at an object, the mutual interest in the object by a caregiver increases "reciprocal attention" (Rosetti, 2001, p. 216) and is a precursor to conversation. This interaction depends on the child's accuracy in gaze and the care-

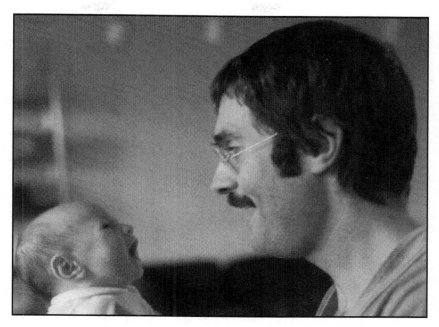

Figure 9–2. Father–child eye contact is the beginning of intentionality.

giver's responsiveness. It appears that increase in joint attention leads to an increase in early use of gesture and an increase in receptive language.

Crais (1990) eloquently discusses the development of "word knowledge from world knowledge" (p. 46). When the child plays with objects, this impacts the semantic component of language. Typically, an adult also labels these objects. This leads to mental representation of the object (McCune, 1995). Children learn about objects during their movement and play. Initially, the object choice during play is based on sensory and perceptual characteristics. As children experiment with toys, generally through movement, they learn other cognitive skills such as object permanence and cause–effect. The semantic component is further developed when children begin to propel themselves through the environment. Just think about an infant's creeping and crawling in, out, on, and under furniture. How about when the child picks up various items under the table? This is often when the child learns the meaning of "no" (Figure 9–3).

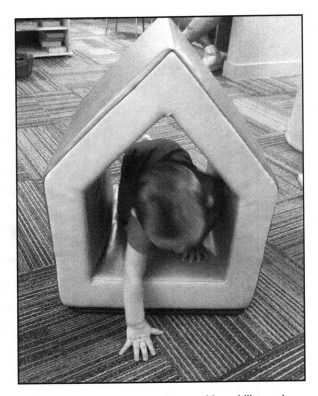

Figure 9–3. An increase in cognitive skills such as object permanence and cause–effect and an increase in the semantic component of language occurs when the child learns about the environment by moving through it.

So many spontaneous interactions take place that enable the young child to feel safe while learning and practicing new skills. The responsivity of the adults in a child's environment is an important aspect of language learning (Pinder, Olswang, & Coggins, 1993). Responsive environments teach children that their actions have specific outcomes: an action leads to a specific response. This has been called contingency experience (Sullivan & Lewis, 2000). In general, it appears that early communication acts performed by both the infant and the infant's caregiver are very important in the development of language (Sigafoos et al., 2000A). All of the items mentioned previously about typical development should be considered when developing an assessment and intervention plan for a child with cerebral palsy.

Early Language and Communication Development in the Child with Cerebral Palsy

The typical development of language skills depends on the intact language areas of the brain. Although children with cerebral palsy have a primary motor disorder, they may also have a primary language disorder. Some consider this an associated problem due to diffuse neuronal damage. However, this needs to be considered with all children with cerebral palsy: Although a language disorder may be secondary, it still may stem directly from the motor impairment. It may also follow cognitive impairments and sensory deficits associated with cerebral palsy. Generally, these children are picked up early for therapy because so many of them begin life in the neonatal intensive care unit (NICU) due to prematurity or respiratory difficulties. But language is not typically addressed as there are so few expectations for infants. Furthermore, medical and feeding issues are the highest priority for them.

Finnie (2001) describes the "dialogue" (p. 107) that develops between an infant and her caregivers during naturally occurring activities. Routines that are developed between mother and child as early as the second month of life set the stage for later play skills, motivation, and independence (Okimoto, Bundy, & Hanzlik, 2000). These routines involve turn-taking, eye contact, and imitation. They occur during dressing, feeding, diaper-changing, getting ready to go out, and play. Many of these routines depend on the motor ability of the infant and the responsiveness of the caregiver to signals from the infant.

One of these early routines is feeding, which leads to early bonding. However, children with cerebral palsy often have feeding issues (Rogers, Arvedson, Buck, Smart, & Msall, 1994) making this bonding difficult. In addition, many children with cerebral palsy began life in the NICU where typical, naturally occurring activities cannot take place.

O'Sullivan (1985) describes early mother–infant attachment as an important interactional component. This author lists several movements that the infant initiates that influence the caregiver's behavior, for example, looking, body orientation, vocalizations, and facial expressions. However, children with cerebral palsy often have difficulty "controlling movements for facial expression, gesture, and speech" (Pennington, Thomas, James, Martin, & McNally, 2009, p. 1121). Infants with motor impairments are often unable to smile and have poor head control, which makes eye contact difficult. They are frequently irritable and have extreme reactions to handling and other stimulation.

A child who is at high risk for developing a motor impairment may require aided communication. As soon as intent is determined, a means of response should be considered. Eye gaze, gesture, and vocalization seem to be important components of determining intentionality (Hetzroni, 2001). Pointing will be an important element for a child requiring aided communication. Although reaching and pointing help the child control his environment, pointing typically occurs at about 10 months of age and requires dissociation of the fingers (Sachs, 2001). It is associated with a shift in eye gaze as well. All of these components of demonstrating communication depend on the child's motor ability. Therefore, determining intent might be "problematic" (Hetzroni, 2001, p. 9).

A child with a neuromotor impairment such as cerebral palsy has difficulty coordinating attention. Hetzroni (2001) notes a strong link between motor impairment and the communication of intent. The clinician then needs to determine if a movement or subtle action by the child with a motor disability is intentional. Studies on the ability of familiar communication partners to understand the communicative intent of a child with a disability showed wide variability in the sensitivity of these adults and their ability to recognize the children's communication cues (Sigafoos, Woodyatt, Tucker, Roberts-Pennell, & Pittendrigh, 2000B; Wilcox, Kouri, & Caswell, 1990).

Although the child with cerebral palsy has atypical motor development, research indicates that parents of children with cerebral palsy have atypical interactional behaviors (Palisano, Chiarello, & Haley, 1993). O'Sullivan (1985) found that parents of children with cerebral palsy tended to work too hard in eliciting a response from their children, often leading to overstimulation. Other researchers (Hanzlik & Stevenson, 1986; Kogan &

Tyler, 1973) have found that the less responsive the child is, the fewer the maternal interactions, and the more directive the parent becomes. Pennington and McConachie (1999) note that, in general, adults tend to dominate and control interactions with nonverbal children who have cerebral palsy.

Traditional Assessment

Every text on language or speech disorders includes a section covering assessment. A comparative examination reveals that most evaluation outlines are similar. However, there is much divergence concerning means of evaluation and selection of protocols. Choices are often based solely on a child's age. Whereas one therapist may employ standardized instruments, another may use informal methods. There are questionnaires and interviews, norm-referenced and criterion-referenced tests, and many developmental checklists. Typical language instruments test the knowledge of symbolic language. They are considered "static" (Snell, 2002, p. 163) because they give us a view of the child at one moment in time. This gives us no idea of what scaffolds may be used to facilitate learning. In addition, all tests of phonology and articulation depend on speech motor control. Many tests of receptive language, syntax, and morphology depend on the ability to point accurately. Some tests assume the child's expressive use reflects the level of receptive knowledge. Some tests require the child to demonstrate through imaginary play. All of these place the child with a motor impairment at a major disadvantage when the standardized test is administered. This section will focus on applications that might improve the accuracy of the assessment of language and early communication skills of a young child with a neuromotor or a suspected neuromotor disability.

Children with cerebral palsy are often described as untestable. This is obviously due to the limitations of the testing instrument in light of the child's motor impairment. However, because this diagnostic group is so heterogeneous, it should not be assumed that a child arriving at your school or clinic is untestable. Some adaptations may be made to standardized instruments to accommodate a child with cerebral palsy, but we would be using them in a nonstandardized manner. Though this will give us some worthwhile information, the data needs to be interpreted with care. We cannot state a score based on the published norms because the test was conducted in a nonstandardized way. However, we can get a general idea about the child's functioning level, and the observation of the test-taking behaviors may be useful. For example, the physical attributes evident during testing will include the child's postural requirements, visual attention skills, and degree of pointing accuracy. In addition, the frustration level and need for external reinforcement can be determined.

Suggested Adaptations for Nonstandardized Test-Taking

1. Enlarge the plates from tests.
2. Provide greater contrast of color.
3. If a test plate has more than one item, copy and cut out items so that they can be presented separately.
4. Consider alternate means of indicating a response such as eye gaze, yes/no, or partner-assisted scanning.
5. Scan test plates into a computer for presentation, and use the child's access system for testing if the child uses aided communication.

Many standardized instruments begin the norming at 2 years of age. However, at-risk children often need to be evaluated earlier. Therefore, developmental checklists that gather information via questionnaire and interview are often used. In general, parents have been found to be accurate reporters. In fact, studies have found that a reliable indicator of a child's need for early intervention is the report of parents (Girolametto, 1997; Rescorla & Alley, 2001). However, definitions of behaviors need to be precise because of the subjectivity involved (Shapiro & Gwynn, 2008).

Informal assessments may be in the form of "anedoctal records, rating scales, checklists, interviews, and language samples" (Lowenthal, 1995) and are typically based on observation of a child's behavior. Observation, in combination with parent/ teacher reporting, may be a better method, because a therapist is able to determine the difference between a delay and a disorder. A delay suggests that the child has not attained a certain milestone within a typical timeframe. On the other hand, a disorder indicates that some atypical or pathological item has been noted that may compromise further development.

For example, some children are considered to be "late talkers." No red flags have been observed in their language production, but they have not attained the expected milestones. In fact, there is controversy concerning the necessity of intervention for these children, because many will develop typical language skills without help (Paul, Hernandez, Taylor, & Johnson, 1996; Paul, Murray, Clancy, & Andrews, 1997). However, when dealing with children who are suspected of developing motor impairments, we need to be aware of their use of abnormal patterns to compensate for a lack of stability or head control. Many of these children use shoulder elevation to stabilize the head, or they may exhibit an abnormal reflex pattern such as an asymmetrical tonic neck reflex (ATNR) when pointing at an object. These patterns may, in fact, interfere with development. This kind of information cannot be determined through a questionnaire.

Assessment of Motor Skills Influencing Language Development

It is likely that a child with a neuromotor disability will be evaluated by a PT, but the SLP needs to be the professional who determines to what extent the child's physical disability has influenced language learning and use. This is a time when the team approach is particularly helpful. The PT examines head control and trunk stability to determine whether the child needs improvement in movement and balance for ambulation. These items are evaluated again by the OT, but this time in the context of hand use for play and self-feeding. The SLP assesses head and trunk for the functions of speech and feeding. The overlap between disciplines is most evident during assessments as everyone studies the child's strengths as well as the pathologies that may be interfering with development or functionality. And an important goal of an evaluation is to determine the direction that treatment should follow. In the past, arena assessments allowed all team members to simultaneously observe a child while one member interacted with the caregiver (Paul, 2007). Although this was considered time-efficient and less stressful for the family, it is not widely used today. It is thought to be more expensive than other models, because all team members are being paid for the same time period. For a successful arena assessment, good communication between team members and adequate preparation are crucial. This approach is admirable and one that should be studied further.

One key item to examine during an evaluation is the child's head control, which can be ascertained either by handling or by observation. This is the basis of oral control for speech sound production. The motor components needed for speech were addressed in Chapter 7. The present chapter describes how the development of motor skills may influence early communication skills. The establishment of head control is essential because it is required for eye gaze, joint attention, and early vocalizations. Head turning also allows for joint attention and the indication of communicative intent. The child can direct a communication partner's attention through eye contact, followed by the turning of the head towards an object. This may mark the initiation of request. Trunk control, characterized by stable sitting and active rotation, allows the child to use the arms for reaching and pointing, a more efficient way to request. However, trunk stability and arm/hand use are also essential for manipulation of objects. This impacts the content of language. Does the child turn to or reach for a bottle when it is labeled? Does the child possess a mental representation of the object? Does the child look when called? Similarly, it is important to observe whether the child is capable of moving through the environment and, if so, how this is accomplished. Again, this influences the child's semantic learning. There may be a reason for the child's decreased vocabulary.

Is the child imitating? Does he know where desired items are? Does the child look for a toy when it drops? These are all signs of cognition that are believed to be necessary for language development. However, the manifestations of these abilities are all motor-based. Another motoric element of language development is play. In the child with cerebral palsy, tactile hypo- or hypersensitivity is often exhibited (Howle, 2002). This limits the child's desire to interact with objects. Therefore, a child with motor impairments cannot readily employ play with objects as a learning method.

We need to consider that a child with a motor disability may also have a primary language disorder or one that is based on intellectual challenges. It is the SLP's task to determine to what extent a language learning problem is based on the child's motor ability.

Communicative Intent and Dynamic Assessment

As noted previously, the perlocutionary period begins very early. It is communication but it is without the intent to communicate. The illocutionary period signifies intent. Although the child is indicating intent, the communication is nonsymbolic. However, this transition to intentionality is a major milestone. It appears to be the beginning of true interaction between a caregiver and infant concerning an object (Olswang & Pinder, 1995; Pinder & Olswang, 1995).

It is vital for the SLP to assess the child during the prelinguistic period. The need for early identification of communicative intent for the child with cerebral palsy is especially important due to the possible need for augmentative and alternative communication (AAC). In the past, the prelinguistic period was ignored or not thought to have prognostic value for later development (Shapiro & Gwynn, 2008). We now know better.

The components of the prelinguistic period are not well documented by typical, standardized, normative, static methods. Researchers and clinicians have recognized that these instruments may not be appropriate for young, nonsymbolic children (Pelligrino, 2007; Snell, 2002). What we really need to know during this period is if the child will communicate. This begins with intent.

The Inventory of Potential Communicative Acts (IPCA) (Sigafoos et al., 2000A) was an attempt to develop a means of determining if the behaviors of a child with a disability indicated a communicative intent. The inventory studied a child's movements in different contexts. This type of structured observation could then be used to teach adults in the child's environment to recognize the underlying communicative intent and react to the child accordingly.

DeVeney, Hoffman, and Cress (2012) discuss the need to use a communication profile based on receptive language and gestural expression to best determine the developmental age of children with physical disabilities. Their findings suggest that the typical multidomain tests administered to infants and young children to qualify for funding and placement underestimate the children's language abilities because of the reliance on higher-level motor output for the formulation of responses. An alternative assessment such as one that is communication-based is a better predictor of cognitive and language development and leads to improved intervention planning.

An alternative to traditional testing is to evaluate via dynamic assessment (DA). There are many variations of DA. Its purpose is to obtain an accurate picture of the child's *potential* for learning (ASHA, 2013; Snell, 2002). Two models of dynamic assessment have been described by Austin (2010). This author targets the evaluation of children who come from linguistically and culturally diverse backgrounds. The goal of this type of assessment is to determine if a child's language performance should be considered a language difference or a disorder. And when working with a population of children with motor impairments, we want to know how much of the child's observed language skills are due to limited motor skills. Therefore, an alternative assessment method such as dynamic assessment can be quite useful.

The first dynamic model is a *test-teach-retest* model. Here we are studying how the child learns and how quickly a behavior can change. I have found that if the client learns quickly, the issue is not one of cognition. This child will learn given the right supports. It is imperative for the clinician to keep up with the child because change will be rapid. Too often, it is assumed that children with motor impairments learn slowly. Such an assumption may lead to a bored child.

The second dynamic model targets the amount and type of cuing that is required for a child to change a behavior. We all have preferred avenues of learning. Some of us are auditory learners, some are visual, and some learn best by doing. Too often, as teachers or therapists, we fall back on what we like, and what we are comfortable with. It is important to employ the type of instructional approach that is best for each child's learning style. Therefore, the kind of information we obtain from this model is really helpful to a clinician who will be working with the client.

Dynamic assessment fits into the Vygotsky concept of development, often popular with educators. It emphasizes learning that is facilitated by an adult who provides supports so that the child can accomplish a task at a difficulty level that could not be achieved without this help. This was described by Vygotsky in 1978 as "the difference between a child's actual developmental level as determined by independent problem solving and the level of potential development as determined through problem solving under adult guidance or in collaboration with more capable peers" (as cited in Schneider & Watkins, 1996, p. 157). This has been called the *zone of proximal development.*

Dynamic Assessment for Children with Cerebral Palsy

After determining the motor and language skills of a child via standardized evaluations (which may be required for funding) and observation, the SLP can predict, based on clinical experience, the influence of the child's motor ability on language performance. Dynamic assessment can then be used to evaluate children's potential as opposed to their performance. A series of language tasks can then be developed from the evaluation previously administered, with each task individualized. The tasks presented would address items either not previously attempted or poorly performed by the child. A hierarchy should then be created to determine the amount of support the child needs to be successful linguistically. Austin (2010) describes hierarchies that have been created for assessing language skills of linguistically diverse children. A hierarchy for a child with a motor impairment would employ similar principles, ranging from the least prompting to maximum support. Here are a few examples: can the child make qualitative and quantitative improvements in pointing, feeding, or vocalizing, if given better postural support through positioning with improved pelvic stability? Can changing the table height or placement of materials improve performance? Does the child's arm move more quickly for aided communication if an arm support is provided? Can the child eat more, fatigue less, or produce bilabial sounds if given oral support?

The success of the SLP in providing these modifications will depend on clinical experience and training. This training will most likely occur in continuing education courses after the master's degree. NDT is one of the avenues for attaining this information.

Dynamic assessment gives the clinician more direction for intervention than a typical standardized evaluation. This is more important for atypical populations. To reiterate, these groups are chronically underrepresented in the collection of normative data and in the development of standardized procedures. Too often, children from culturally diverse backgrounds or those with motor impairments get token representation.

Intervention for Early Interactive Communication Skills

Although we acknowledge the importance of early intervention, treatment to improve early communication skills for children with cerebral palsy is typically provided long after children have not developed speech at an age-appropriate time. Unfortunately, this is a little like closing the barn door after the horse has bolted. Part of the reason for this is the naïve hope that these at-risk children will develop speech on their own. A more valid reason may be the need to focus on immediate medical issues. Because so little is expected from infants concerning communication, diagnosing such a disorder is challenging. Compounding this problem is the difficulty of working with an infant with a severe motor disorder. It is therefore not surprising that intervention and research in this area have been sparse.

One goal for a child with cerebral palsy may be to improve functional speech production through speech therapy. Intervention addressing speech sound production was addressed in Chapter 7 of this book. In that chapter methods to improve the coordination of the subsystems of speech, the type of sounds to encourage, and NDT handling techniques were discussed.

However, improving intelligibility alone does not automatically improve interaction (Pennington et al., 2009). Difficulties involving lack of initiation and passivity in interactions may continue to exist despite significant improvements in the means of communication. The concept of specificity of learning applies here. If interaction is a goal, then it needs to be taught and used. For example, the SLP might facilitate a sound and then encourage the child to practice it in different sound environments while using it in a functional context. A functional communicative context involves interaction. This might be the use of the sound for a request, comment, greeting, or question in a functional setting such as the home or school. The speech therapy room is *not* a functional setting! But it is a good place for functional practice.

The combining of goals during an activity requires creativity on the part of the SLP, as does the ability to make practice interesting. In addition, the SLP needs to provide the supports necessary for functioning and the fading of those prompts as the child takes over more actively and performs more independently. We are reminded that the focus of early intervention is actually to enhance "development within the context of parent-infant interaction" (Palisano, Chiarello, & Haley, 1993, p. 59).

Direct/Child-Oriented Approaches

The functions of language are varied. We use language to get and give information, avoid or reject an item, request an object or person, make a comment, and be social. However, requesting and rejecting are two of the earliest functions to develop (Sigafoos, Drasgow, Reichle, O'Reilly, & Tait, 2004) and, therefore, are the ones that have been studied in children with cerebral palsy. In addition, they encourage functional communication and are contingent-based, which makes a communication immediately salient to the child

We can learn about the ingredients of a good program from studies investigating early interaction interventions. For example, a single-subject study presented by Pinder, Olswang, and Coggins (1993) demonstrates that a severely impaired child with cerebral palsy can be taught the early communication skills of choice and request. Choices were indicated by active looking and reaching before the child was given a toy. Eye gaze first to the object and then to the adult indicated a request that had been elicited by an adult tempting the child with a toy and then stopping. This program was multidisciplinary, employing both a PT and SLP. It incorporated NDT principles of stability, posture, head control, positioning of materials, and handling. It also shaped the child's communicative behaviors along a hierarchy from passive to active. The authors noted that the child developed early communication skills from the simplest to the most motorically complex. As the child demonstrated more complex motor skills, he needed to be encouraged to demonstrate consistent use of communicative intent. It is also interesting to note that active looking was established in the choice context first, followed by the request.

The importance of providing play opportunities with an adult for children with cerebral palsy was emphasized by Olswang and Pinder (1995) as a means of improving interactive communication. These authors studied a program to develop requesting skills during a play situation with an adult. A definite developmental sequence was found. The four children in the study, about 1 year of age, first focused on either the adult or the object and then began to coordinate the two elements. Each child began to have more control over the play situation and engaged the adult increasingly, with the adult better able to read the intent of the child. The authors noted the value of this "shared reciprocal learning" (p. 289) in a program for children with cerebral palsy.

In this study, the sessions with the children were all conducted by Pinder who is an NDT speech instructor. She provided shaping of behaviors along with extra time for the children to respond. These are typical therapy techniques used for most children with language disorders. However, she also provided postural stability and "facilitation of shoulders, arms, and hands" (p. 283) to enhance the child's play. These prompts were individualized for each child and changed over time as the child took over actively.

Rejecting is another early communication function, and children with cerebral palsy often indicate rejection in unacceptable, negative ways. We have all seen children push aggressively or throw tantrums to indicate, in no uncertain terms, that they do not want something. Just because a child has been taught the appropriate words and can point to the correct icon on an aided communication system does not mean that the child knows when, or how, to use the vocabulary. Teaching this function is important because it is used often throughout the day (Sigafoos et al., 2004). Think of how often you have wanted to get out of a situation, stop an event from happening, or tell someone that you have had enough. For children with cerebral palsy communicating these feelings can be frustrating, because their signals are not always easy to interpret.

Sigafoos et al. (2004) note that procedures employed to teach rejection often include techniques that are used routinely in therapy such as physical guidance, which is faded over time, and motivating materials. Their tutorial also stresses that a new behavior should be as efficient as the one it replaces. Typically, using AAC to reject an aversive action will take much too long a time. Sigafoos et al. cite the need to elicit a well-defined behavior so that everyone recognizes when it occurs and can offer appropriate and consistent reinforcement. It is important for the SLP to make sure that the child has increased opportunities to practice this new behavior.

Assistive technology can also be used to promote a more responsive environment and improve attention to objects and exploration in play (Sullivan & Lewis, 2000). SLPs should embrace technology as a means of facilitating the child's ability to learn cause–effect and to demonstrate communicative intent. The use of switches to activate toys and sounds can aid in early language learning and teach children to control their environment. Later, it can be used for turn-taking in play and conversation.

Indirect/Communication-Partner Intervention

Most of this book has been geared to SLPs, providing direction and suggestions to enhance direct intervention for children with cerebral palsy. However, we need to help parents, teachers, and other caregivers as well to become more responsive to infants' and young children's behaviors indicating communicative intent. This can be accomplished using a modified process described by Sigafoos et al. (2000). The SLP can interview caregivers to arrive at a consensus to determine which behaviors show intent, along with an indication of their linguistic functions. For example, did the change in facial expression represent a social greeting or a protest? Was the arm movement a request or a choice? Did the sound mean "hi" or "more"? Subsequently, the SLP should observe the child directly.

An additional element that should be studied carefully in children with cerebral palsy is the motor component. Does the attempt of communication lead to hypertonicity? Head extension? Does the child use an asymmetrical tonic neck reflex (ATNR) to reach? Parent and staff training should be provided so that there is consistency of expectations regarding the child's communication attempts among the caregivers. Training should also include information regarding that specific child's need for symmetry, stability, and alignment; and methods to meet these needs should be implemented so that the child may communicate successfully.

It is particularly important that practice take place outside the therapy room. This is necessary for learning a skill, generalizing it, and maintaining it. Caregivers at home and in school are wonderful resources for this. There are a number of approaches focusing on caregivers that were developed to help children with language disorders. Although these approaches are considered child-centered (Lowenthal, 1995) because they stress the child's attempts to communicate, the techniques actually target the adult as a communication partner. These include milieu teaching, parallel talk, self-talk, and expansions of the child's communicative attempts. These can be taught to parents of young children as well as to teachers in preschool classrooms.

Pennington, Goldbart, and Marshall (2004) reviewed four studies that targeted the training of communication partners to improve the quality of interaction between caregivers and children with cerebral palsy. These authors concluded that, although little research is available, this type of approach may be worthwhile for improved outcomes for children with cerebral palsy.

The goal of this training is to enhance input for children by teaching their parents to become coaches and to show them ways to become more responsive and less directive, in general. Caregivers are taught methods of scaffolding a child's interaction that will increase the likelihood of comprehension and a successful exchange. Some of these techniques include speaking more slowly, using less complex language, and balancing turn-taking during interactions. And many of these are done automatically by most parents.

In an effort to create a more responsive environment for typically developing children in daycare centers, Girolametto, Weitzman, and Greenberg (2003) studied the Hanen program, which focuses on caregivers. Hanen was provided to the staff in daycare centers and then studied to determine if it changed the verbal input to children. The program involved group discussions as well as individual video analyses. Concepts emphasized the reduction of both the rate and the complexity of speech, and causing interactions to be less directive and more responsive. Results indicated that the caregivers improved their ability to be more child-centered and their effectiveness in turn-taking skills. However, the use of strategies by the caregivers was context-selective, and they did not adjust the complexity of their language to the children's level. This was an interesting study concerning caregivers of typical children. However, as we have noted previously, this dynamic changes when a child has a disability.

Pennington et al. (2009) studied the effects of the Hanen program for a heterogeneous group of mothers of 10 children with cerebral palsy aged 19 to 36 months. Results indicated that the pattern of mothers' dominance did not change, but the children became less passive. Mothers' language input did not change significantly, a result similar to the findings of Girolametto et al. with typical children. However, Pennington et al. noted that the mothers became more responsive. In general, it was felt that the program had positive effects on interaction patterns. Although the dyads in the study included children with cerebral palsy, no training to specifically address this motor disability was included.

An earlier randomized, controlled study by Palmer et al. (1990) compared two parent-administered programs for children with diplegia cerebral palsy. One program included NDT intervention for 1 year; the second provided infant stimulation for 6 months, followed by NDT for 6 months. The infant stimulation program targeted sensory, fine-motor, and language activities.

Both programs were administered by parents and supervised by therapists. It was hypothesized that the infant stimulation program would modify the ways parents related to their children with cerebral palsy. However, the results indicated that the inclusion of an infant stimulation program did not improve the outcomes. In fact, the program with the full year of NDT led to small but significant gains in the emotional and verbal responsivity of the mother.

Conclusions

In my view, the most important contribution of indirect therapy is its acknowledgment of the importance of the family. Parents and other caregivers should be taught specific techniques to improve their responsivity and their child's interactive abilities. NDT has always acknowledged the importance of the family in the carryover of skills into daily life, incorporating the teaching of techniques for carrying, bathing, playing, feeding, and speech sound production. Here are some basic techniques that can be used frequently: become more child-centered and talk about what the child is interested in; allow more time for the child to respond; place desired objects by your face to improve eye gaze; and simplify your verbal output to the child's level. A few basic *motor* suggestions to teach caregivers might include: provide the child with a stable base; position toys so that abnormal reflexes and head extension are not likely to occur; and give just enough support to facilitate the next level of play and exploration.

However, to think that the role of the SLP should be limited only to teaching parents how to be SLP coaches is a mistake. This role should be but one component of a comprehensive program for a child with cerebral palsy. Too many of the studies reviewed suggest that direct and indirect therapy approaches are mutually exclusive. They are not. They can and should be combined in a clinical setting. If a therapist knows that teaching caregivers specific techniques will enhance early communication and interaction, the therapist is ethically bound to teach these techniques. This is true of handling techniques for positioning to enhance vocalization, speech, and play. But clinicians should also provide individual therapy to facilitate the next step in learning and development. This might be described as a two-pronged approach.

A case in point is an interesting study conducted by three occupational therapists investigating parent–child interactions during play. Okimoto et al. (2000) studied tapes used for earlier research to examine playfulness in two groups of children with cerebral palsy. One group had 1 hour of parent training in social interaction, and the other group had 1 hour of NDT occupational therapy in which no social interaction techniques were demonstrated. On one hand the authors state that the improvement in playfulness between the groups was exactly the same. But they subsequently conclude that the interaction program was more effective. This expressed preference, lacking significant data to support it, suggests a bias that will be discussed in a later chapter. However, these authors do reasonably recommend that a program to improve mother–child interaction should supplement the provision of direct intervention.

The young child with cerebral palsy may, in fact, require a three-pronged approach. This would involve the elements of a direct communication program and an indirect program of parent training that have been described above. However, one other component is required to account for the unique motor aspects involved in communication for the child with this motor impairment. In order to provide efficient communication, adequate head and trunk alignment with normal muscle tone is required. This entails additional knowledge and skills on the part of the SLP. It should be noted that greater improvement in outcomes in many of the studies discussed previously might have been achieved had the programs included a comprehensive home training program along with the provision of direct speech therapy incorporating NDT techniques.

The last point I'd like to emphasize is that SLPs need to recognize that children with cerebral palsy have a motor impairment. If the SLP is providing treatment, clearly there is a language, speech, or feeding problem as well. Often, it is assumed that speech is too difficult for a child with this type of disability. This, in fact, is sometimes the case for young children. But do not assume that speech therapy should be postponed forever. Instead, sign language is often presented to nonverbal children with cerebral palsy as an alternative means of communication. However, signing is a motor-based skill. As professionals we need to ask, how accurately and rapidly can a child make manual signs? Also, the child's audience must be considered. Do the people in the child's environment know sign language? Are we inadvertently limiting this child's ability to communicate to a small community? Nonetheless, signs that are gesture-based and universal, comprehended by most people, are definitely worthwhile. These might include all-done, come, go, or stop.

It is important for us to use common sense along with our clinical expertise and knowledge of research evidence to determine what is best to teach each child. We also need to plan for and anticipate the next step in this child's development. The work we do today to enrich our clients' communication skills will have a major impact on the lives they live tomorrow.

Ten Items to Improve Intervention

1. Individualize assessment procedures.
2. Don't be afraid to use standardized instruments in a nonstandardized manner. Just report it the way you did it.
3. Be aware of specific motor skills necessary for language development.
4. Monitor and understand the subtle communicative signals of the child.
5. Do not assume that the child is untestable.
6. Use dynamic assessment.
7. Teach caregivers to be alert to *possible* indications of intent.
8. Be consistent and repetitive during daily routines.
9. Wait (time-delay) expectantly for a response from the child.
10. Try to have a balance of communication between yourself and the child. You should not do all the talking. Teach this to the caregiver.

Think Critically for Self-Study or Classroom Discussion

1. How does the infant communicate without intent?
2. How is this different from the illocutionary stage?
3. How might you adapt the *Peabody Picture Vocabulary Test* for a 3-year-old with spastic quadriplegia?
4. How does dynamic assessment differ from typical informal assessment?
5. How would you begin intervention with a child who spent 2 months in a NICU and is suspected of developing cerebral palsy?

References

Accardo, P. J., Accardo, J. A., & Capute, A. J. (2008). A neurodevelopmental perspective on the continuum of developmental disabilities. In P. J. Accardo (Ed.), *Capute & Accardo's neurodevelopmental disabilities in infancy and childhood. Volume I: Neurodevelopmental diagnosis and treatment* (3rd ed., pp. 3–26). Baltimore, MD: Paul H. Brookes.

American Speech, Language, and Hearing Association. (2013). *Dynamic assessment.* Retrieved from http://www.asha.org/practice/multicultural/issues/Dynamic-Assessment.htm

Austin, L. (2010). Dynamic assessment: Whys and hows. *Perspectives on School-Based Issues, 11,* 80–87.

Bates, E. (1976). *Language in context: Studies in acquisition of pragmatics.* New York, NY: Academic Press.

Bell, R. (1971). Stimulus control of parent or caretaker behavior by offspring. *Developmental Psychology, 4,* 63–72.

Berko-Gleason, J. (2001). *The development of language* (5th ed.). Boston, MA: Allyn & Bacon.

Billeaud, F. P. (1998). *Communication disorders in infants and toddlers: Assessment and intervention* (2nd ed.). Boston, MA: Butterworth-Heinemann.

Bloom, L., & Lahey, M. (1978). *Language development and language disorders.* New York, NY: Wiley.

Crais, E. R. (1990). From world knowledge to word knowledge. *Topics in Language Disorders, 10,* 45–62.

DeVeney, S. L., Hoffman, L., & Cress, C. J. (2012). Communication-based assessment of developmental age for young children with developmental disabilities. *Journal of Speech, Language, and Hearing Research, 55,* 695–709.

Drominey, P. F., & Dodane, C. (2004). Indeterminancy in language acquisition: The role of child directed speech and joint attention. *Journal of Neurolinguistics, 17,* 121–145.

Finnie, N. R. (2001). *Handling the young child with cerebral palsy at home* (3rd ed.). Oxford, UK: Butterworth-Heinemann.

Girolametto, L. (1997). Development of a parent report measure for profiling the conversational skills of preschool children. *American Journal of Speech-Language Pathology, 6,* 25–33.

Hanzlik, J. R., & Stevenson, M. B. (1986). Interaction of mothers with their infants who are mentally retarded, retarded with cerebral palsy, or nonretarded. *Journal of Mental Deficiency, 90,* 513–520.

Hetzroni, O. E. (2001). Identifying intentional communication in children with severe disabilities. *Perspectives on Language Learning and Education, 8,* 8–11.

Howle, J. M. (2002). *Neurodevelopmental treatment approach: Theoretical foundations and principles of clinical practice.* Laguna Beach, CA: NDTA.

Kogan, K. L., & Tyler, N. (1973). Mother-child interactions in physically handicapped children. *American Journal of Mental Deficiency, 77,* 492–497.

Lowenthal, B. (1995). Naturalistic language intervention in inclusive environments. *Intervention in School and Clinic, 31,* 114–118.

McCune, L. (1995). A normative study of representational play at the transition to language. *Developmental Psychology, 31,* 198–206.

Mueller, H. A. (2001). Speech. In N. R. Finnie (Ed.), *Handling the young child with cerebral palsy at home* (3rd ed., pp. 112–117). Oxford, UK: Butterworth-Heinemann.

Mundy, P., & Newell, L. (2007). Attention, joint attention, and social cognition. *Current Directions in Psychological Science, 16,* 269–274.

Okimoto, A. M., Bundy, A., & Hanzlik, J. (2000). Playfulness in children with and without disability: Measurement and intervention. *The American Journal of Occupational Therapy, 54,* 73–82.

Olswang, L. B., & Pinder, G. L. (1995). Preverbal functional communication and the role of object play in children with cerebral palsy. *Infant-Toddler Intervention, 5,* 277–299.

O'Sullivan, S. B. (1985). Infant-caregiver interaction and the social development of handicapped infants. *Physical & Occupational Therapy in Pediatrics, 5,* 1–12.

Palisano, R. J., Chiarello, L. A., & Haley, S. M. (1993). Factors related to mother-infant interaction in infants with motor delays. *Pediatric Physical Therapy, 5*, 55–60.

Palmer, F. B., Shapiro, B. K., Allen, M. C., Mosher, B. S., Bilker, S. A., Harryman, S. E., . . . Capute, A. J. (1990). Infant stimulation curriculum for infants with cerebral palsy: Effects on infant termperament, parent-infant interaction, and home environment. *Pediatrics, 85*, 411–415.

Paul, R. (2007). *Language disorders from infancy through adolescence: Assessment and intervention* (3rd ed.). St. Louis, MO: Mosby.

Paul, R., Hernandez, R., Taylor, L., & Johnson, K. (1996). Narrative development in late talkers: Early school years. *Journal of Speech and Hearing Research, 39*, 1295–1303.

Paul, R., Murray, C., Clancy, K., & Andrews, D. (1997). Reading and metaphonological outcomes in late talkers. *Journal of Speech, Language, and Hearing Research, 40*, 1037–1047.

Pelligrino, L. (2007). Cerebral palsy. In M. L. Batshaw, L. Pelligrino, & N. J. Roizen (Eds.), *Children with disabilities* (pp. 387–408). Baltimore, MD: Paul H. Brookes.

Pennington, L., Goldbart, J., & Marshall, J. (2004). Interaction training for conversational partners of children with cerebral palsy: A systematic review. *International Journal of Language & Communication Disorders, 39*, 151–170.

Pennington, L., & McConachie, H. (1999). Mother–child interaction revisited: Communication with non–speaking physically disabled children. *International Journal of Language & Communication Disorders, 34*, 391–416.

Pennington, L., Thomson, K., James, P., Martin, L., & McNally, R. (2009). Effects of It Takes Two to Talk—The Hanen program for parents of preschool children with cerebral palsy: Findings from an exploratory study. *Journal of Speech, Language, and Hearing Research, 52*, 1121–1138.

Pinder, G. L., & Olswang, L. B. (1995). Development of communicative intent in young children with cerebral palsy: A treatment efficacy study. *Infant-Toddler Intervention, 5*, 51–70.

Pinder, G. L., Olswang, L., & Coggins, K. (1993). Development of communicative intent in a physically disabled child. *Infant-Toddler Intervention, 3*, 1–17.

Rescorla, L., & Alley, A. (2001). Validation of the Language-Development Survey (LDS). *Journal of Speech, Language, and Hearing Research, 44*, 434–445.

Rogers, B., Arvedson, J., Buck, G., Smart, P., & Msall, M. (1994). Characteristics of dysphagia in children with cerebral palsy. *Dysphagia, 9*, 60–73.

Rossetti, L. M. (2001). *Communication intervention: Birth to three* (2nd ed.). Albany, NY: Singular.

Sachs, J. (2001). Communication development in infancy. In J. Berko Gleason (Ed.), *The development of language* (pp. 40–69). Boston, MA: Allyn & Bacon.

Schneider, P., & Watkins, R. V. (1996). Applying Vygotskian developmental theory to language intervention. *Language, Speech, and Hearing Services in Schools, 27*, 157–170.

Shapiro, B. K., & Gwynn, H. (2008). Neurodevelopmental assessment of infants and young children. In P. J. Accardo (Ed.), *Capute & Accardo's neurodevelopmental disabilities in infancy and childhood. Volume I: Neurodevelopmental diagnosis and treatment* (3rd ed., pp. 367–382). Baltimore, MD: Paul H. Brookes.

Sigafoos, J., Drasgow, E., Reichle, J., O'Reilly, M., & Tait, K. (2004). Tutorial: Teaching communicative rejection to children with severe disabilities. *American Journal of Speech-Language Pathology, 13*, 31–42.

Sigafoos, J., Woodyatt, G., Keen, D., Tait, K., Tucker, M., Roberts-Pennell, D., . . . Pittendreigh, N. (2000A). Identifying potential communicative acts in children with developmental and physical disabilities. *Communication Disorders Quarterly, 21*, 77–86.

Sigafoos, J., Woodyatt, G., Tucker, M., Roberts-Pennell, D., & Pittendrigh, N. (2000B). Assessment of potential communicative acts in three individuals with Rett syndrome. *Journal of Developmental and Physical Disabilities, 12*, 203–216.

Snell, M. E. (2002). Using dynamic assessment with learners who communicate nonsymbolically. *Augmentative and Alternative Communication, 18*, 163–176.

Sullivan, M., & Lewis, M. (2000). Assistive technology for the very young: Creating responsive environments. *Infants & Young Children, 12*, 34–52.

Wilcox, M. J., Kouri, T. A., & Caswell, S. (1990). Partner sensitivity to communication behavior of young children with developmental disabilities. *Journal of Speech and Hearing Disorders, 55*, 679–693.

CHAPTER 10

AAC for Children with Cerebral Palsy

Cindy Geise Arroyo

Introduction

Augmentative and alternative communication (AAC) has transformed the lives of children with various types and severity levels of cerebral palsy. Because communication is considered the essence of life (ASHA, 2005), AAC has created opportunities never thought possible before. Prior to the 1980s individuals with severe communication impairments, such as those associated with cerebral palsy, struggled to communicate in a functional manner.

It is obvious that technology has expanded the field of speech-language pathology greatly, but changes in the underlying philosophy of AAC have evolved as well. Children using an AAC system can now choose the clothes to wear or buy, tell a sibling what game to play or video to watch, go to the neighborhood school, take a test with the rest of the class, or even tell a parent to "cool it." These are things we take for granted but change the way society views children with cerebral palsy and how they view themselves.

However, misconceptions kept the field of speech-language pathology from fully embracing AAC, especially for young children. This included the notion that AAC would hinder the development of speech. Both clinical observations and research indicate that this was wrong. As a speech-language pathologist working in a cerebral palsy center in the 1970s and 1980s, I observed the evolution of AAC, which was considered a part of assistive technology (AT). This significantly expanded the scope of practice in our field.

In many cases, it was not until the 1990s that courses in AAC were included in university programs. The results of a survey conducted by Ratcliff, Koul, and Lloyd (2008) indicated that the number of speech-language pathology university programs offering a separate course in AAC has increased over the last decade. However, only about 50% of the respondents reported that AAC was a *required* course in their program. ASHA's special interest division in AAC (SID 12) is rapidly growing, and it is evident that AAC is not a "specialty fringe area," but rather an integral part of the speech-language pathologist's scope of practice (Ratcliff et al., 2008).

Legislation such as the Individuals with Disabilities Education Act (IDEA) and the amendments of 2004 continue to support the need for communication and assistive technology to be available and documented as part of a child's individualized education plan or individualized family service plan. ASHA defines AAC as an "attempt to compensate and facilitate, temporarily or permanently, for the impairment and disability patterns of individuals with severe expressive and/or language comprehension disorders" (1993). However, Dowden (1999) feels this definition is too "formal" (p. 345). It is so much more than that for the children and families of children with cerebral palsy.

Communicative competence is developed over time through a complex integration of knowledge, judgment, and skills (Light, 1988). The child with cerebral palsy who uses AAC is constrained in the development of communicative competence by issues that the typically developing child does not have to face. Whereas natural speech is a fast, dynamic, and socially accepted method of communication, the use of alternative methods (AAC) may be considerably slower. It also takes more effort and is often not readily accepted or understood by the mainstream population. Children may need to learn how to use a communication system without the benefit of observing models of competent communicators who use AAC.

Cerebral Palsy and AAC

It is crucial to consider implementing AAC methods and strategies early, because children with cerebral palsy are generally considered to be at risk for being nonverbal or for having a severe speech impairment (Hustad & Miles, 2010). Motor impairment resulting from damage to the central nervous system is often the primary characteristic that impacts communication in cerebral palsy, but deficits in language, cognition, and sensory functioning (e.g., vision, hearing) may also be associated with cerebral palsy. These vary in severity from child to child, resulting in a heterogeneous population (Pennington, Goldbart, & Marshall, 2005). The individual and unique characteristics of children with cerebral palsy need to be considered when implementing AAC. There is no single strategy or AAC recommendation that will fit the needs of all children.

It has been estimated that about 20% of children diagnosed with cerebral palsy are considered nonverbal (Pennington et al., 2005). Parkes, Hill, Platt, and Donnelly (2010) found that speech impairments affect approximately 36 to 40 % of children with cerebral palsy. A report from a large population-based sample in Europe indicated that 60% of children with cerebral palsy have some type of communication impairment (Bax, Tydeman, & Flodmark, 2006). Additionally, there is an increased prevalence of communication disorders associated with increased degree of motor and intellectual impairment.

There is a relationship between expressive language function, speech production, and gross motor function in children diagnosed with cerebral palsy. Sigurdardottir and Vik (2011) found that 88% of the nonverbal children had multiple disabilities, compared with only 18% of verbal children. They found a strong correlation between a diagnosis of spastic quadriplegia and dyskinesia, and nonverbal or severely unintelligible speech. Hustad and Miles (2010) identified 21 of their 22 participants with cerebral palsy as needing some form of AAC. It is interesting that although almost half of these children also used some natural speech, they still benefited from AAC as an interim, augmentative, or secondary strategy.

The need for AAC is great for children with cerebral palsy, due to the primary motor impairment affecting the oral mechanism for speech, and this impairment makes access to AAC challenging. In addition, the development of communicative competence that occurs over time through a complex integration of knowledge, judgment, and skills is difficult because of the many constraints that need to be addressed.

Definitions

AAC has evolved as a multidisciplinary and international field (Beukelman & Miranda, 2013). This has led to differing vocabularies (Lloyd, Fuller, & Arvidson, 1997). It might be worthwhile at this point to define the terms. We've already read ASHA's definition of AAC, but what is the difference between augmentative and alternative? The term *augmentative* communication refers to strategies used to supplement and enhance speech/vocalizations, whereas *alternative* is used when speech is not functional as a primary communication mode.

AAC falls under the broader term of *assistive technology* (AT), which is defined as any product or service that is used to maintain or improve the functional capabilities of individuals with disabilities. Other examples of assistive technology are mobility aids, such as wheelchairs, and hand splints or pointers that may improve an individual's access for technology such as AAC. What we need to keep in mind is that the primary purpose of AAC is to facilitate efficient and effective communicative interactions in a variety of environments, in order to communicate wants and needs, transfer information, and establish social relationships (Beukelman & Mirenda, 2013; Light, 1988).

AAC systems may be characterized as *unaided* or *aided*. The use of *unaided* strategies involves the user's body conveying the message, such as gestures, facial expressions, or sign language. It is important to consider that sign language may not be an effective strategy for children with cerebral palsy because of their fine motor impairments. In addition, it is limiting for those whose family and peers are not fluent in sign.

Aided systems require tools or equipment in addition to the user's body. This may range from simple communication boards and books to sophisticated, speech-generating, computer-based devices. When we consider any aided system, we need to remember that it requires the use of symbols to represent concepts and messages (ASHA, 2002). Children's ability to understand and identify the meaning of symbols may be affected by concreteness, context, and familiarity. Cultural and experiential backgrounds and developmental age may also influence understanding and acceptance of symbols (Beukelman & Mirenda, 2013). Many children with cerebral palsy and significant communication impairments will require implementation of some form of aided AAC (Treviranus & Roberts, 2003).

Technology and Aided AAC

Advances in the area of technology have increased the range of options for aided communication systems. They are often viewed on a continuum. For example, a "no-tech" system typically displays symbols on a communication board or book and does not generate voice output. A "light-tech" system usually refers to a simple, battery-operated device that utilizes digitized (recorded) voice output. Light-tech devices generally have static (or fixed) displays of symbols, which require physical changing of paper overlays/displays. "High-tech" usually indicates the use of a speech-generating device (SGD) with more advanced, computer-based technology. High-tech devices as seen in Figure 10–1 have dynamic displays that electronically change the selection set. We then further categorize SGDs as either dedicated or nondedicated. A dedicated SGD is used solely for communication, whereas a nondedicated one may run additional software for other purposes such as gaming or watching videos.

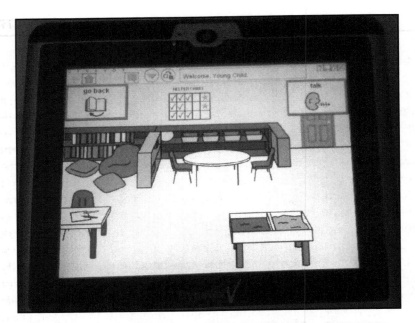

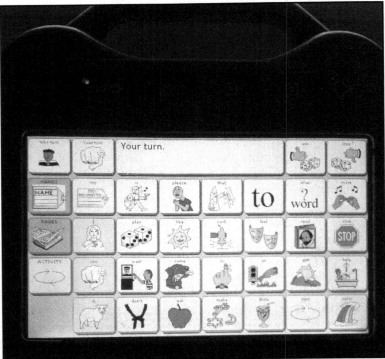

Figure 10–1. Two examples of dedicated high-tech, speech-generating communication devices.

Access

In order to effectively use or activate an AAC system or device, a consistent mode of access, or selection technique must be determined. Children with cerebral palsy present with significant challenges that include: motoric limitations, the presence of abnormal reflexes and muscle tone, and vision and hearing impairments. These may significantly impact access options. Establishing a consistent mode of access is essential to achieving *operational competence*, which Light (1989) defines as "the ability to effectively control the tool or tools used to communicate . . . " (p. 140).

Selection techniques are generally divided into two categories: direct selection and indirect selection, which is typically called scanning. When direct selection is employed, the AAC user indicates the desired items in the selection set specifically. This process is not time dependent (Dowden & Cook, 2002; Johnston & Feeley, 2012) and may be accomplished by touching with some body part. We typically think of pointing to an item or depressing a key or switch. This can also be accomplished without physical contact by using eye gaze or a light pointer that may be placed on the user's glasses or headband (Beukelman & Mirenda, 2013; Lloyd et al., 1997).

Direct Selection

Most clinicians and researchers agree that direct selection is the fastest method of selection. It is also noted for its ease of learning and natural occurrence, because pointing is a common form of prelinguistic communication (Dowden & Cook, 2002). However, a significant disadvantage of direct selection for children with cerebral palsy is the demand it places on the user's motor abilities. Direct selection requires an extensive range of motion to allow the individual to access all of the items in a selection set. The size of the symbol display is also an important consideration in order to maximize effective communication. Fewer symbols/messages on a page may minimize physical/visual demands, but it limits the available vocabulary for the AAC user. Therefore, the decision with regard to layout must be individualized, and the number of symbols on a display may be increased gradually as motor proficiency increases (Dowden & Cook, 2002).

Interface adjustments can often be made to enhance access. Keypad sensitivity is an adjustment than can be made so that a child whose touch is very light due to lack of strength can still select the item. In addition, different forms of feedback can be activated for children with visual and auditory impairments, and adjustments may be made to acceptance and release timing (Cook & Hussey, 1995; Dowden & Cook, 2002; Johnston & Feeley, 2012).

Equipment that can be constructed or may be commercially available can facilitate improved motor control for AAC use as well as other activities. These are called *control enhancers* (Cook & Hussey, 1995; Dowden, 1999) and they are very useful for children with cerebral palsy. They include items such as splints for fingers and wrists, head pointers, and seating modifications.

Scanning

Many children with cerebral palsy cannot use direct selection due to motor or sensory disorders. These children will need indirect selection. Scanning is the most common type of indirect selection (Beukeleman & Mirenda, 2013; Cook & Hussey, 1995). In scanning, the words/messages in the selection set are presented by a communication partner or on an electronic display on an AAC device. The child must wait until the desired message is presented and then indicate a choice. This is generally accomplished by activating a switch (Beukelman & Mirenda, 2013).

There are many considerations when implementing this method for a child with cerebral palsy. Scanning imposes significant visual and cognitive demands. We need to determine what switch will be used based on ease of use and accuracy of activation. This may be a comprehensive assessment in itself. There is a wide array of commercially available switches. Typically, young children use some type of mechanical switch that requires applying movement with pressure, but other more sophisticated switches are available (Dowden & Cook, 2012).

Then a place on the body, which is called the "control site," must be established so that the switch can be activated. Researchers have developed a hierarchy of anatomic control sites (Cook & Hussey, 1995; Dowden & Cook, 2012) with fingers, arms, head, and foot suggested frequently. However, the choice will be determined by the child's range of movement, strength, and preferences (Dowden & Cook, 2012).

Switches, as a type of assistive technology, can be used for more than AAC. They can be used to activate an adapted toy or computer software. A switch may also produce voice output that can command the attention and influence the actions of communication partners. Initially, emerging communicators should be taught to use a switch in tasks with a direct one-to-one relationship between the motor movement and the consequence/output (Dowden & Cook, 2012). For example, single switches with digitized speech capabilities such as the "Big Mack" can speak a recorded message when activated by a single motor movement as seen in Figure 10–2.

Scanning Patterns

As mentioned previously, in scanning the child needs to be able to wait until the correct message is available and then activate a switch (Beukelman & Mirenda, 2013). This activation signals the

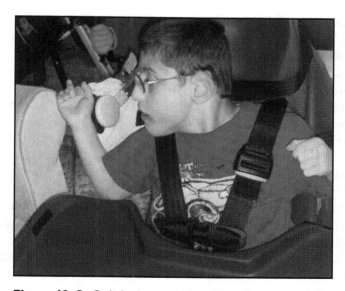

Figure 10–2. Switch placement for activation by a consistent movement. This switch plays a recorded message indicating a desire for the child to play with a specific toy.

child's choice. In a no-tech, partner-assisted visual scanning, the communication partner points to each item on the display, one at a time, and the child uses a predetermined signal when the partner arrives at the desired item/symbol. The response may be unaided, such as a smile or an eye blink, or the response may be aided, where the child activates a switch to emit a positive response such as a beep or a recorded message.

Computer-based scanning options are typically highlighted by a moving cursor or light, with the child activating a switch when the desired symbol is reached. When using scanning, the most efficient pattern must be determined. Patterns of scanning refer to the way items in the display are systematically presented (electronically or nonelectronically) (Johnston & Feeley, 2012). Linear scanning displays items one at a time, usually from left to right. Although it is the slowest scanning method, it is less cognitively demanding and is, therefore, a good choice for beginning communicators or younger children. There are other possible scanning patterns that are configured so that multiple symbols are scanned simultaneously to increase the rate of communication. Examples of these patterns include group-item scanning and group-row-column scanning (Treviranus & Roberts, 2003). Scanning speeds can be adjusted and it is generally better to start at a slower rate for learning purposes and to reduce error rate.

Directed scanning is another scanning method, in which a multifunction switch (e.g., a joystick) controls the direction of the cursor movement. This method requires the AAC user to visually locate the desired symbol and then plan and implement a scanning path to reach the symbol. This method may reduce the number of cursor movements required to reach a symbol, but it requires the motor ability to operate a multifunction switch (Dropik & Reichle, 2008) and the ability to motor plan.

If we search the literature for guidance in determining the most efficient scanning pattern, there have been a number of studies that compared the accuracy and efficiency of directed scanning versus group-item scanning (Dropik & Reichle, 2008; White, Carney, & Reichle, 2010) and linear versus row-column scanning (Peterson, Reichle, & Johnston, 2000). Results indicate that directed scanning yields better accuracy but is slower than group-item scanning. When comparing linear and row-column scanning, there is no significant difference in scanning errors. It is important to note, however, that all of the studies were conducted with young, typically developing children. It would be difficult to generalize these results to children with cerebral palsy who are likely to have different perceptual, cognitive, or motor abilities.

Scanning with Feedback

Because cerebral palsy is often associated with multiple disabilities including a high risk for visual impairment (Kovach & Kenyon, 2003), some children may require the implementation of auditory scanning techniques (Clarke & Price, 2012). Auditory scanning is a method for accessing AAC systems where choices are presented using a verbal auditory cue, typically consisting of a word, phrase, or sentence. This also can help children learn the names of the symbols, help maintain attention, and enhance interaction with communication partners by allowing them to listen to the scanning pattern (Kovach & Kenyon, 2003).

Case Study—John

John is a 6-year-old child with spastic quadriplegia cerebral palsy. His only vocalizations are grunts, yells, and occasional vowel sounds. His limited fine motor skills have precluded the use of sign language or pointing to symbols on a communication board or device. John also has a significant visual impairment, but his hearing is normal and he responds to some verbal commands and receptive identification tasks. In order to provide John with a means to communicate basic wants and needs and make choices, a switch assessment was conducted that would provide a method of "auditory scanning." A traditional placement of a "jelly bean switch" in front of John on his laptray yielded a repetitive "raking" motion with his right hand, which was not functional for consistent switch activation. After trying several other sites, John is able to consistently activate the switch by moving his right forearm perpendicular to the laptray to where the switch is mounted on an extension to the back of his adaptive chair as seen in Figure 10–2. John is using his switch to play recorded messages to indicate his preference for activities.

Principles of AAC Assessment

Decisions regarding AAC assessment and intervention processes should be dynamic and ongoing, taking into consideration the individual's strengths and needs; their present method of communication and the effectiveness of that method; as well as future communication needs. The processes should also be conducted with a variety of communication partners in a variety of contexts and natural environments (ASHA, 2004; Beukelman & Mirenda, 2013). Assessment of children with cerebral palsy who have communicative limitations can be complex and challenging. Often, the cognitive and receptive language skills of emerging communicators with significant motor impairments may be underestimated or misrepresented, especially when using standardized testing. Motor limitations may preclude the use of typically expected responses for traditional testing, such as isolating a finger to point to a picture or providing a verbal response. Significant motor limitations may also affect a child's ability to be assessed through nonverbal or manipulation tasks, typically used to assess cognitive functioning (Dowden & Cook, 2012).

Historically, when AAC services and systems emerged in the 1970s and 1980s, some individuals were excluded from being considered a "candidate." Criteria such as a minimum age, cognitive level, or prerequisite skills were often considered a requirement. In order to eliminate this form of discrimination, ASHA (2004) and the National Joint Commission for Persons with Disabilities (2002) established a "zero exclusion" criterion, meaning that no one may be excluded from being considered for AAC assessment and intervention. The emphasis should not be on eligibility rather than on identifying the individual's "participation patterns and communication needs" as a starting point (Beukelman & Mirenda, 2013, p. 111).

Feature Matching

It is important to employ the concept of *feature matching* in the assessment process. This involves selecting an appropriate AAC system based on its components or features in relation to the individual's communication needs and skill (Lloyd et al., 1997).

It is important for SLPs who are either evaluators or clinicians to be aware of the features on the different aided systems in order to meet the individual needs of the AAC user (Johnston & Feeley, 2012). Multiple features may be available on systems that need to be considered. Some have both visual display and speech output. Some have a variety of symbol displays and selection techniques. Additionally, high-tech systems may have options for rate enhancement such as word and phrase prediction and the ability to act as an environmental control (e.g., to turn on the TV or video player).

Principles of Intervention

Light and Drager (2002) provide some important considerations when implementing AAC for young children. They note that systems should be appealing, motivating, and integrated easily into all aspects of daily living. The available symbols and messages also need to be sensitive to the linguistic and cultural backgrounds of the family. The systems should also support the development of communication, language, and literacy. In addition, they should be easy for the child to learn and use and also be easy for family and professionals to learn and maintain. Too often, AAC is not used because families have not had sufficient training and practice with the system in order to be comfortable using it.

Positioning

Children with cerebral palsy are often considered for AAC because of their motor limitations affecting respiratory, phonatory, and articulatory systems for intelligible speech. The child's muscle tone, lack of stability, and poor head and trunk alignment affect the use of the hands as well as the mouth. In order to have the child function optimally on the selected device, stable positioning is crucial (Beukelman & Mirenda, 2013; Cook & Hussey, 1995).

Knowledge of positioning is included in ASHA's (2002) list of competencies for SLPs providing AAC services. The first principle that has been noted repeatedly in this book includes the need for optimal stability, usually at the pelvis, in order to allow for the possibility of accurate distal functioning. In this case, we are talking about the accurate use of an arm or the head for selection. The best starting positioning is hip and knee flexion at 90 degrees with a solid footrest. Trunk support should be considered to ensure that the head and arms have a stable base on which to move, so that the individual can focus on the motor task, rather than on maintaining posture (McEwen & Lloyd, 1990).

Head control and head/trunk alignment are vital for attention, communication, and successful arm/hand function (Carlberg & Hadders-Algra, 2005). Costigan and Light (2010, 2011) cite the importance of addressing the seating/positioning needs of children with cerebral palsy to increase the accuracy of their target selection on AAC devices. Equipment may be used to facilitate stability and symmetry of the AAC user. This may take the form of a footrest, laptray, or lateral supports. Sometimes physical assistance is provided by a caregiver or a therapist during an activity. This may take the form of stabilizing an arm (York & Weimann, 1991).

Tray height is another important variable that can affect trunk stability and hand usage. A tray that is too high may restrict arm movements, whereas one that is too low may restrict the user's reach and cause increased neck and trunk flexion. Tray height is a variable that is difficult to predict and needs to be adjusted during function. Additionally, implementing a slant to a lap-tray may facilitate arm extension, visual attention, and trunk stability. This will enhance the accuracy of reach (McEwen & Lloyd, 1990).

Positioning of Equipment

Positioning of the AAC system should also be a consideration. Smith, McCarthy, and Benigna (2009) suggest that aligning an AAC device with the communication partner's eye gaze may facilitate learning and communication, because children using the system will not have to shift their gaze from the device to the communication partner. Also, switches and other targets should be placed to optimize function but must not reinforce abnormal patterns of movement (McEwen & Lloyd, 1990). For example, if a child has a strong asymmetrical tonic neck reflex (ATNR) to the right, placing the switch to the right will reinforce that abnormal movement and lead to increased muscle tone throughout the body. In summary, positioning should enhance the ability to use the AAC system. Any equipment used should provide support without restricting necessary movement. It must also promote the child's ability to attend to presented tasks (Cook & Hussey, 1995; Dowden & Cook, 2012; York & Weimann, 1991).

Early Intervention and AAC

For clinicians, a primary focus of early intervention should be building a relationship of trust and partnership with parents. The introduction of AAC may be a difficult concept for parents of a young child with a disability to understand and accept (Blockberger & Sutton, 2003). We must introduce the interventions with sensitivity, acknowledge the parents' fears, and answer all questions. Parents should be involved in every stage of the AAC process: assessment, decision-making, system selection, and implementation (Goldbart & Marshall, 2004). Parette, Brotherson, and Huer (2000) conducted interviews with families of children who used or needed AAC interventions. The families expressed their desire for professionals to understand them better and to respect their ethnicity and family values. They were concerned with the terminology used to describe their children and the possible stigma associated with it. They also expressed a desire for more information and training in the use of AAC devices, requested support in using the devices, and indicated an interest in contacting other families with children using AAC.

The importance of implementing AAC strategies as early as possible has been well documented (Cress & Marvin, 2003; Hustad & Miles, 2010; Romski & Sevcik, 2005). Implementation of augmentative strategies such as gestures/signs or simple picture communication boards with very young children can facilitate intentional communicative behavior with caregivers. The caregiver, in turn, can respond to these behaviors, thereby reinforcing them and fostering further development of intentional communication (Cress & Marvin, 2003). Branson and Demchak (2009) conducted a systematic review and found strong evidence for the use of AAC with infants and toddlers. All of the children in the reviewed studies showed an improvement in their communication skills following AAC interventions (aided and unaided). These improvements were observed with young children across many disabilities, including cerebral palsy. These authors conclude that training parents to respond to nonsymbolic and symbolic acts facilitates children's communication and language development.

Unfortunately, many young children with cerebral palsy who have significant communication and physical disabilities are often not considered for AAC early in their development. This results in a loss of valuable time and learning opportunities. Research has shown that AAC interventions can have a significant impact on the development of language skills in young children who have significant communication impairments (Drager, Light, & McNaughton, 2010). AAC interventions can support the development of pragmatics (social communication); semantics (meaning of words); and syntax (combining words to form sentences). Light and Drager (n.d.) report significant increases in turn-taking behaviors, expression of wants and needs, vocabulary, and length of utterance in young children with cerebral palsy following AAC interventions. The authors suggest initiating AAC interventions by the age of 6 to 9 months, when children have been diagnosed with a disability that puts them at risk for communication impairments such as cerebral palsy.

One reason for the delay in implementing AAC services may be the myths or misconceptions that have been associated with early intervention. For many years, it was felt that children had to be a certain age or have cognitive prerequisites in order to be considered for AAC intervention (Cress & Marvin, 2003; Romski & Sevcik, 2005). In the past, parents and professionals often assumed that the use of AAC could inhibit the development of natural speech in young children. None of these myths is supported either by research or clinical experience. In fact, research indicates that AAC facilitates verbal communication and reduces challenging behaviors often seen with nonverbal children (Millar, Light, & Schlosser, 2006). This may be attributed to the fact that the use of speech-generating devices (SGDs) provides the child with both a visual representation (symbol/picture) and auditory feedback/model in the spoken message from the device.

Another myth associated with the early introduction of AAC is that it is being used as a "last resort" when other interventions have been unsuccessful at improving communication. AAC is sometimes regarded as a separate area of practice (Romski & Sevcik, 2005) when it should be a strategy that is part of a more comprehensive intervention plan. Romski and Sevcik (2005) emphasize that AAC can play a variety of roles in early intervention, depending on the child's individual needs and characteristics. These may include: augmenting existing verbal output; providing the primary output mode for communication; providing an input and an output mode for communication; and acting as a language intervention strategy. AAC strategies, devices, and systems should be viewed as important tools in intervention to provide a foundation for the development of early communication skills.

"Multimodal" communication is often encouraged as part of communication intervention programs. When working with young children, therapists and caregivers must acknowledge and reinforce all forms of communication including facial expressions, gestures, and vocalizations. At an early age, symbol representations such as photographs of family members and favorite toys or line drawings representing words can be introduced. This supports language learning and facilitates expressive communication. Words should always be included on the pictures to enhance preliteracy skills. One little boy whom I worked with had learned 30 sight words by the time he was 2½ years old, because they were included on the visual display of his communication board.

Vocabulary

An important consideration for young children is the selection of vocabulary and the organization of that vocabulary on the AAC system. Light and Drager (2002) emphasize that AAC systems are designed and programmed by adults and therefore usually reflect the conceptual knowledge and judgment of adults without disabilities. Characteristics of first lexicons in typically developing children may be used to guide decisions in choosing vocabulary (Light, 2003). However, words identified in the first lexicons of typically developing children may not be appropriate for children with severe communication and physical impairments such as those with cerebral palsy. I have often emphasized the importance of including vocabulary/messages that enable children with cerebral palsy to negotiate their environment (e.g., "go outside," "come here!") and to request activities they may not be able to physically do themselves (e.g., "read me a book").

Vocabulary words or messages must also be represented graphically. In many high-tech systems, the symbol sets are inherent in the systems, thus limiting the choices. However, no-tech and low-tech systems are, again, usually dependent on adults making the choices. Consequently, the clarity of the symbol (iconicity) must be considered. Digital photography and the ability to download photographs into a system, or print them out for a communication board or book, have resulted in increased options for improved iconicity and realistic representations. Many high-tech systems have built-in cameras.

Additional choices must be made with regard to the organization of vocabulary on aided AAC systems. Vocabulary on the pages of a communication board, book, or screen of a high-tech device can be organized according to frequency of use. For example, the most frequently used words and messages can be placed in an area of the display that is highly accessible. Displays can also be organized categorically (e.g., people, places, things) or schematically (a page/board for a designated activity such as circle time or snack). When it is developmentally appropriate, displays can also be organized syntactically, using a left to right orientation to develop the appropriate syntax for phrase and sentence construction (e.g., noun + verb) (Beukelman & Mirenda, 2013; Lloyd et al., 1997).

AAC systems with vocabulary emphasizing basic nouns, wants, and needs is appropriate for emerging communicators. But many interventionists/families keep the child at this stage longer than necessary (Cress & Marvin, 2003). Expansion of communicative functions should include vocabulary for greetings, protests, requests for attention, and termination of an activity (Reichle, Halle, & Johnston, 1993). Young children who have limited control over their environment feel empowered when they can say, "all done" or "I'm mad!" A message such as "see you later, alligator" has been more appealing than the typical "good-bye" for many of the young children I have worked with. There is also a need to expand beyond basic wants and needs for the AAC use. This can help to establish social closeness and exchange information with communication partners such as parents, siblings, peers, and teachers.

Children need a variety of vocabulary words, verb tenses, and morphological endings to develop their syntactic, semantic and morphological skills. Ultimately, these skills will enhance their reading and writing (Beukelman & Ray, 2010). Initially, the ability to generate a narrative, such as telling a story in preschool, is an important milestone in communication development. But the child who uses AAC can only succeed if the necessary vocabulary is available.

Imagine what it would be like to be unable to communicate your emotions, preferences, or basic wants and needs. If you had significant physical and communication impairments, you would be dependent on others to provide you with a method to communicate and the symbols/vocabulary to do so. Typically developing preschoolers add five words every day to their vocabularies. In many cases, we are not doing this for our children who use AAC.

Other Considerations for Displays

When organizing displays, physical characteristics also need to be considered, including symbol size and overall dimensions. The background color and the color of the symbols can enhance or diminish attention, and the spacing and arrangement of symbols will influence the accuracy of selection (Beukelman & Mirenda, 2013; Lloyd et al., 1997). Additionally, navigation between pages or displays should be considered on no-tech, low-tech, and high-tech devices. No-tech displays such as communication boards or books may need to be organized with colored tabs or labels for ease of locating specific pages. This will assist the communication partner in accessing the appropriate page if the child with cerebral palsy is unable to physically turn the pages. Similarly, low-tech systems need to have the paper overlays physically changed by a caregiver or communication partner. High-tech systems have the capability of dynamically changing pages, but the user must achieve the operational competence to navigate the computer-based system. This includes cognitive skills such as memory as well as motor ability and can be seen in Figure 10–3.

Augmented Input

In typical development, children are exposed to the model of spoken language for almost a year before they begin to produce their own verbal utterances. Young children who use AAC do not experience this type of linguistic input/modeling with AAC (Romski & Sevcik, 2003). The importance of teaching parents and other communication partners to model AAC use in

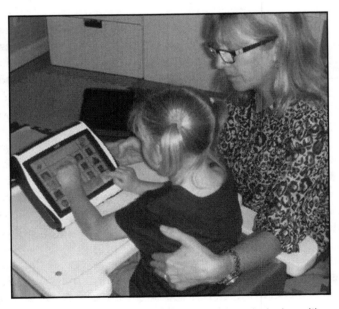

Figure 10–3. A young child using a high-tech device with a dynamic display.

a variety of contexts has been recognized in the intervention literature (Blockburger & Sutton, 2003; Light, 1997; Romski & Sevcik, 2003). Light (1997) noted that young children who use AAC are limited in their exposure to communication partners using AAC modeling. Unfortunately, the opportunity for them to observe other children using AAC functionally and proficiently is rarer still. Furthermore, children with significant physical limitations like cerebral palsy are not able to independently gain access to their environment and communication partners, and this limits the experience on which their language is mapped (Light, 1997).

AAC modeling is incorporated into intervention strategies that are collectively known as *augmented input interventions* (Romski & Sevcik, 2003). Binger and Light (2007) define aided AAC modeling as any model of AAC use provided for an individual with a significant communication impairment by a communication partner during an interaction. The System for Augmenting Language (SAL) (Romski & Sevcik, 1996) and Aided Language Stimulation (ALS) (Goossens', 1989; Goossens', Crain, & Elder, 1992) are examples of intervention strategies that use augmented input as part of an AAC intervention program. SAL involves the use of an SGD by the user and the communication partner while teaching through natural communicative exchanges (Harris & Reichle, 2004). ALS (Goossens' et al., 1992) involves a communication partner pointing to specific symbols on the AAC user's communication display simultaneously providing verbal language stimulation.

There is some empirical evidence to support the use of augmented input (Dada & Alant, 2009; Romski & Sevcik, 1996; Schlosser, Belfiore, Nigam, Blischak, & Hetzroni, 1995). Harris and Reichle (2004) found that aided language stimulation facilitated object labeling and symbol comprehension. If this type of intervention is going to be used with a child with cerebral palsy, it is important to train communication partners, whether they are teachers or parents, and motivate them to use the AAC system in all interactions (Jones & Bailey-Orr, 2012). Parents and professionals are often overwhelmed by the charge of implementing AAC strategies; therefore, I often start by focusing on a preferred activity.

Case Study—Katie

Katie's parents expressed that "bath-time" was her favorite activity, and it was also their favorite, because she typically goes to bed right afterward. We developed vocabulary and symbols related to bath-time (e.g., rubber duck, towel, bubbles, dry), and her parents began implementing aided language stimulation using Katie's AAC system during bath-time. Katie's successful use of the vocabulary during this favored activity motivated the family to expand the AAC strategies to other activities throughout the day.

AAC for Interaction

Many researchers have noted that children with cerebral palsy, especially those using AAC systems, tend to be passive communicators, rarely initiating conversation. They tend to respond only when their communication partners direct the conversational exchanges (Clark & Wilkinson, 2007; Pennington, Goldbart, & Marshall, 2004; Pennington & McConachie, 2001). Additionally, parents and other communication partners interacting with children using AAC have been observed to integrate AAC use with spoken language less than 10% of the time (Romski & Sevcik, 1996). Observations of peer interactions between children using AAC and typically developing peers have revealed that, unlike verbal children, AAC users interact more frequently with adults than with their peers (Clarke & Wilkinson, 2007).

Parents of children with significant communication impairments are often most secure in directing them to respond to yes/no questions. Therefore, the children may have limited opportunities to use communication for other purposes (Pennington & McConachie, 2001; Pennington, Thomson, James, Martin, & McNally, 2009). The concept of "learned helplessness" is often referred to in the AAC literature. An example of this is the tendency for young children with significant disabilities to have a limited range of communication partners due to their dependence on caregivers and the tendency for the caregiver to anticipate their needs. They also may have limited opportunities to learn strategies for skills such as conversational turn-taking and maintaining conversational exchanges, because they primarily interact with familiar communication partners who direct and control the conversation. It is therefore important to give the child varied opportunities, in natural contexts, to interact with a variety of communication partners. Parents can schedule play dates, participate in a preschool class for children with special needs, or take the child with the AAC system to the local playground or fast-food restaurant.

Children with a motor impairment such as cerebral palsy also have a more limited range of communication environments and play activities they can access, due to their physical limitations (Reichle & Brady, 2012). Programs such as "It Takes Two to Talk—The Hanen Program for Children with Cerebral Palsy" were designed to help parents adopt a more responsive approach to communication interactions. This program teaches them to modify their own behaviors to promote the child's engagement in, and ability to control, conversation. This includes allowing children sufficient time to initiate and uses the acronym "OWL" (observe, wait, listen). It also recognizes all forms of communication, including vocalizations, gestures, and AAC systems (Pennington et al., 2009). Pennington et al. (2004) found evidence to support a relationship between interaction training for communication partners of children with cerebral palsy and some positive changes in their communication patterns. Too often, well-meaning communication partners anticipate or try to "fill in" a child's intended message instead of giving the child time to formulate and physically initiate a message using AAC. Typically developing children learn through repetition and from making mistakes. In my experience, parents and professionals often limit opportunities for these experiences when they are interacting with a child who has a significant physical and communication impairment.

The mother of a nonverbal child with cerebral palsy whom I treated using an AAC device commented that she was so happy to hear me talking to him throughout the session. She said that the child's previous therapist worked on the use of a switch to activate his AAC device, but the therapist never talked *to* her son. Sometimes, we get so focused on the technology and the task at hand that we forget to treat the person as a person!

New Directions for AAC

Historically, the availability of dedicated AAC devices emerged slowly and were developed, produced, and supported by a small number of AAC manufacturers. Recently, the field has been impacted by a rapid proliferation of mobile technologies such as tablets, iPads, and an ever-increasing proliferation of "apps." Mobile technologies are appealing because of their portability, availability, social acceptance, and options for multifunctions.

Mobile technology development, however, has been driven by the preferences and needs of the mass market. Therefore, many devices are not equipped to meet the complex needs of individuals with significant communication and physical impairments, like children with cerebral palsy (McNaughton & Light, 2013). Motor access limitations have been noted in many of the mobile devices and popular communication applications (Flores et al., 2012). Additionally, a number of the available AAC apps address only one aspect of communication such as making requests or responding to yes/no questions (McNaughton & Light, 2013).

The application of mobile technologies must be guided by evidence-based practice that includes client preferences and clinical expertise, along with what we have already learned in the area of AAC (McNaughton & Light, 2013). Some professionals have attempted to develop strategies such as "feature-matching charts" that can be used to evaluate the large number of "apps" that claim to support and facilitate communication. It is also crucial that developers of these technologies and applications investigate options to improve access and support for individuals with complex communication needs. If these new technologies cannot adequately accommodate the needs of individuals with disabilities, what may result is a phenomenon called the "digital divide—the gap between those who either have easier access to the technology or are able to make effective use of it, and those who do not have access or are unable to make effective use of these technologies" (Garcia et al., 2011, p. 136).

The area of augmentative and alternative communication is "clearly at a crossroads" (McNaughton & Light, 2013, p. 114). Mobile technologies and apps have brought new recognition to the area of AAC. However, substantial research, development, and collaboration are imperative to determine and provide the most effective intervention applications for individuals who require AAC. "It is important to keep the focus on communication, not on technology" (McNaughton & Light, 2013, p. 110).

Ten Items for Improving AAC Interventions

1. Implement/explore AAC strategies as early as possible. There are no age limitations or cognitive prerequisites.
2. Evaluate seating and positioning to maximize functional access of AAC systems.
3. When using scanning, establish a consistent site for functional switch activation.
4. Assessment should be dynamic and ongoing and should not rely on standardized testing.
5. When programming AAC devices, go beyond requests involving basic needs and labeling, and develop a range of communicative functions to achieve communicative competence.
6. Teach parents and other communication partners to model AAC use in a variety of contexts.
7. Limit use of yes/no questions and encourage children to initiate conversation by giving them sufficient time to create a message and control conversation.
8. Recognize and respond to all forms of communication including vocalizations, gestures, and AAC use.
9. Build a relationship of trust and partnership with parents/caregivers and provide them with adequate support and training.
10. Respect cultural and linguistic diversity, ethnicity, and family values and incorporate them into AAC interventions.

Think Critically for Self-Study or Classroom Discussion

1. Identify the difference between unaided and aided modes of communication.
2. What are some of the myths/misconceptions associated with implementing AAC use with the Early Intervention population, and how can we address them?
3. What are the different options for indirect selection when working with individuals who have physical and/or visual limitations?
4. What components contribute to the development of communicative competence?
5. What are some of the advantages and challenges of the new mobile technologies for the field of AAC and AAC users?

References

American Speech-Language-Hearing Association (ASHA). (1993). *Definitions of communication disorders and variations* (Relevant Paper). Retrieved August 5, 2013, from http://www.asha.org/policy/RP1993-00208.htm

American Speech-Language-Hearing Association (ASHA). (2002). *Augmentative and alternative communication: Knowledge and skills for service delivery. Special Interest Division 12, Augmentative and Alternative Communication.* Retrieved August 12, 2013, from http://www.asha.org/policy/KS2002-00067.htm

American Speech-Language-Hearing Association (ASHA). (2004). *Roles and responsibilities of speech-language pathologists with respect to augmentative and alternative communication: Technical report* (Technical report). Retrieved August 13, 2013, from http://www.asha.org/policy/TR2004-00262.htm

American Speech-Language-Hearing Association (ASHA). (2005). *Roles and responsibilities of speech-language pathologists with respect to augmentative and alternative communication: Position statement* (Position statement). Retrieved August 5, 2013, from http://www.asha.org/policy/PS2005-00113.htm

Bax, M., Tydeman, C., & Flodmark, O. (2006). Clinical and MRI correlates of cerebral palsy: The European cerebral palsy study. *Journal of American Medical Association, 13*, 1602–1608.

Beukelman, D., & Mirenda, P. (2013). *Augmentative and alternative communication* (4th ed.). Baltimore, MD: Paul H. Brookes.

Beukelman, D., & Ray, P. (2010). Communication supports in pediatric rehabilitation. *Journal of Pediatric Rehabilitation Medicine, 3*(4), 279–288.

Binger, C., & Light, J. (2007). The effects of aided AAC modeling on the expression of multi-symbol messages by preschoolers who use AAC. *Augmentative and Alternative Communication, 23*, 30–43.

Blockberger, S., & Sutton, A. (2003). Toward linguistic competence: Language experiences and knowledge of children with extremely limited speech. In J. Light, D. Beukelman, & J. Reichle (Eds.), *Communicative competence for individuals who use AAC: From research to effective practice* (pp. 63–106). Baltimore, MD: Paul H. Brookes.

Branson, D., & Demchak, M. (2009). The use of augmentative and alternative communication methods with infants and toddlers with disabilities: A research review. *Augmentative and Alternative Communication, 25*(4), 274–286.

Carlberg, E., & Hadders-Algra, M. (2005). Postural dysfunction in children with cerebral palsy: Some implications for therapeutic guidance. *Neural Plasticity, 12*, 221–228.

Clarke, M., & Price, K. (2012). Augmentative and alternative communication for children with cerebral palsy. *Paediatrics and Child Health, 22*(9), 367–371.

Clarke, M., & Wilkinson, R. (2007). Interactions between children with CP and their peers 1: Organizing and understanding VOCA use. *Augmentative and Alternative Communication, 23*(4), 336–348.

Cook, A. M., & Hussey, S. M. (1995). *Assistive technologies: Principles and practice.* St. Louis, MO: Mosby.

Costigan, F. A., & Light, J. (2010). The effect of seated position on access to augmentative communication for children with cerebral palsy: Preliminary investigation. *American Journal of Occupational Therapy, 64*, 596–604.

Costigan, F. A., & Light, J. (2011). Functional seating for school-aged children with cerebral palsy: An evidence-based tutorial. *Language, Speech, and Hearing Services in Schools, 42*, 223–236.

Cress, C., & Marvin, C. (2003). Common questions about AAC services in early intervention. *Augmentative and Alternative Communication, 19*(4), 254–272.

Dada, S., & Alant, E. (2009). The effect of aided language stimulation on vocabulary acquisition in children with little or no functional speech. *American Journal of Speech-Language Pathology, 18*, 50–64.

Dowden, P. A. (1999). Augmentative and alternative communication for children with motor speech disorders. In A. J. Caruso & E. A. Strand (Eds.), *Clinical management of motor speech disorders in children* (pp. 345–384). New York, NY: Thieme Medical.

Dowden, P. A., & Cook, A. M. (2002). Choosing effective selection techniques for beginning communicators. In J. Reichle, D. R. Beukelman & J. C. Light (Eds.), *AAC series: Exemplary practices for beginning communicators: Implications for AAC* (pp. 395–432). Baltimore, MD: Paul H. Brookes.

Dowden, P. A., & Cook, A. M. (2012). Improving communicative competence through alternative selection methods. In S. Johnston, J. Reichle, K. Feeley, & E. Jones (Eds.), *AAC strategies for individuals with moderate to severe disabilities* (pp. 81–117). Baltimore, MD: Paul H. Brookes.

Drager, K., Light, J., & McNaughton, D. (2010). Effects of AAC intervention on communication and language for young children with complex communication needs. *Journal of Pediatric Rehabilitative Medicine: An Interdisciplinary Approach, 3*, 303–310.

Dropik, P. L., & Reichle, J. (2008). Comparison of accuracy and efficiency of directed scanning and group-item scanning for augmentative communication selection techniques with typically developing preschoolers. *American Journal of Speech-Language Pathology, 17*, 35–47.

Flores, M., Musgrove, K., Renner, S., Hinton, V. Strozier, S., Franklin, S., & Hil, D. (2012). A comparison of communication using the Apple iPad and a picture-based system. *Augmentative and Alternative Communication, 28*(2), 74–84.

Garcia, T. P., Loureira, J. P., Ing, C. S., Gonzalez, B. G., Riveiro, L. N., & Sierra, A. P. (2011). The use of computers and AAC devices by young children with cerebral palsy. *Assistive Technology, 23*, 135–149.

Goldbart, J., & Marshall, J. (2004). "Pushes and pulls" on the parents of children who use AAC. *Augmentative and Alternative Communication, 20*(4), 194–208.

Goossens', C. (1989). Aided communication intervention before assessment: A case study of a child with cerebral palsy. *Augmentative and Alternative Communication, 5*, 14–26.

Goossens', C., Crain, S., & Elder, P. (1992). *Engineering the preschool environment for interactive symbolic communication 18 months to 5 years developmentally.* Birmingham, AL: Southeast Augmentative Communication.

Harris, M. D., & Reichle, J. (2004). The impact of aided language stimulation on symbol comprehension and production in children with moderate cognitive disabilities. *American Journal of Speech-Language Pathology, 13*, 155–167.

Hustad, K. C., & Miles, L. K. (2010). Alignment between AAC needs and school-based speech-language services provided to young children with cerebral palsy. *Early Childhood Services, 4*(3), 129–140.

Johnston, S., & Feeley, K. (2012). AAC systems features. In S. Johnston, J. Reichle, K. Feeley, & E. Jones (Eds.), *AAC strategies for individuals with moderate to severe disabilities* (pp. 51–79). Baltimore: MD: Paul H. Brookes.

Jones, E., & Bailey-Orr, M. (2012). Using AAC to support language comprehension. In S. Johnston, J. Reichle, K. Feeley, & E. Jones (Eds.), *AAC Strategies for individuals with moderate to severe disabilities* (pp. 311–345). Baltimore, MD: Paul H. Brookes.

Kovach, T. M., & Kenyon, P. B. (2003). Visual issues and access to AAC. In J. C. Light, D. R. Beukelman, & J. Reichle (Eds.), *Communicative competence for individuals who use AAC.* (pp. 277–319). Baltimore, MD: Paul H. Brookes.

Light, J. (1988). Interaction involving individuals using augmentative and alternative communication systems: State of the art and future directions. *Augmentative and Alternative Communication, 4,* 66–82.

Light, J. (1989). Toward a definition of communicative competence for individuals using augmentative and alternative communication systems. *Augmentative and Alternative Communication, 5,* 137–144.

Light, J. (1997). "Let's go starfishing": Reflections on the contexts of language learning for children who use aided AAC. *Augmentative and Alternative Communication, 13,* 158–171.

Light, J. (2003). Shattering the silence: Development of communicative competence by individuals who use AAC. In J. Light, D. Beukelman, & J. Reichle (Eds.), *Communicative competence for individuals who use AAC* (pp. 3–38). Baltimore, MD: Paul H. Brookes.

Light, J., & Drager, K. (n.d.). *Early intervention for young children with autism, cerebral palsy, Down Syndrome and other disabilities.* Retrieved August 13, 2013, from http://aackids.psu.edu/index.php/page/show/id/8

Light, J., & Drager, K. (2002). Improving the design of augmentative and alternative technologies for young children. *Assistive Technology, 14*(1), 17–32.

Lloyd, L., Fuller, D., & Arvidson, H. (1997). *Augmentative and alternative communication: A handbook of principles and practices.* Boston, MA: Allyn & Bacon.

McEwen, I., & Lloyd, L. (1990). Positioning students with cerebral palsy to use augmentative and alternative communication. *Language, Speech, and Hearing Services in Schools, 21*(1), 15–21.

McNaughton, D., & Light, J. (2013). The iPad and mobile technology revolution: Benefits and challenges for individuals who require augmentative and alternative communication. *Augmentative and Alternative Communication, 29*(2), 107–116.

Millar, D. C., Light, J., & Schlosser, R. W. (2006). The impact of augmentative and alternative communication intervention on the speech production of individuals with developmental disabilities: A research review. *Journal of Speech, Language, and Hearing Research, 49*, 248–264.

National Joint Committee for the Communication Needs of Persons with Severe Disabilities. (2002). Access to communication services and supports: Concerns regarding the application of restrictive "eligibility" policies. *Communication Disorders Quarterly, 23*(3), 145–153.

Parette, H. P., Brotherson, M. J., & Huer, M. B. (2000). Giving families a voice in augmentative and alternative communication decision-making. *Education and Training in Mental Retardation and Developmental Disabilities, 35*, 177–190.

Parkes, J., Hill, N., Platt, M., & Donnelly, C. (2010). Oromotor dysfunction and communication impairment in children with cerebral palsy: A register study. *Developmental Medicine and Child Neurology, 52*, 1113–1119.

Pennington, L., Goldbart, J., & Marshall, J. (2004). Interaction training for conversational partners of children with cerebral palsy: A systematic review. *International Journal of Language and Communication Disorders, 39*(2), 151–170.

Pennington, L., Goldbart, J., & Marshall, J. (2005). Direct speech and language therapy for children with cerebral palsy: Findings from a systematic review. *Developmental Medicine and Child Neurology, 47*, 57–63.

Pennington, L., & McConachie, H. (2001). Interaction between children with cerebral palsy and their mothers: The effects of speech intelligibility. *International Journal of Language and Communication Disorders, 36*, 371–393.

Pennington, L., Thomson, K., James, P., Martin, L., & McNally, R. (2009). Effects of It Takes Two to Talk—The Hanen Program for parents of preschool children with CP: Findings from an exploratory study. *Journal of Speech, Language and Hearing Research, 52*, 1121–1138.

Peterson, K., Reichle, J., & Johnston, S. (2000). Examining preschoolers' performance in linear and row-column scanning techniques. *Augmentative and Alternative Communication, 16*, 27–36.

Ratcliff, A., Koul, R., & Lloyd, L. (2008). Preparation in augmentative and alternative communication: An update for speech-language pathology training. *American Journal of Speech-Language Pathology, 17*, 48–59.

Reichle, J., & Brady, N. (2012). Teaching pragmatic skills to individuals with severe disabilities. In S. Johnston, J. Reichle, K. Feeley, & E.

Jones (Eds.), *AAC for individuals with moderate to severe disabilities* (pp. 3–24). Baltimore, MD: Paul H. Brookes.

Reichle, J., Halle, J., & Johnston, S. (1993). Developing an initial communicative repertoire: Applications and issues for persons with severe disabilities. In A. P. Kaiser & D. B. Gray (Eds.), *Enhancing children's communication: Research foundations for intervention* (pp. 105–138). Baltimore, MD: Paul H. Brookes.

Romski, M. A., & Sevcik, R. A. (1996). *Breaking the speech barrier: Language development through augmented means.* Baltimore, MD: Paul H. Brookes.

Romski, M. A., & Sevcik, R. A. (2003). Augmented input: Enhancing communication development. In J. Light, D. Beukelman, & J. Reichle (Eds.), *Communicative competence for individuals who use AAC: From research to effective practice* (pp. 147–161). Baltimore, MD: Paul H. Brookes.

Romski, M. A., & Sevcik, R. A. (2005). Augmentative communication and early intervention: Myths and realities. *Infants and Young Children, 18*(3), 174–185.

Schlosser, K. W., Belfiore, P. J., Nigam, R., Blischak, D., & Hetzroni, O. (1995). The effects of speech output technology in the learning of graphic symbols. *Journal of Applied Behavior Analysis, 28,* 537–549.

Sigurdardottir, S., & Vik, T. (2011). Speech, expressive language, and verbal cognition of preschool children with cerebral palsy in Iceland. *Developmental Medicine and Child Neurology, 53,* 74–80.

Smith, J. L., McCarthy, J. W., & Benigna, J. P. (2009). The effect of high tech AAC system position on the joint attention of infants without disabilities. *Augmentative and Alternative Communication, 25*(3), 165–175.

Treviranus, J., & Roberts, V. (2003). Supporting competent motor control of AAC systems. In J. C. Light, D. R. Beukelman, & J. Reichle (Eds.), *Communicative competence for individuals who use AAC: From research to effective practice* (pp. 199–240). Baltimore, MD: Paul H. Brookes.

White, A., Carney, E., & Reichle, J, (2010). Group-item and directed scanning: Examining preschoolers' accuracy and efficiency in two augmentative communication symbol selection methods. *American Journal of Speech-Language Pathology, 19,* 311–320.

York, J., & Weimann, G. (1991). Accommodating severe physical disabilities. In J. Reichle, J. York, & J. Sigafoos (Eds.), *Implementing augmentative and alternative communication: Strategies for learners with severe disabilities* (pp. 239–255). Baltimore, MD: Paul H. Brookes.

CHAPTER 11

Literacy Challenges and Early Intervention for Children Using Aided Communication: Starting Well

Martine M. Smith

Introduction

As you made your way through this book, you may have encountered some new ideas, or gained a new perspective on some things you already knew; you may have found yourself disagreeing with some of the issues raised or perspectives offered, or thinking of specific clients you have worked with; at times you may have found it hard to keep track of ideas and have taken notes to support your retention of what you have read. It is far less likely that at any point you found yourself thinking about how you were doing any of those things—how you were reading. It's only wh#n w# d# str#ng# th#ngs t# t#xt that competent readers and writers have to focus on the *process* of reading and writing. It is only then that the complexity of these skills and the scale of the achievement of becoming literate are apparent.

As competent readers and writers, we take these skills for granted. If you are reading this text, it is likely that there is nothing exceptional about your abilities in relation to your peers. However, if you had a medical diagnosis of cerebral palsy and limited speech intelligibility and were reading this text, you would be exceptional. Despite the impressive progress that has been made in technology, in diagnosis, and in our understanding of what is needed to learn to read and write, little has changed in the prevalence of literacy difficulties in this group over the past 3 decades. The rate of these difficulties is estimated to be as high as 90% for children with severe physical involvement (Andrade, Haase, & Oliveira-Ferreira, 2012).

The vulnerability of this group was recognized as long ago as 1956, when Schonell reported a clear and negative correlation between extent of physical impairment associated with cerebral palsy and reading achievement (Schonell, 1956). Over 20 years ago, Berninger and Gans profiled the literacy difficulties of children with severe speech impairments secondary to cerebral palsy, highlighting the disproportionate nature of these difficulties when literacy-related skills such as language and cognitive skills were taken into account (Berninger & Gans, 1986). Since then, many other studies have provided evidence that children with cerebral palsy and severe speech impairments seem uniquely vulnerable to difficulties in learning to read and write (Dahlgren Sandberg, 1998, 2001, 2006; Dahlgren Sandberg & Hjelmquist, 1996b; Foley, 1993; Koppenhaver & Yoder, 1992; McNaughton, 1998; Smith, 1989). However, there is also evidence that some individuals can achieve full literacy skills, despite similar levels of physical and speech impairments (Bishop & Robson, 1989; Dahlgren Sandberg, Smith, & Larsson, 2010; Erickson, Koppenhaver, & Yoder, 2002; Foley & Pollatsek, 1999; Smith, 1992; Smith, Dahlgren Sandberg, & Larsson, 2009).

It seems clear that children with cerebral palsy and dysarthria are at significant risk for literacy difficulties, but that neither the presence of cerebral palsy nor limited speech intelligibility necessarily prevents these children from learning to read and write. Understanding what makes literacy learning so challenging and how best to support these skills in this group is particularly important. Children with severe dysarthria often require the use of augmentative and alternative communication (AAC) techniques to supplement or replace their natural speech so that they can communicate functionally. The motor impairments of the groups discussed in this book mean that they frequently rely on aided communication (i.e., use of an external support, such as a communication board, a speech generating device, or a keyboard) where vocabulary is stored external to the user. Because the vocabulary exists external to the user, it is typically chosen by someone else, organized and arranged in space by someone else, and operates under capacity limitations that are very different from the internal structure of lexical organization of natural speakers. Vocabulary is limited to what can be displayed or organized and accessed at any one point.

Learning to read and spell unlocks access to an unlimited vocabulary store that can be selected directly by an aided communicator. Although spelling may be a very slow method of communication, being able to spell means an aided communicator can independently select and store vocabulary, prepare messages in advance, and retain unambiguous authorship of communication messages. Learning to read and write therefore has particular significance for children with cerebral palsy and severe speech impairments.

This chapter will start by outlining briefly the multilayered processes involved in reading and writing. Some of what we know about the challenges experienced by children with cerebral palsy will then be explored, leading to some suggestions about intervention approaches that have an established evidence base for speaking children. The main focus in this chapter is on the early stages of becoming literate, partly because this represents the foundation of later skill development and partly because this is the stage that has received the most research attention with this group. Two caveats are important at this point. One is that there is no such thing as a "typical" user of AAC or aided communicator. Children with cerebral palsy who use aided communication are a heterogeneous group, whose physical similarities should not blind us to the different cognitive, sensory, motivation, and attention abilities they present, not to mention the diverse personal interests that each brings to the task of learning to read and write (Smith, 2005). The second caveat is that much of what we have learned about the challenges and successes they may experience is based on the study of small numbers of individuals, often with contradictory findings.

Reading, Writing, and Development

Reading is often described as a multilayered process, meaning there are several interrelated activities that must work seamlessly together. Cunningham (1993) outlines three sets of interrelated constructs involved in silent reading comprehension—the kind of reading you are likely engaging in here. In this model, word identification, language comprehension, and print processing must integrate together. Each of these constructs is also multi-layered. Words can be identified directly (as single wholes) or through part-to-whole assembly, where each component sound/group of letters is identified and assembled to create the whole word. Test your word identification skills.

Word Identification Activities

As a fluent reader, you are probably seldom aware of having to identify words. The next few tasks demonstrate the many skills you draw on, usually unconsciously, but that can become explicit if needed. The solution to these activities is presented at the end of the chapter.

See how easily you can decode the following sentences:

1. d#l#t#ng v#w#ls fr#m w#rds d##sn't #ff#ct r##d#ng n##rly #s m#ch #s l##v#ng ##t c#ns#n#nts

2. #ea#i## #o### #i## #o #o##o#a### #s #u## #o#e #i##i#u##

3. Using the key below, decode the following short sentence:

   Φ§¡¢ΔΨ¶ Ψ§∩ ∩ξΦ¢φ #¡Ψ €§ †¡Φ¢

   Key:

   a = ¡   b = €   c = #   d = ¢   e = §   g = ¶
   h = †   i = Δ   n = Ψ   o = ξ   r = Φ   s = φ   w = ∩

   If all your reading were like this, you probably would choose to read as little as possible.

4. See if you can pronounce the following nonsense word. As you pronounce it, think about how you are managing to construct a pronunciation.

agroughtfercationalisationing

Language comprehension involves comprehension of individual words, comprehension of the relationships of words to each other within a given sentence, comprehension of sentence relationships in the context of a text structure, and integration of all of these elements with comprehension of the content domain. The Comprehension Activities that follow illustrate some of these processes.

Reading and Language Comprehension Activities

1. The text below contains a word in Irish (Gaelic). If you can read Irish, you can skip this task. If not, see if you can work out the meaning of the word "peann"—pronounced *pee-own*, rhyming with "town." When you work it out, think about all the resources you drew on to work out the word puzzle. The meaning of "peann" is presented at the end of the chapter.

   Gerard put the peann in his mouth. He rolled it between his teeth and chewed slowly. Something wasn't quite right. He needed more ideas. Suddenly a strong taste almost took his breath. He quickly pulled the peann back out. It was leaking! Blue ink dripped onto his fingers.

2. Read the following two sentences:

   I like to read crime fiction
   The last book I read was the best in the series

   You probably pronounced "read" differently in the two sentences. What triggered the change in pronunciation for you?

Finally, print processing "consists of everything that reading requires beyond word identification and language comprehension" (Cunningham, 1993, p. 36). This construct has at least four subconstructs: eye movement strategies, print-to-meaning links, inner speech, and integration.

Print Processing Activities

Look at the following sentence:

A woman without her man is nothing

Can you position commas in two different points to create contrasting meanings? Then consider the attention to print that is necessary to distinguish these contrasting meanings. A discussion is found at the end of this chapter.

Each of these layers develops over time, in response to specific experiences, both incidental and strategically structured. Some of the processes are often described as "bottom-up," that is, involving the assembly of a whole from individual subunits, as happens in mediated word identification. Other elements (particularly language comprehension) are regarded as "top-down," where higher level processing guides and limits decisions, such as when knowledge of syntax allows a reader to fill in gaps or predict elements within a text to support word identification.

Explanations of Literacy Difficulties

Vellutino and colleagues (2004) categorized explanations of reading and writing difficulties in children with dyslexia under four broad themes. Biological explanations focus on neuroanatomical and neurobiological similarities and differences between good readers and struggling readers. Cognitive explanations focus on the processing capacity of the child, addressing issues such as language processing, phonological processing, and working memory capacities that are known to underpin effective and efficient reading and writing. Both of these major themes place the child in center focus, understanding literacy problems in terms of factors intrinsic to the child that may make the task of learning to read and write more difficult. However, literacy development rarely happens spontaneously. Children are born into cultures where literacy is assigned a particular role (and in Western cultures that role is strategically important), and they experience literacy in culturally determined ways. Reading and writing are skills that do not simply emerge—they are specifically taught. Vellutino and colleagues suggest that far too little attention has focused on experiential and instructional explanations of literacy difficulties, especially as these explanations address factors that are extrinsic to the child, are amenable to explicit manipulation, and that therefore offer particular opportunities for intervention.

Although these four themes have been described in relation to children with dyslexia, they resonate well with what we know about the literacy difficulties of children with cerebral palsy. They will serve to structure the discussion in the remainder of this chapter. As with children with dyslexia, the emphasis in research for children with cerebral palsy using AAC has focused initially on within-child explanations of their difficulties. Less emphasis has been placed on the external factors associated with the experience and instruction themes.

Biological Explanations of Reading and Writing Difficulties

Reading and writing are cognitive activities, but they also rely on integration of sensory and perceptual information. All cognitive activities are closely linked to brain function, and considerable research efforts have been invested in understanding the specific neurological bases of reading difficulties. Brain structure and function along with the genetic endowment of the reader influence the task of becoming literate (Vellutino et al., 2004). One brain structure, in particular, has been studied. It is the planum temporale, on the temporal lobe, which has been reported as being atypically symmetrical in the brains of individuals with dyslexia. This area of the brain supports language functions, and so the structural symmetry noted for some individuals with dyslexia is viewed as a partial cause of language difficulties resulting in dyslexia (Vellutino et al., 2004). From the point of view of brain function, neuroimaging studies have suggested differences in activation of areas of the angular gyrus during reading tasks in individuals with dyslexia, when compared to their typically developing peers (Vellutino et al., 2004). There is also a growing body of evidence that reading skills are strongly influenced by genetics, again hinting at a neurological bases for written language difficulties.

Taken together, these three strands offer a convincing argument that brain function and structure are important factors in determining the potential of any individual to attain mastery of a complex cognitive skill such as reading. Children with cerebral palsy, by definition, present with notable structural and functional differences in their brains. In all likelihood, the greater the extent of the damage (as evidenced by more significant motor impairment), the greater the risk of reading difficulties. This is well-documented by Schonell (1956) and supported by others (Andrade et al., 2012). Thus we can argue that children with cerebral palsy have a high risk of brain structure and function differences that may pose specific challenges for them in learning to read. However, given the lack of consensus on the specific neuroanatomical structures or functions that are essential in learning to read, and the widely varied profile of neurological differences presented by children with cerebral palsy, it seems unlikely that these differences represent the only explanation for the pervasive difficulties in learning to read that are reported for this group.

Cognitive Explanations of Reading and Writing Difficulties in Cerebral Palsy

The question of cognitive differences is probably the area that has received the greatest attention in relation to the reading difficulties of children and adults with cerebral palsy. Research efforts have focused on language processing, speech processing, and working memory differences that have been explored as explanations of literacy difficulties.

Language Processing and Literacy Difficulties in Children with Cerebral Palsy

As reading and writing involve the construction of meaning from print, oral language and communication skills are fundamental in the process of becoming a reader–writer. Difficulties with oral language skills impact particularly on reading comprehension (Nation & Snowling, 2000; Vellutino et al., 2004). The language and communication experiences of children with cerebral palsy who use AAC are very different from those of their naturally speaking peers. We know that these children tend to have fewer opportunities to communicate than their peers (Kraat, 1987; Smith, 1998), and that they are generally less successful than their speaking partners in conversations (Basil, 1992; Light, Collier, & Parnes, 1985a; Udwin & Yule, 1991). Speaking partners tend to dominate conversations, so that aided communicators may have limited opportunities to develop narrative skills or to make extended contributions within dialogues (Björck-Åkesson, 1990; von Tetzchner & Martinsen, 1996). Such narrative and discourse skills may provide an important base for written language development.

The output of many aided communicators is characterized by a reliance on single symbol selections (e.g., Basil, 1992; Brekke & von Tetzchner, 2003). And there is a developmentally slow transition to multisymbol utterances with an apparent lack of development of internal linguistic structure in symbol output (Blockberger & Sutton, 2003; Hjelmquist & Dahlgren Sandberg, 1996; Smith, 1998; Udwin & Yule, 1991) This raises concerns about underlying syntactic and morphological skills.

In many cases it is almost impossible to work out whether these differences: (i) reflect performance constraints (i.e., limited vocabulary and slow rates of communication prompt aided communicators to maximize efficiency by using only single symbol selections and relying on their partner to fill in the gaps); (ii) are an accurate reflection of their underlying language abilities (i.e., if they could speak, their output would be very similar); or (iii) are linked to the unique features of communicating using graphic symbols (Smith & Grove, 2003). It is also unclear what impact these different language experiences might have on the language system that aided communicators construct internally:

Is practice in using language structure important in becoming masters of those language structures? This question is far too wide-ranging to be explored further here, but it is worth bearing in mind that many theories of language acquisition stress the important role of children themselves in constructing their own language systems (e.g., Tomasello, 2003).

There is some evidence that children with very limited speech experience specific difficulties with acquiring aspects of syntax and morphology, at least in relation to English (Binger & Light, 2008; Blockberger & Johnston, 2003) and that similar morphological and syntactic processing problems have been linked to specific difficulties with reading comprehension in children who are speaking (Snowling, 2000). So it may be that even if children who use aided communication come to the task of learning to read and write with biological bases that are comparable in all respects to their peers, their language learning experiences create barriers that interrupt their progress. Some of these barriers may be directly linked to language skills (e.g., having limited knowledge of syntactic structures may make it more difficult to use sentence structure to guide word identification). Other barriers may be indirect, in that children's access to language may affect the learning experiences they are offered and the ways in which they can access those experiences.

One final point to remember is that as children progress through the primary school years, much of their later language learning of complex syntax and of vocabulary comes from their reading (Nagy & Anderson, 1984; Nippold, Allen, & Kirsch, 2001; Rasinski, 2003). Whereas language difficulties may create barriers to literacy learning, literacy difficulties may constrain later language development, creating a negative cycle of mutual influence.

Speech Processing and Literacy Difficulties in Children with Cerebral Palsy

One of the most obvious differences that sets children with cerebral palsy who use aided communication apart from their peers is their speech impairment, and early research focused primarily on this aspect as a possible explanation for literacy difficulties. In particular, attention has focused on aspects of phonological processing and the relationship between severe speech difficulties and the ability to consciously think about phonological structure. In part, this interest is driven by the overwhelming evidence that the ability to think about the sound structure of language and to link those skills to letter knowledge is critically important in learning to read and write within an alphabetic orthography (e.g., National Institute of Child Health and Human Development, 2000; Shanahan & Lonigan, 2010). These skills are crucially important for word identification, particularly in English, where the relationship between sounds and letters is not always predictable. For example, the letter sequence "-ed" can be pronounced /t/ (as in kicked), /d/ (as in peeled), or /ud/ as in "wanted," whereas the sequence "-ough" offers even more variation (think of cough, bough, enough, through, though, thought). Without word identification skills, comprehension cannot proceed. Although children must develop a set of words they can recognize as wholes, or sight words, the sheer range of words they are likely to encounter means that they must also be able to tackle new words strategically, through breaking words down into their component sounds or syllables, and re-synthesizing those elements into a recognized word.

Most of the research that has been carried out with English-speaking children with cerebral palsy and severe speech impairments has highlighted problems in the development of the ability to segment words into phonemes, or into larger units such as onsets (i.e., all the sounds before a vowel in a syllable) and rimes (the sounds that come after the vowel) or syllables (e.g., Smith, 1989, 2001; Smith et al., 2009; Vandervelden & Siegel, 1999, 2001). Comparable difficulties have been reported for many Swedish-speaking children (Dahlgren Sandberg & Hjelmquist, 1996a, 1996b, 1997, 2002; Larsson & Dahlgren Sandberg, 2008b). If children cannot "sound out" letters of words, or convert letters into phonological representations, then word identification is challenging, and the inner speech referred to by Cunningham (1993) may not develop.

One of the ways in which speaking children are thought to develop these sounding out, blending, and segmenting skills is through subvocal articulation. One hypothesis that has been explored is whether the presence of a severe speech impairment might constrain the development of subvocal articulation. Findings have been equivocal, with some studies finding that articulatory coding is not contingent on speech production ability (e.g., Bishop & Robson, 1989; Foley & Pollatsek, 1999), whereas other studies have pointed to a relationship between the degree of speech impairment and phonological processing skills (Peeters, Verhoeven, de Moor, & van Balkom, 2009). These latter findings seem to suggest that severe speech difficulties represent an important risk factor, but of themselves do not preclude the development of phonological processing skills.

Many of the studies with these children have highlighted the fact that, although as a group they tend to do more poorly on tests of phonological processing than their speaking peers, there is a wide range of abilities (Card & Dodd, 2006; Dahlgren Sandberg et al., 2010; Foley & Pollatsek, 1999; Smith et al., 2009). Moreover, some studies have hinted that, even with relatively strong phonological processing skills, children with cerebral palsy who use aided communication do not always seem to reap the benefits of these strengths in terms of positive impacts on reading and spelling (e.g., Dahlgren Sandberg, 2006). For example, in the study reported by Smith et al. (2009), phonological awareness skills were strongly correlated with reading and spelling for the naturally speaking group of children, but this pattern was not replicated for the children with cerebral palsy. In Dahlgren Sandberg's (2006) longitudinal study, children with cerebral palsy using aided communication made progress in developing phonological processing skills, but these gains were not reflected in improved reading or spelling—unlike their peers who were matched for mental age. Phonological awareness skills may be necessary, but they are certainly not sufficient to allow word identification skills to develop.

Working Memory and Literacy Difficulties in Children with Cerebral Palsy

Working memory is another cognitive process that is known to be important in reading and spelling (Baddeley, 2003; Cohen-Mimran & Sapir, 2007; Vanderberg & Swanson, 2007) and difficulties with working memory have been found to distinguish between good and poor readers (e.g., Alloway, 2009; Gathercole, Alloway, Willis, & Adams, 2006; Muter & Snowling, 1998). Although work in this area is still only emerging, there is some evidence to suggest that children with severe speech impairments are also vulnerable to difficulties with working memory (Dahlgren Sandberg, 2001; Larsson & Dahlgren Sandberg, 2008a; Taibo, Iglesias, Mendez, & Raposo, 2009). It seems plausible that the ability to subvocally rehearse supports working memory, and therefore severe speech difficulties may constrain working memory by impacting articulatory processes (Hulme, Thomson, Muir, & Lawrence, 1984). However, this hypothesis has only limited support from research evidence to date (e.g., Bishop & Robson, 1989).

So far it seems clear that cognitive processes related to language, speech, and working memory are all important to reading and writing development and that difficulties with these cognitive skills are likely to impact a child's ability to achieve full literacy skills easily. We also know that children with cerebral palsy who use AAC are particularly vulnerable to difficulties with these cognitive skills and so are at high risk of poor literacy development. There is some evidence to indicate that even if they do develop these foundation skills, the predicted benefit for learning to read and write does not always materialize. Finally, these statements, of course, are only generalizations. There are many individuals with cerebral palsy and severe speech impairments who are expert, even gifted reader–writers (e.g., Nolan, 1987). Furthermore, many children without cerebral palsy who have language or speech processing difficulties nonetheless learn to read and write. They do so because their needs are recognized, and specific instructional and environmental supports are put in place to scaffold their learning. Cognitive explanations therefore can only be part of the picture.

Experiential Explanations of Reading and Writing Difficulties in Cerebral Palsy

Reading and writing are learned skills—they rarely, if ever, emerge spontaneously. Instead, children encounter particular experiences that pique their interest in print; they become enculturated into a particular literacy community, and they become reader–writers according to culturally dictated norms. As pointed out by Vellutino and colleagues (2004, p. 21), "research suggests that the brain and the environment, either through instruction or some other form of early literacy support, *interact* to produce the neural networks that must be in place to mediate the unique component of reading—word recognition" (italics added). What is particularly important about environmental and instructional explanations of literacy difficulties is that these are arenas where changes can be made, and the impact of these changes can be monitored. Unlike neuroanatomical or cognitive explanations, experiential and instructional explanations are amenable to direct manipulation and examination, and they therefore offer a more productive starting point for redirecting the literacy learning pathways of children who are struggling with literacy.

Emergent literacy researchers (Clay, 1991; Sulzby & Teale, 1991; Teale & Sulzby, 1989) have drawn attention to the many ways in which very young children are immersed in reading and writing. These children learn about the many purposes of print, the conventions such as orientation, the distinction between words and pictures, the scripts of storybook reading, and the unique features of the printed word. Many young children come to formal education already able to recognize many single words, recite the alphabet, identify some letters, and distinguish between writing and drawing. They have absorbed this information through natural interactions with adults and older siblings. Shared storybook reading is argued by many to represent a particularly important context for this learning (Teale & Sulzby, 1987; van Kleeck, 2008; Yaden, Smolkin, & Conlon, 1989).

These learning experiences may differ in important ways for children who have limited speech and who rely on aided communication, including many children with cerebral palsy. At a very basic level, even if these children are immersed in the same learning contexts, they may not be able to access the learning opportunities. Physical impairments may mean that a child cannot independently take a pencil or crayon and scribble, and through that scribbling come to recognize and master the difference between letters, numbers, and drawing. Visual impairments may mean that even if these opportunities are potentially available, a child may not be able to access the learning. Visual acuity and visuomotor difficulties are very common in cerebral palsy (Costa & Ventura, 2012; Duckman, 1987), with estimates ranging as high as 70% (Fazzi et al., 2012).

These challenges may also be difficult to identify and manage. Even if a child is positioned on an adult's lap for story reading, the print information from the book may not be visible or accessible, due either to visual difficulties or to poor head control, so that the incidental learning that is so important for typically developing children may not be available. Finally, communication difficulties may further constrain the learning experiences of children with cerebral palsy who use aided communication. Naturally speaking children play an important role in directing the behavior of the adults around them. As anyone who interacts with preschool children can attest, children can be very assertive about what they choose to have read to them, and how, when, and where it is read. Adults may plead for a change of storybook, but often unsuccessfully. This drive to read the same story multiple times is not simply a reflection of desiring control over adults. In their initial encounter with a new story, children tend to be quiet listeners. It is only when they have heard the story several times that they can engage in talk about and around the story, ask questions, seek clarifications, make predictions, take on roles within the story, and generally create the rich language environment that is pivotal to the learning experience and to the emergence of proto-reading (Clay, 1991; Teale & Sulzby, 1987; van Kleeck, 2008).

Creating comparable opportunities for young children with cerebral palsy is difficult. For one thing, every activity throughout the day takes longer if a child has a significant physical impairment—washing, dressing, eating, drinking, and playing as well as reading. There are also far more time constraints, with a range of ancillary needs to be considered, and many other pulls on caregivers' priorities (Light & Kelford-Smith, 1993; Peeters, Verhoeven, van Balkom, & de Moor, 2009). Within storybook reading, it is extraordinarily difficult to maintain an interactive dialogue while at the same time trying to position a child who has high physical dependency needs, support access to aided communication, and position a book so that it is visible. The greater the level of physical involvement, the harder the juggling act (Peeters Verhoeven, de Moor, van Balkom, & van Leeuwe, 2009), whereas the greater the level of speech impairment, the greater the challenge of scaffolding the dialogue to ensure effective participation in storybook reading (Light, Binger, & Kelford-Smith,

1994; Peeters, Verhoeven, de Moor, van Balkom, & van Leeuwe, 2009). If the child is using aided communication, predicting what vocabulary might be needed to interact around a particular story and ensuring that that vocabulary is available and understood by the child is often simply impossible. Similar practical difficulties emerge with writing, which creates even higher motor demands. Coordinating physical positioning and writing materials and encouraging independent writing activities at the same time stretches the abilities of even the most skilled facilitators.

Given the many demands and pressures, parents of children with both motor and speech impairments may postpone expectations for literacy until a child has started school, prioritizing communication and physical needs in the early years (Light et al., 1994). Alternatively, they may simply not be aware of what is reasonable to expect in terms of how children might participate in literacy activities such as storybook reading (Peeters, Verhoeven, van Balkom, et al., 2009).

When Light et al. (1994) compared the home literacy experiences of children with severe developmental disabilities using aided communication with their age-matched speaking peers, one of the most noticeable differences was that parents of children using AAC were less likely to engage in repeated readings of stories, compared to the parents of typically developing children. If these repeated readings are important to enable a child to exploit the language and literacy learning opportunities of storybook reading, then it is important to ensure that children with cerebral palsy using aided communication can be as assertive as their speaking peers in insisting on repeated readings of the same stories. Caregivers need to be encouraged to offer choices of books, even those that they really hope a child will not pick. Their role as literacy models and tutors needs to be recognized and valued to the same extent as their role as communication partners.

Furthermore, we need to exploit the environmental adaptations that can be made to maximize the literacy learning opportunities that can emerge naturally. In light of the above research findings, a number of intervention recommendations suggest themselves, including:

1. *Prioritize the creation of a print-rich learning environment to maximize the incidental literacy learning opportunities*

for children with cerebral palsy who use aided communication. A key step toward building literacy learning experiences involves ensuring that children have access to a range of different books and writing materials. Some books offer repeated lines that can easily be recorded onto single message devices if the child uses AAC. In this way, the child can actively participate in the story. Other books offer rhyming or alliteration experiences so that children can access enjoyable sound play activities. Yet others scaffold narrative skills or factual information, important for language and learning. Children benefit from many different kinds of books, so they need access to a range of learning opportunities.

Writing is equally important. Caregivers may need encouragement to support children in drawing, scribbling, and writing, using whatever materials are accessible. Some children can manipulate thick crayons if their seating is well supported and if they have access to some physical support. Others may need total physical support but may still benefit from the direct experience of seeing a mark appear on a page as they physically move a pen. These experiences are unlikely to be sufficient to replicate the writing experiences of their typically developing peers. Therefore, alternative access to generating print through keyboard or drawing activities or through eye gaze to visually displayed letters should also be considered. Low-tech or no-tech solutions are more likely to be manageable within a home environment or in instances where there is only a short period of time available and should always be part of the range of solutions put in place to maximize access to writing.

2. *Emphasize the importance of shared storybook reading.* Storybook reading is enjoyable for parents and children alike. Ironically that very factor may lead parents to overlook its power to foster interest and motivation in reading and to build language and print skills that can have lifelong benefits (Shanahan & Lonigan, 2010). Reinforcing the value of this activity and validating caregiver roles in supporting early literacy, as well as encouraging caregivers to set aside specific time each day to savor the pleasure of reading with their child, may enhance the range and frequency of literacy experiences available to young aided communicators.

3. *Consider the physical and visual needs of the aided communicator.* To offer an increasing range of literacy experiences in and of itself is pointless, unless those experiences are accessible to the developing child. It's important therefore to think about the physical and visual challenges to be faced. Adaptations including enlarged print, page separators, alternative formats, and print settings may be necessary. Careful positioning is always important, as has been highlighted elsewhere within this book. Often, optimal positioning for physical functioning involves supported seating, perhaps with hip and head supports. However, such positions may not work well in supporting the intimacy that is part of shared storybook reading. Finding a balance between the physical needs and the communication intimacy that is a hallmark of shared storybook reading may involve some element of compromise and guidance from many members of the team.

Team support may also be essential in order to work out the optimal positioning to facilitate visual access. We cannot presume that materials are visually accessible, and often it is important to ensure that auditory input is provided (e.g., naming letters in an array; labeling elements in a picture or on a page) to compensate for possible visual difficulties.

4. *Maximize active participation in literacy activities.* Children participate actively through their physical engagement (holding the pen, turning the page) but more crucially through their communication. Supporting this kind of active engagement involves flexibility and creativity on the part of interventionists and caregivers alike. One strategy involves ensuring that children have access to the vocabulary they need to participate and to talk about storybooks being read to them. It is unrealistic to expect to provide all potential vocabulary for the wide range of books children may access. However, as noted above, children often seek to return to particular books multiple times, and it is these books that should be prioritized when developing text-specific vocabulary displays.

There is an important set of vocabulary that is linked to the script or process of storybook reading, a set that is generic and predictable and that can transfer across many different books—vocabulary for control of the process (e.g., *more, stop, turn the page, read it again, what's that?, my turn*). These vocabulary elements can be incorporated into a storybook reading vocabulary chart, onto which story-specific vocabulary may or may not be added. Having multiple copies of such vocabulary charts located where books are housed may take one more burden off the caregivers.

Repeated lines in storybooks may be recorded quickly and easily onto single-message speech-generating devices, to allow a child to play the role of the narrator or a key character in a book. Finally, evidence from speaking children suggests that it is the repeated reading experience that enables them to change and extend their active participation in storybook reading (Teale & Sulzby, 1987). Supporting adults to offer repeated opportunities with the same text to children is important. Caregivers should be reminded that each repetition provides an opportunity to add another piece to the overall picture—the "repetition with variety" advocated so eloquently by Erickson and Carter (2006).

Instructional Explanations of Reading and Writing Difficulties in Cerebral Palsy

Reading and writing abilities emerge in response to very specific environmental and instructional supports. It has been argued that the literacy difficulties encountered by children with dyslexia reflect teaching failures as much as learning difficulties, and it seems likely that similar factors are at play in the case of many children who use aided communication. Many teachers may only encounter one child who uses aided communication within their classroom and may feel unprepared for the unique requirements of that child. Expectations for a child's literacy progress may be limited (Peeters, Verhoeven, & de Moor, 2009) and become self-limiting (Mirenda, 2003). However, research evidence suggests that children with severe physical impairments and who use aided communication *can* learn early core literacy skills, including phoneme segmentation and blending (Clendon, Gillon, & Yoder, 2005; Johnston, Davenport, Kanarowski, Rhodehouse, & McDonnell, 2009) and can learn to map these skills to word identification and generation (Fallon, Light, McNaughton, & Hammer, 2004). What is important, therefore, is that we draw on the available evidence to construct interventions that scaffold early literacy learning experiences.

There is now a substantial body of evidence that indicates that for children learning an orthography such as English, a specific emphasis on phonemic awareness and building sound-letter knowledge is an important building block for effective word identification skills (Adams, 1990; Shanahan & Lonigan, 2010). In the early literacy interventions reviewed by the National Early Literacy Panel (2008), code-focused interventions that help children to understand and apply the alphabetic principle (i.e., that sounds in words are represented by unique letter representations) demonstrated moderate to strong effects on literacy outcomes, particularly word identification and phonological awareness. In other words, these are skills that are important for reading and spelling, and they are skills that can be targeted successfully in focused interventions. Improving skills in these areas has a positive impact on reading and spelling (National Institute of Child Health and Human Development [NICHHD], 2000) for all children.

Furthermore, the National Reading Panel (2000) identified the characteristics of successful intervention programs. The interventions that demonstrated the greatest effects were characterized by a focus on specific skills—especially phoneme segmentation and analysis. Interventions delivered in small groups were more effective than those that involved large groups of children. They also found that interventions did not need to be prolonged. The greatest effect sizes were found for interventions that ranged between 5 and 18 hours, in total, across a school year. In other words, more was not necessarily better. This finding dovetails nicely with the idea that children need a critical mass of awareness of sounds and letters, but then they must move on. They need to apply this knowledge to more sophisticated word skills as well as to other dimensions of reading and writing that emphasize comprehension and fluency. The specific time required to reach this "critical mass" may vary, particularly for children with cerebral palsy. However, the principle to remember is that the acquisition of these skills is but one step along the pathway to literacy.

Code-focused instruction is not a literacy intervention program, but it is an important ingredient within such a program. Finally, The Reading Panel noted that computer-supported interventions demonstrated similar effects to teacher-delivered programs, but only when physical access was not a problem. In other words, as long as children did not need to focus on *how* they engaged in computer-assisted instruction, they could garner the benefits of playing sound and letter games mediated through technology. However, if physical access was difficult, the benefits were significantly reduced.

What do these findings mean for our interventions with young children with cerebral palsy who use aided communication? Given the evidence of a high risk of phonological processing difficulties in children with severe speech impairments, the inclusion of focused interventions addressing these skills seems particularly important. Preliminary studies (Clendon et al., 2005; Johnston et al., 2009; Truxler & O'Keefe, 2007) with children using AAC suggest that following these same principles, that is, structuring interventions carefully to address specific phonological processing skills and linking these interventions to print activities, can be effective. They are effective whether incorporated into naturalistic learning opportunities (Johnston et al., 2009) or through specific instruction (Blischak, Shah, Lombardino, & Chiarella, 2004), even for children with significant speech and physical impairments. Such interventions can also benefit word identification and early spelling skills (Fallon et al., 2004), provided that the targets are carefully selected and intervention is structured and consistent. In addition, adaptations to materials and response modalities must ensure that children can focus their attention on the cognitive task of learning, rather than the physical demands of participating in learning activities.

Two caveats are in order. One is that not all children seem to benefit equally, even with well-structured and focused interventions. Each of the studies cited above included participants who made surprisingly little progress when compared with their coparticipants. In most cases, researchers suggested that additional cognitive difficulties made the challenge of integrating print and phoneme processing skills more complex for these participants. This finding highlights the importance of constant monitoring of learning. It also underscores the importance of recognizing the many different challenges that young aided communicators may face when learning to read and write and hence the need for differentiated and individualized intervention planning.

A second caveat is that, at least in the study reported by Clendon et al. (2005), successful participants tended to learn only the specific targets presented, with little evidence of transfer of this knowledge to new words. This finding resonates with the preliminary evidence that building phonological awareness skills does not automatically translate into enhanced reading and spelling for aided communicators in the way that we might expect with typically developing children (Dahlgren Sandberg, 2006; Smith et al., 2009). Clearly, what is important is not that children learn to identify specific words, but that they acquire strategies to attempt to identify all words.

It is only when children have consolidated a critical mass of knowledge about strategies that they are in a position to actively engage in independent word identification, starting them off on the track of self-teaching proposed by Share (1995). The implications of this caveat are similar to the first—presumptions based on naturally speaking children may not apply to children with cerebral palsy who use aided communication. Vigilance must be exercised concerning what children are learning and how they can apply what they have learned. Nonetheless, the studies above provide an important road map. They suggest that by addressing our attention to instruction and by drawing on the substantial evidence base that now exists about the kind of instruction that is most effective, we can support children with cerebral palsy who use aided communication. We can guide them along the path toward word identification skills that can serve as the foundation for effective reading and spelling.

Conclusions and Summary

There is no question that children with cerebral palsy who use aided communication face many challenges in developing effective reading and writing skills. Some of these challenges reflect the underlying set of resources they bring to the task of becoming literate—the physical, sensory, perceptual, cognitive, and linguistic resources available to them. Vellutino et al. (2004) argue for a model of gradation of risk factors for reading difficulties, incorporating the particular assortment of reading-related cognitive (and sensory) abilities with which the child is endowed, and the degree to which the child's home and school environments tailor supports to scaffold that unique skill-mix and configuration of needs. The more heavily weighted the risk factors, the greater the need for strong environmental scaffolds. For children in the early stages of engaging with literacy learning, key elements of that scaffolding include generating interest in print and fostering motivation to learn by maximizing exposure to pleasurable literacy experiences in the privileged context of shared storybook reading. Building language and communication skills is fundamental to increasing access to participation in those experiences.

Part of the process of engaging with print is learning about the sound structure of the target language. The risk factor in relation to phonological processing skills may be particularly heavily weighted for children with severe speech impairments. Structured interventions targeting these skills are important, and there is emerging evidence that they can be successful. However, phonological awareness is not reading; it is simply one (important) strut in the scaffold. The scaffold is also not the end goal—scaffolds serve a purpose related to some other structure; they are a means to an end. It is important, therefore, to pay attention also to that end goal and to monitor the impact of our interventions and scaffolds on the final prize of effective literacy development.

10 Principles for Improving Intervention

1. Children with cerebral palsy who use aided communication are at high risk for reading and spelling difficulties because of their physical, sensory, perceptual, language, and cognitive vulnerabilities.
2. The presence of a severe speech impairment does not necessarily limit a child's progress in learning to read and spell.

3. Environmental and instructional adaptations must be configured to reflect the unique set of skills presented by each child, tailored to reflect each child's physical, sensory, language, and cognitive abilities.

4. Reading and writing are language-based skills. Intervention must target building language and communication skills to support transition to written language.

5. Shared storybook reading offers a privileged context to support language and literacy development. Multiple opportunities to engage with the same text offer repetition with variety and should be a key target of intervention.

6. Participation in storybook reading should be active. Active participation requires access to appropriate communication resources.

7. Children learning to read and write English need to be able to consciously reflect on sounds and letters, to analyze the sound structure of words, and to map that analysis onto letter knowledge. These skills are crucial for word identification.

8. Building phonological awareness requires focused, structured intervention. This intervention should target both phonological awareness and letter knowledge, simultaneously.

9. Phonological awareness is not reading. It is one important component of effective reading instruction. Skills in phonological awareness should be linked to authentic literacy experiences to ensure that the benefits of enhanced phonological awareness skills are realized in terms of improved word identification and spelling. Writing is an important support for building phonological awareness and letter knowledge.

10. Reading and writing are multilayered, complex activities. Developing mastery can take a long time. Children will only persist with the journey if literacy learning is enjoyable, rewarding, and motivating. Building motivation and interest in literacy is the most important step on the journey.

Think Critically for Self-Study or Classroom Discussion

1. Some studies have found that children using aided communication have particular difficulties with morphology. Why might this be relevant to literacy learning?
2. How might severe dysarthria impact the development of phonological awareness?
3. Name two ways in which active participation in storybook reading might be scaffolded for children with cerebral palsy who use aided communication.
4. Why should an SLP attend to letter knowledge in working with a young child with cerebral palsy who uses aided communication?
5. What are three critical ingredients of an early literacy intervention program for a child with cerebral palsy who uses aided communication?

SOLUTIONS

Word Identification Solutions

1. Deleting vowels from words doesn't affect reading nearly as much as leaving out consonants
2. Reading words with no consonants is much more difficult
3. Reading new words can be hard
4. You probably pronounced it in segments ag-rought-fer-cation-al-is(-)ation-ing, using the groupings of known letter patterns to segment the word into manageable chunks. This strategy involves a sophisticated use of orthographic knowledge.

Comprehension Solutions

1. "Peann" is the Irish word for pen. You may have initially thought that it was a kind of food, but probably quickly

discarded that hypothesis on the basis of the first couple of sentences.

2. The morphological markers of tense were the likely cues for you to change pronunciation from "read" (rhyming with reed) to "read" (rhyming with red). Most likely, by the time you had read the first two words of the second sentence, you were already "hearing" the correct pronunciation in the second sentence. Consider the range of language skills that you drew on for this task.

Print Processing Solutions

A woman without her man, is nothing

A woman, without her, man is nothing

References

Adams, M. J. (1990). *Beginning to read: Thinking and learning about print.* Cambridge, MA: MIT Press, A Bradford Book.

Alloway, T. P. (2009). Working memory, but not IQ, predicts subsequent learning in children with learning difficulties. *European Journal of Psychological Assessment, 25*(2), 92–98.

Andrade, P. M., Haase, V. G., & Oliveira-Ferreira, F. (2012). An ICF-based approach for cerebral palsy from a biopsychosocial perspective. *Developmental Neurorehabilitation, 15,* 391–400.

Baddeley, A. D. (2003). Working memory and language: An overview. *Journal of Communication Disorders, 36,* 189–208.

Basil, C. (1992). Social interaction and learned helplessness in severely disabled children. *Augmentative and Alternative Communication, 8,* 188–199.

Berninger, V., & Gans, B. (1986). Language profiles in nonspeaking individuals of normal intelligence with severe cerebral palsy. *Augmentative and Alternative Communication, 2,* 45–50.

Binger, C., & Light, J. (2008). The morphology and syntax of individuals who use AAC: Research review and implications for effective practice. *Augmentative and Alternative Communication, 24,* 123–138.

Bishop, D. V. M., & Robson, J. (1989). Unimpaired short-term memory and rhyme judgment in congenitally speechless individuals: Implications for the notion of "Articulatory Coding." *The Quarterly Journal of Experimental Psychology, 41A*(1), 123–140.

Björck-Åkesson, E. (1990, August 12–16). *Communicative interaction of young physically disabled nonspeaking children and their parents.* Paper presented at the Fifth Biennial Meeting of the International Society of Augmentative and Alternative Communication (ISAAC), Stockholm, Sweden.

Blischak, D., Shah, P., Lombardino, L., & Chiarella, K. (2004). Effects of phonemic awareness instruction on the encoding skills of children with severe speech impairment. *Disability and Rehabilitation, 26*, 1295–1304.

Blockberger, S., & Johnston, J. (2003). Grammatical morphology acquisition by children with complex communication needs. *Augmentative and Alternative Communication, 19*, 207–221.

Blockberger, S., & Sutton, A. (2003). Toward linguistic competence: Language experiences and knowledge of children with extremely limited speech. In J. Light, D. Beukelman, & J. Reichle (Eds.), *Communicative competence for individuals who use AAC* (pp. 63–106). London, UK: Paul H. Brookes.

Brekke, K. M., & von Tetzchner, S. (2003). Co-construction in graphic language development. In S. von Tetzchner, & N. Grove (Eds.), *Augmentative and alternative communication: Developmental issues* (pp. 176–210). London, UK: Whurr.

Card, R., & Dodd, B. (2006). The phonological awareness abilities of children with cerebral palsy who do not speak. *Augmentative and Alternative Communication, 22*, 149–159.

Clay, M. M. (1991). *Becoming literate.* Portsmouth, NH: Heinemann Education Books Limited.

Clendon, S., Gillon, G., & Yoder, D. E. (2005). Initial insights into phoneme awareness intervention for children with complex communication needs. *International Journal of Disability, Development and Education, 52*(1), 7–31.

Cohen-Mimran, R., & Sapir, S. (2007). Deficits in working memory in young adults with reading disabilities. *Journal of Communication Disorders, 40*, 168–183.

Costa, M. F., & Ventura, D. F. (2012). Visual impairment in children with spastic cerebral palsy measured by psychophysical and electrophysiological grating acuity tests. *Developmental Neurorehabilitation, 15*, 414–424.

Cunningham, J. W. (1993). Whole-to-part reading diagnosis. *Reading and Writing Quarterly, 9*, 31–49.

Dahlgren Sandberg, A. (1998). Reading and spelling among nonvocal children with cerebral palsy: Influences of home and school literacy environment. *Reading and Writing, 10*, 23–50.

Dahlgren Sandberg, A. (2001). Reading and spelling, phonological awareness and short-term memory in children with severe speech production impairments—a longitudinal study. *Augmentative and Alternative Communication, 17*, 11–26.

Dahlgren Sandberg, A. (2006). Reading and spelling abilities in children with severe speech impairments and cerebral palsy at 6, 9, and 12 years of age in relation to cognitive development: A longitudinal study. *Developmental Medicine and Child Neurology, 48*, 629–634.

Dahlgren Sandberg, A., & Hjelmquist, E. (1996a). A comparative, descriptive study of reading and writing skills among non-speaking children: A preliminary study. *European Journal of Disorders of Communication, 31*, 289–308.

Dahlgren Sandberg, A., & Hjelmquist, E. (1996b). Phonologic awareness and literacy abilities in nonspeaking preschool children with cerebral palsy. *Augmentative and Alternative Communication, 12*, 138–154.

Dahlgren Sandberg, A., & Hjelmquist, E. (1997). Language and literacy in nonvocal children with cerebral palsy. *Reading and Writing: An Interdisciplinary Journal, 9*, 107–133.

Dahlgren Sandberg, A., & Hjelmquist, E. (2002). Phonological recoding problems in children with severe congenital speech impairments —the importance of productive speech. In E. Witruk, A. Friederici, & T. Lachmann (Eds.), *Basic mechanisms of language and language disorder*. Dordrecht, The Netherlands: Kluwer Academic.

Dahlgren Sandberg, A., Smith, M., & Larsson, M. (2010). An analysis of reading and spelling abilities of children who use AAC: Understanding a continuum of competence. *Augmentative and Alternative Communication, 26*(3), 191–202.

Duckman, R. (1987). Visual problems in cerebral palsy. In E. McDonald (Ed.), *Treating cerebral palsy* (pp. 105–132). Austin, TX: Pro-Ed.

Erickson, K., & Carter, J. (2006). *Reading, writing, and word study for adolescents and adults with significant disabilities who are beginning readers and writers*. Retrieved Februrary 15, 2013, from http://www.med.unc.edu/ahs/clds/files/conference-hand-outs/Rte66Presentation.pdf

Erickson, K., Koppenhaver, D., & Yoder, D. E. (2002). *Waves of words: Augmented communicators read and write*. Toronto, Canada: ISAAC Press.

Fallon, K., Light, J., McNaughton, D., & Hammer, C. (2004). The effects of direct instruction on the single-word reading skills of children who require augmentative and alternative communication. *Journal of Speech, Language, and Hearing Research, 47*, 1424–1439.

Fazzi, E., Signorini, S., La Piana, R., Bertone, C., Misefari, W., Galli, J., . . . Bianchi, P. E. (2012). Neuro-ophthalmological disorders in cerebral palsy: Opthalmological, oculomotor and visual aspects. *Developmental Medicine and Child Neurology, 54,* 730–736.

Foley, B. E. (1993). The development of literacy in individuals with severe congenital speech and motor impairments. *Topics in Language Disorders, 13,* 16–32.

Foley, B. E., & Pollatsek, A. (1999). Phonological processing and reading abilities in adolescents and adults with severe congenital speech impairments. *Augmentative and Alternative Communication, 15,* 156–173.

Gathercole, S. E., Alloway, T. P., Willis, C., & Adams, A. M. (2006). Working memory in children with reading disabilities. *Journal of Experimental Child Psychology, 93,* 265–281.

Hjelmquist, E., & Dahlgren Sandberg, A. (1996). Sounds and silence: Interaction in aided language use. In S. von Tetzchner & M. Jensen (Eds.), *Augmentative and alternative communication: European perspectives* (pp. 137–152). London, UK: Whurr.

Hulme, C., Thomson, N., Muir, C., & Lawrence, A. (1984). Speech rate and the development of short-term memory span. *Journal of Experimental Child Psychology, 38,* 241–253.

Johnston, S., Davenport, L., Kanarowski, B., Rhodehouse, S., & McDonnell, A. (2009). Teaching sound letter correspondence and consonant-vowel-consonant combinations to young children who use augmentative and alternative communication. *Augmentative and Alternative Communication, 25,* 123–135.

Koppenhaver, D., & Yoder, D. E. (1992). Literacy learning of children with severe speech and physical impairments in school settings. *Seminars in Speech and Language, 12,* 4–15.

Kraat, A. (1987). *Communication interaction between aided and natural speakers: A state of the art report.* Madison, WI: Trace Research and Development Center.

Larsson, M., & Dahlgren Sandberg, A. (2008a). Memory ability of children with complex communication needs. *Augmentative and Alternative Communication, 24,* 139–148.

Larsson, M., & Dahlgren Sandberg, A. (2008b). Phonological awareness in Swedish-speaking children with complex communication needs. *Journal of Intellectual and Developmental Disabilities, 33*(1), 22–35.

Light, J., Binger, C., & Kelford Smith, A. (1994). Story reading interactions between preschoolers who use AAC and their mothers. *Augmentative and Alternative Communication, 10,* 255–268.

Light, J., Collier, B., & Parnes, P. (1985a). Communicative interaction between young nonspeaking physically disabled children and their primary caregivers: Discourse patterns. *Augmentative and Alternative Communication, 1,* 74–83.

Light, J., & Kelford-Smith, A. (1993). The home literacy experiences of preschoolers who use augmentative communication systems and of their nondisabled peers. *Augmentative and Alternative Communication, 9,* 10–25.

McNaughton, S. (1998). *Reading acquisition of adults with severe congenital speech and physical impairments: theoretical infrastructure, empirical investigation, education implication.* (Unpublished doctoral dissertation). University of Toronto, Toronto, Canada.

Mirenda, P. (2003). "He's not really a reader . . . " Perspectives on supporting literacy development in individuals with autism. *Topics in Language Disorders, 23*(4), 271–282.

Muter, V., & Snowling, M. (1998). Concurrent and longitudinal predictors of reading: The role of metalinguistic and short-term memory skills. *Reading Research Quarterly, 33*(3), 320–343.

Nagy, W. E., & Anderson, R. C. (1984). How many words are there in printed school English? *Reading Research Quarterly, 19,* 304–330.

Nation, K., & Snowling, M. (2000). Factors influencing syntactic awareness skills in normal readers and poor comprehenders. *Applied Psycholinguistics, 21,* 229–241.

National Early Literacy Panel. (2008). *Developing early literacy: Report of the National Early Literacy Panel.* Washington DC: National Institute for Literacy.

National Institute of Child Health and Human Development. (2000). *National Reading Panel. Teaching Children to Read: An evidence-based assessment of the scientific research literature on reading and its implications for reading instruction* (NIH Publication No. 00-4769). Washington DC: Government Printing Office.

Nippold, M., Allen, M., & Kirsch, D. (2001). Proverb comprehension as a function of reading proficiency in preadolescents. *Language Speech and Hearing Services in Schools, 32,* 90–100.

Nolan, C. (1987). *Under the eye of the clock: The life story of Christopher Nolan.* New York, NY: St Martin's Press.

Peeters, M., Verhoeven, L., & de Moor, J. (2009). Teacher literacy expectations for kindergarten children with cerebral palsy in special education. *International Journal of Rehabilitation Research, 32*(3), 251–259.

Peeters, M., Verhoeven, L., de Moor, J., & van Balkom, H. (2009). Importance of speech production for phonological awareness and word decoding: The case of children with cerebral palsy. *Research in Developmental Disabilities, 30,* 712–726.

Peeters, M., Verhoeven, L., de Moor, J., van Balkom, H., & van Leeuwe, J. (2009). Home literacy predictors of early reading development in children with cerebral palsy. *Research in Developmental Disabilities, 30,* 445–461.

Peeters, M., Verhoeven, L., van Balkom, H., & de Moor, J. (2009). Home literacy environment: characteristics of children with cerebral palsy. *International Journal of Language and Communication Disorders*, 44(6), 917–940.

Rasinski, T. (2003). *The fluent reader*. New York, NY: Scholastic Professional Books.

Schonell, F. E. (1956). *Educating spastic children: The education and guidance of the cerebral palsied*. London, UK: Oliver & Boyd.

Shanahan, T., & Lonigan, C. (2010). The National Early Literacy Panel: A summary of the process and the report. *Educational Researcher*, 39, 279–285.

Share, D. L. (1995). Phonological recoding and self-teaching: *Sine qua non* of reading acquisition. *Cognition, 55*, 151–218.

Smith, M. (1989). Reading without speech: A study of children with cerebral palsy. *Irish Journal of Psychology, 10*, 601–614.

Smith, M. (1992). Reading abilities of nonspeaking students: Two case studies. *Augmentative and Alternative Communication, 8*, 57–66.

Smith, M. (1998). *Pictures of language: The role of picture communication symbols in the language acquisition of children with severe speech impairments.* (Unpublished doctoral dissertation). Trinity College Dublin, Dublin, Ireland.

Smith, M. (2001). Literacy challenges for individuals with severe congenital speech impairments. *International Journal of Disability, Development and Education, 48*, 331–353.

Smith, M. (2005). *Literacy and augmentative and alternative communication*. London, UK: Elsevier Academic Press.

Smith, M., Dahlgren Sandberg, A., & Larsson, M. (2009). Reading and spelling in children with severe speech and physical impairments: A comparative study. *International Journal of Language and Communication Disorders, 44*(6), 864–882.

Smith, M., & Grove, N. (2003). Asymmetry in input and output for individuals who use AAC. In J. Light, D. R. Beukelman, & J. Reichle (Eds.), *Communicative competence for individuals who use AAC: From research to effective practice.* (pp. 163–195). Baltimore, MD: Paul H. Brookes.

Snowling, M. (2000). Language and literacy skills: Who is at risk and why? In D. V. M. Bishop & L. B. Leonard (Eds.), *Speech and language impairments in children* (pp. 245–260). Hove, East Sussex, UK: Psychology Press.

Sulzby, E., & Teale, W. (1991). Emergent literacy. In R. Barr, M. Kamil, P. Mosenthal, & D. Pearson (Eds.), *Handbook of reading research* (Vol. 2, pp. 727–757). New York, NY: Longman.

Taibo, M., Iglesias, P., Mendez, M., & Raposo, M. (2009). A descriptive study of working memory, phonological awareness and literacy performance of people who use AAC. *International Journal of Special Education, 24*(1), 1–20.

Teale, W., & Sulzby, E. (1987). Literacy acquisition in early childhood: The roles of access and mediation in storybook telling. In D. A. Wagner (Ed.), *The future of literacy in a changing world* (pp. 111–130). New York, NY: Pergamon Press.

Teale, W., & Sulzby, E. (1989). Emergent literacy: New perspectives on young children's reading and writing. In D. Strickland & L. M. Morrow (Eds.), *Emerging literacy: Young children learn to read and write* (pp. 1–15). Newark, DE: International Reading Association.

Tomasello, M. (2003). *Constructing a language: A usage-based theory of language acquisition.* Cambridge, MA: Harvard University Press.

Truxler, J., & O'Keefe, B. (2007). The effects of phonological awareness instruction on beginning word recognition and spelling. *Augmentative and Alternative Communication, 23*(2), 164–176.

Udwin, O., & Yule, W. (1991). Augmentative communication systems taught to cerebral palsy children—a longitudinal study. 1: The acquisition of signs and symbols and syntactic aspects of their use over time. *British Journal of Disorders of Communication, 25,* 295–309.

van Kleeck, A. (2008). Providing preschool foundations for later reading comprehension: The importance of and ideas for targeting inferencing in storybook-sharing interventions. *Psychology in the Schools, 45*(7), 627–643.

Vanderberg, R., & Swanson, L. H. (2007). Which components of working memory are important in the writing process? *Reading and Writing, 20,* 721–752.

Vandervelden, M., & Siegel, L. (1999). Phonological processing and literacy in AAC users and students with motor speech impairments. *Augmentative and Alternative Communication, 15,* 191–211.

Vandervelden, M., & Siegel, L. (2001). Phonological processing in written word learning: Assessment for children who use augmentative and alternative communication. *Augmentative and Alternative Communication, 17,* 11–26.

Vellutino, F. R., Fletcher, J. M., Snowling, M., & Scanlon, D. (2004). Specific reading disability (dyslexia): What have we learned in the past four decades? *Journal of Child Psychology and Psychiatry, 45*(1), 2–40.

von Tetzchner, S., & Martinsen, H. (1996). Words and strategies: Communicating with young children who use aided language. In S. von Tetzchner & M. H. Jensen (Eds.), *Augmentative and alternative communication: European perspectives* (pp. 65–88). London, UK: Whurr.

Yaden, D. B., Smolkin, L. B., & Conlon, A. (1989). Preschoolers' questions about pictures, print convention, and story text during reading aloud at home. *Reading Research Quarterly, 24*(2), 188–214.

CHAPTER 12

Commentary on Evidence-Based Practice and NDT

Fran Redstone

Evidence-Based Practice

In 2000 Sackett and his colleagues devised a system that scrutinized studies to determine their level of evidence for medicine. Through this system the authors propose that the best evidence is produced by randomized controlled trials (RCT) (Dijkers, Murphy, & Krellman, 2012) whereas lower levels of evidence are found in case reports and expert opinions (Tomlin & Borgetto, 2011). The American Speech, Language, and Hearing Association (ASHA) cites evidence-based practice (EBP) as an approach to clinical decision making in which research evidence is used along with practitioner expertise and client values (Elman, 2007). However, Steele (2004) notes that in medicine there is actually only evidence for about 30% of a physician's activities.

In 2005 ASHA stated that the impetus for EBP was the perceived limitation of expert opinion. More recently, though,

ASHA (2013) cited "expert opinion" first in its statement advocating EBP. In addition, Sackett makes it quite clear that external "evidence can inform, but can never replace, individual clinical expertise" (1997, p. 4). It is important to keep this in mind when evaluating interventions for a group that is chronically understudied, such as children with cerebral palsy. In addition, there is little evidence at this point in time that EBP is effective (Dijkers et al., 2012; Jenicek, 2006; Larner, 2004).

A positive aspect of EBP is that it encourages professionals to question why techniques are employed (Jenicek, 2006) and suggests areas that require more study (Butler & Darrah, 2001). Some authors have proposed a broadening of the definition of "evidence" to include experience and observation, along with experimental research (Jenicek, 2006) whereas others have suggested changing the model. Tomlin and Borgetto (2011) describe a research pyramid that includes a method of evaluating qualitative research often used in clinical disciplines. These authors "assert that trustworthy evidence of different types can be discovered through disciplined inquiry, and all are important to the profession" (p. 193).

As clinicians we need to remember that some perceived truths and standard treatments that seemed well founded in evidence were later determined to be equivocal or untrue. Ratner (2006) reminds us of the inconsistent findings regarding nutrition and health over the last several years. In the early 1990s the intake of wine was discouraged. By the mid-1990s, however, it appeared that moderate consumption could be beneficial. More recent research indicates that red wine may reduce the incidence of breast cancer in women (DeAmicis et al., 2011). We need to exercise sound clinical judgment in making decisions in both our professional as well as our private lives.

The purpose of this chapter is to discuss the benefits and drawbacks of EBP in our field. It is not a balanced review of all NDT literature. This has been attempted elsewhere by others. I will be presenting evidence from a clinician's point of view, elucidating the drawbacks of using only Level I evidence for clinical decision making for children with cerebral palsy. This chapter should be considered a commentary on EBP and NDT rather than a comprehensive review.

EBP and Speech Pathology

Have you ever read an article in our field where the authors did not say that "more research is needed"? It's like a mantra. Evidence is apparently lacking or equivocal for speech intervention for childhood apraxia of speech (Ballard, 2001) and for augmentative and alternative communication (Clark & Clark, 2002). There is also widespread controversy concerning intervention approaches for speech sound disorders (Kamhi, 2006). Even studies of the benefits of early intervention in general have found few or modest results (Blauw-Hospers & Hadders-Algra, 2005; Majnemer, 1998). Steele (2004) asserts that there are very few worthwhile studies in many areas of our discipline to support our field's practice of them. Ratner (2006) states that our best evidence-supported treatments only demonstrate improvement for 50 to 70% of participants in the studies. There are those who claim that evidence is lacking to support speech therapy in general (Glogowska, Roulstone, Enderby, & Peters, 2000). It has even been suggested that practice (repetition of movement) may not be effective (Fetters & Kluzik, 1996). Others say that practice is essential. Clinical fields are rife with contradictions.

Evidence Regarding Interventions for Children with Cerebral Palsy

Evidence for treatments for individuals with cerebral palsy is lacking (Schertz & Gordon, 2009; Yorkston, 1996). In 2001 Butler and Darrah reviewed evidence for NDT in a report for the American Academy of Cerebral Palsy and Child Neurology (AACPCN). It is interesting to note that this is perhaps the most cited study about NDT. Butler and Darrah stated that their review "did not confer any advantage of NDT over the alternatives to which it was compared" (p. 789).

These authors qualify this statement and note that "an absence of evidence . . . should not be construed as proof that a treatment is not effective" (p. 778). It is particularly important for SLPs to note that this review included no studies of communication, respiration, language, speech, or feeding. Investigations of other treatments for children with cerebral palsy have found, as in the case of NDT, that there is no good published evidence to support or refute them (Darrah, Watkins, Chen, & Bonin, 2004; Salario et al., 2008).

Studies Supporting NDT

There are studies that demonstrate that NDT is supported for physical and occupational therapy outcomes. Some of these studies addressed outcomes that are important to SLPs. For example, the effect of NDT intervention on reaching was studied by Kluzik, Fetters, and Coryell (1990). Functional improvement was found after one session of treatment in five children with cerebral palsy. The ability to reach is an important component for SLPs in relation to aided communication use as well as object manipulation for language learning.

Trunk and postural control are often addressed by SLPs for both improved respiration for speech and increased head control for better oral functioning for speech and feeding. Trunk control was studied by Arndt and colleagues (2008) who compared infants in an NDT-based program with those in a structured parent/infant playgroup and found significant positive outcomes in children in the NDT program. Improved postural control was found by Girolami and Campbell (1994) in premature infants after being treated with NDT. Other studies addressing outcomes more specific to physical therapists have found positive improvements after NDT intervention (Adams, Chandler, & Schuhmann, 2000; Emby, Yates, & Mott, 1990; Knox & Evans, 2002; Trahan & Malauin, 1999). In fact, a meta-analysis by Ottenbacher and colleagues (1986) found small but positive changes using NDT.

Evidence for Non-NDT SLP Interventions for Children with Cerebral Palsy

SLP outcomes for children with cerebral palsy may be related to feeding, speech, respiration, and receptive language. A Cochrane

Review (Pennington, Marshall, & Goldbart, 2003) of techniques used to improve communication in children with cerebral palsy indicates that "evidence of their effectiveness is limited."

Traditional breath support interventions developed for physically typical children were used with children with cerebral palsy from 10 to 18 years of age (Pennington, Smallman, & Farrier, 2006). Although minimal results were found, these authors conclude that traditional interventions may be effective for some children. An adult-oriented, cognitive approach to improved phonation found significant improvement after an intensive 6-week program (Pennington, Miller, Robson, & Steen, 2010). These results were impressive but the techniques used are not appropriate for young children.

Pennington and her associates (2009) also studied the Hanen program to improve the interaction between mothers and children with cerebral palsy. After the training, positive results were found in the mothers' responsiveness whereas no changes were found in their dominance and the complexity of language. It is admirable that the authors acknowledged that adaptations should be made to the program for children with cerebral palsy.

Lee Silverman Voice Treatment (LSVT) was developed for adults with Parkinson's disease. Fox and Boliek (2012) studied the use of LSVT with children with cerebral palsy. Improvement in vocal functioning was found in two of the four children after intervention.

Evidence for NDT Speech Interventions

Is NDT effective? This is the $64,000 question. NDT, like other protocols for children with cerebral palsy, has scant evidence. However, perhaps one of the best ways to provide evidence for an approach such as NDT is to study specific NDT techniques. A colleague once told me, "Don't attempt to find the TRUTH, look for the truth." The point is to ask and answer smaller, clinically significant questions such as, "If I do this, will the child eat better?" Or be able to speak more words on one breath? Or be able to use direct selection for aided communication? There is evidence for the effectiveness of NDT speech techniques *but* NDT itself is seldom credited.

In the Cochrane Review of communication interventions for children with cerebral palsy (Pennington et al., 2003), NDT was not mentioned as a strategy studied, but several of the authors included in the analysis were NDT trained, NDT instructors, or used NDT principles in their research. Similarly, the review of respiratory treatment strategies for children with cerebral palsy by Solomon and Charron (1998) has one section on body positioning and another on NDT. Perhaps the authors were unaware that NDT practitioners were among the first speech professionals to emphasize positioning of children with cerebral palsy for the improvement of respiratory/phonatory development. They cite an important study by Nwaobi, Brubaker, Cusick, and Sussman (1983) that includes an NDT therapist and a chapter by Workinger and Kent (1991) that includes an NDT SLP. In addition, the article cites Redstone (1991), Folkman (1992), Alexander (1987), and Boehme (1988), all of whom have been certified as NDT instructors.

Feeding Therapy for Children with Cerebral Palsy

NDT feeding techniques were used long before ASHA acknowledged that swallowing was in the scope of practice for SLPs. The developer of the basic NDT speech treatment techniques was Helen Mueller who began her work in the 1960s and first wrote about NDT techniques for feeding and speech in 1972. Morris and Davis were two of the first NDT SLPs in the United States. They began writing in 1985 and 1987, respectively.

Prior to ASHA's embrace of feeding and swallowing, OTs met the need for feeding therapy. This explains why some very good scholarship has been provided by OTs in this area. However, in the 1970s and 1980s, SLPs who treated children with cerebral palsy who had feeding disorders began to gather and publish information about the anatomy, development, and process of swallowing.

It is important to note that many feeding techniques originally developed by NDT are now considered part of good practice. Most of what Arvedson and Brodsky (2002) cover in their section on management of feeding problems was initially developed by Mueller. Another example is Wolf and Glass (1992) who are occupational therapists who wrote about postural control for feeding and included many oral techniques developed by Mueller, including jaw control, oral stimulation, and vibration. These are all techniques documented by Mueller (1972) and taught in NDT courses. They are the basis of NDT speech therapy.

NDT Alignment for Feeding and Speech

Earlier in this book the importance of having a sound fundamental knowledge of both development and the assessment of head/trunk alignment for communication, language learning, and oral functioning were stressed. This is an area of overlap for OTs, PTs, and SLPs treating children with cerebral palsy. The need for positioning to provide adequate alignment has been acknowledged by our field, but rarely has NDT been recognized for pioneering its use by SLPs providing therapy to children with cerebral palsy. For example, in their book on pediatric feeding/swallowing, Arvedson and Brodsky (2002) write about development of oral skills for feeding and readily discuss posture for treatment but do not credit NDT.

Typically, the articles in ASHA journals addressing communication or feeding issues of children with cerebral palsy give lip service (pun intended) to its importance (Arvedson, Clark, Lazarus, Schooling, & Frymark, 2010; Pennington et al., 2009; Sheppard, 2005). However, Sheppard (2005) underscores the importance of postural support in sensori-motor therapy, and she, admirably, gives both Bobath and Mueller credit for being among the first to employ this principle in feeding and speech.

AAC is an area for which positioning has been emphasized. Several authors (Costigan & Light, 2011; McDonald & Schultz, 1973; McEwen & Lloyd, 1990) discuss seating, posture, the importance of pelvic stability, weight-bearing, and body alignment for AAC use. However, most authors give OTs and PTs primary responsibility for this. It is important that the speech professional be capable of making independent decisions concerning seating. A team approach is ideal but, in reality, it is not always possible on a daily basis. Additionally, if the treatment goals include language, speech, or feeding, the SLP should have the knowledge and skills to accomplish them.

There are a number of studies supporting the NDT principle of good positioning for various aspects of communication and feeding. Redstone (2005) researched respiratory patterns and syllable production, in upright and in semireclining, for both physically typical children and preschoolers with cerebral palsy. Although reclining made speech difficult for both groups, it was more difficult for the children with cerebral palsy. Hulme and her associates (1987, 1989) studied the effects of positioning on vocalization and feeding using adaptive equipment developed from NDT principles. The authors found a greater number of vocalizations and greater intake of food with improved posture resulting from the use of these NDT-inspired seating devices.

Pinder and her colleagues (1993, 1995) along with Olswang (1995) studied techniques to develop early language concepts for successful communicative interaction in children with cerebral palsy. They emphasized the influence of a motor foundation for the development of communication signals. Their treatment sessions included input from both a PT and SLP. Although Pinder, an NDT speech instructor, is quite capable herself of providing the stability and movement transitions needed during a session, she notes the benefits of cotreatment. But it is a rare luxury to have a PT or OT facilitate appropriate alignment, stability, and movements while an SLP focuses on communication. This is seldom available in the real world and typically not funded.

NDT-Oral Control

The significance of the development of jaw stability has been addressed in many articles. Because of the jaw's importance, the technique of jaw control, which is now called oral control, was developed by Mueller for NDT. The name change indicates that so much more is controlled when the jaw is stable. Oral control is used to provide stability to the jaw and aid in the maintenance of head/trunk alignment during feeding or speech therapy. It has been studied and found to be effective by several investigators (Boiron, Da Nobrega, Roux, Henrot, & Saliba, 2007; Einarsson-Backes, Deitz, Price, Glass, & Hays, 1994; Hill, Kurkowski, & Garcia, 2000) who credit NDT practitioners including Bobath, Mueller, and Morris for this approach.

Bias

Bias in research is defined as a systematic distortion of findings (Finn, 2006). This can take many forms. This section will present some areas of bias that have influenced the acceptance of NDT in academia. The preference for evidence from Level I studies, along with publication, editorial, funding, and interpretive biases is presented.

Preference for Level I Evidence

EBP states that Level I research such as randomized controlled trials (RCT), meta-analyses, and reviews are the best. However, these may not be appropriate for a clinical discipline such as speech-language pathology. Schlosser and Raghavendra (2004) note that there are concerns over the "tendency to declare research evidence to be the 'authority'" (p. 17). This diminishes the client and the clinician in decision making and neglects the benefits of qualitative research (Tomlin & Borgetto, 2011). Reviews and RCT are beneficial but should be considered as guideposts only (Kent, 2006; Montgomery & Turkstra, 2006).

In addition, Level I "meta-analysis is only as good as the studies that go into it" (Law, Garrett, & Nye, 2004, p. 935). Barry (2001) notes that the articles chosen for meta-analysis are based on subjective decisions, as is the interpretation of the results. This is highlighted by McCauley, Strand, Lof, Schooling, and Frymark (2009) in their review of oral motor exercises (OME). They note that a similar article (Lass & Pannbacker, 2008) was published during the time they were preparing their manuscript and only three articles overlapped. Clearly, the differing selections were based on subjective interpretation. Although both groups found insufficient evidence, one article recommended not using OME, whereas the other stated more impartially that there was insufficient evidence to support or refute OME use.

Another example of subjective bias in selection of articles is Arvedson et al.'s (2010) review of oral motor interventions for preterm infants. They do not include oral support as a target for their review although it is a technique that has long been recommended for infants in the NICU (Arvedson & Brodsky, 2002). It was developed by Mueller and found to be successful (Boiron et al., 2007; Einarsson-Backes et al., 1994; Hill et al., 2000; Hwang, Lin, Coster, Bigsby, & Vergara, 2010). However, it is not included in Arvedson et al.'s publication.

Level I studies have also been criticized because they do not provide sufficient clinically relevant information (Autti-Ramo, 2011). This may be one reason that RCTs are rarely performed in speech therapy. RCTs only reveal what is statistically significant, not what is clinically relevant (Dijkers et al., 2012; Montgomery & Turkstra, 2006). In addition, there is disagreement within the results of published RCTs (Ratner, 2006). McCullough (2006) also reminds us that just because clinical trials do not exist does not mean that evidence does not exist. This, then, suggests a corollary: just because a clinical trial exists does not mean that it provides any clinically important information.

A number of authors (ASHA, 2004; Bartlett & Palisano, 2000; Blauw-Hospers & Hadders-Algra, 2005; Fetters & Kluzik, 1996; Majnemer, 1998; Pennington, Marshall, & Goldbart, 2005) cite typical problems in producing Level I investigations. These include the need for large samples of homogeneous subjects and the measurement of easily quantifiable outcomes without regard to quality or improved function. These are central to research dealing with NDT and children with cerebral palsy.

Although evidence from case studies is considered a low level of evidence (ASHA, 2004), they still may be quite valuable in our field. They reveal individual differences among clients, which was demonstrated by Baker and Mcleod (2004). Their two case studies described the great variation of outcomes among similar children. This would not have been evident in a large Level I RCT.

Publication Bias

Elman (2007) notes that evidence may be lacking in certain fields due to funding and publication bias, which makes it difficult for researchers outside the "mainstream view" to get published or funded. Journals in our field address many types of disorders, their descriptions, assessments, and interventions. However, it appears that *treatment* of children with cerebral palsy is not a favored topic for publication.

Bias in Treatment Articles Dealing with Cerebral Palsy

In an editorial, Justice (2008) states that ASHA publishes far fewer articles covering treatment than in other areas, despite the fact that 81% of the members of the organization describe themselves as clinicians. Only 1% are researchers (Scott, Bahr, & Reardon-Reeves, 2009). Although the *American Journal of Speech-Language Pathology (AJSLP)* is considered to be the premier journal of SLP intervention in the United States, there is a lack of clinically relevant research published in this journal (Justice, 2008).

To further highlight this point, Bahr (2008) notes that although 78% of clinicians surveyed by ASHA said they deal with phonological disorders, only 4% of the articles published in *AJSLP* from 2004 to 2007 addressed phonology. There was a similar discrepancy for motor speech disorders. The only area in which this was reversed was for language/communication in which 47% of clinicians said they provide this service to clients, while 74% of the articles covered this area.

An examination of the reference list of Solomon and Charron's (1998) respiratory review article demonstrates this type of bias as it relates to treatment of children with cerebral palsy. In this article there are 104 references. Of these, 17 (16%) were published in ASHA journals after 1972. Only one of these dealt with treatment: an abstract from 1992 regarding inspiratory checking by Netsell and Hixon. All other articles referenced in this article from ASHA journals addressed normal function or general assessment—not treatment.

In addition, although there are many convention presentations and posters indicating an interest in cerebral palsy by ASHA members, only a few articles addressing treatments for children with cerebral palsy are published by ASHA. A search of ASHA's publications indicates that there are articles that describe or compare the speech and language of children with cerebral palsy to typical children (Ansel & Kent, 1992; Hustad, Gorton, & Lee, 2010; Hustad, Schueler, Schultz, & DuHadway, 2012) but few that address treatment approaches. For example, is it really necessary to conduct and *fund* a study to determine that the intelligibility of children with cerebral palsy is poorer than that of age-matched physically typical children (Hustad et al., 2012)? This seems like common sense. To their credit, the researchers explored other questions. However, this was their major finding.

There are a number of SLPs who are experts in the field of cerebral palsy, and although ASHA publishes a lot of expert opinion (Duffy, 2005; Duffy & Josephs, 2012; Kamhi, 2006; Kuehn, 1997), this does not occur in the area of cerebral palsy. It appears that feeding and communication for children with cerebral palsy has been ceded to other disciplines.

The one area that ASHA does address regarding children with cerebral palsy is AAC. An example is the article by Costigan and Light (2011) on the importance of proper seating. The article cited 61 references. But only two of these were from ASHA, and one was a policy statement. The second reference was also an article about seating for AAC (McEwen & Lloyd, 1990). It is notable that both of these articles are first-authored by an OT and a PT, respectively. Costigan and Light note that an SLP may "notice changes" (p. 234) but subsequently recommend that the SLP seek a professional who may be able to fix this. Although the team approach is indispensable, the ability to position a client for a communication function should be the responsibility of the SLP. The SLP must have the skills necessary to make adjustments in a child's posture so that the child may improve within a speech/feeding context.

I am reminded of a second-grade class observation I conducted recently of a child with spastic diplegia. This child was in a small class and was helped with a one-to-one aide. The youngster began to demonstrate frustration stemming from a lack of intelligibility. This resulted from a loss of stability, which led to poor trunk support. I quietly asked the aide if I could intervene and adjusted the foot support and pelvic positioning. The child sat upright and communicated better immediately. This probably took 1 minute. After the lesson, the aide thanked me and said she would remember what I showed her. There was no need to make a referral to another professional.

Editorial Bias

Necessarily, there are a small number of people who are journal editors and associate editors. However, this may lead to a
type of bias because all publication decisions are subjective.
Elman (2007) suggests that term limits be placed on this position in all ASHA journals. Another way to mitigate such bias is
to have reviewers unaware of the identity of the author. This is
called blind review and is employed by organizations such as the
American Occupational Therapy Association. This is not ASHA's
editorial procedure unless specifically requested. However, if
you are a new researcher, or one writing on a controversial topic,
how likely would you be to request a special editorial accom-
modation? Interestingly, the process in our field is half-blind,
which means that the authors of articles do not know who is
reviewing their submissions, but the reviewers are aware of the
authors' identities.

Again, using the references in the Solomon and Charron
(1998) article as an example, there is one writer who was either
first or second author in almost half of the 17 cited articles (47%)
from ASHA. In addition, the authors of the 17 articles from ASHA
publications were heavily represented on the editorial boards
of ASHA journals. For example, Hixon and colleagues, Hoit and
associates, Kent, Netsell, and Strathopoulos are represented in 13
of the 17 articles (76%). All have served on the editorial boards
of ASHA journals for several years. Another article addressing
descriptive, nontreatment issues of cerebral palsy (Hustad et
al., 2012) cites 16 articles published by ASHA. Thirteen of these
articles (81%) were by authors who had served on ASHA's editorial boards.

The reference list in Pennington et al.'s (2009) article studying an interaction treatment approach for children with cerebral
palsy also suggests bias. This article lists 100 references, only
12 of which were published in ASHA journals. None of these
articles deal with cerebral palsy directly, although several deal
with various developmental delays. Of the 12 ASHA articles, 9
(75%) had either first or second authors who were also editors
of ASHA journals.

Another recent article regarding LSVT for children with
cerebral palsy (Fox & Boliek, 2012) cites 54 articles. Thirteen
appeared in ASHA journals after 1970. Of these 13, nine (69%)

were authored by individuals on ASHA's editorial boards. Of the 13, only 3 were about cerebral palsy, and 2 of these were authored by individuals on ASHA's editorial boards. Do we see a pattern here?

The need for an editorial board is apparent, and I would like to acknowledge the work and time commitment that this entails. However, whether intentionally or otherwise, it appears that some authors are repeatedly published in ASHA journals. The editorial boards of ASHA publications heavily represent researchers who have laboratories and funding. And the problem becomes cyclical: realistically, no one is going to be funded without a reasonable number of publications. Herein lies the problem: Readers of ASHA journals are presented with a narrow range of viewpoints.

At ASHA, clinicians who attempt to share their considerable knowledge formed by years of observation and direct treatment with children, as opposed to those whose work is principally limited to conducting 12-week research studies, are rarely published, funded—or even recognized.

Interpretive/Confirmatory Bias

One insidious form of bias according to Feeney (2006) is when researchers evaluate data in favor of their hypotheses while ignoring its shortcomings or suggesting reasons why the expected results did not occur. We know from market research how much one can be influenced by the method of presentation. Again, it is important for both authors of articles and consumers of these articles to remember that lack of evidence for an intervention does not mean that the approach is ineffective.

Two examples of appropriate use of neutral terminology when no positive results are found are Cirrin et al.'s (2010) review of service provision models and Law et al.'s (2004) meta-analysis of language interventions. However, the use of bias in terminology has been noted in publications evaluating NDT. For example, Butler and Darrah (2001) did NOT report that NDT was ineffective. However, others cite their article as evidence of its ineffectiveness.

Stanger and Oresic's article (2003) demonstrates the power of terminology in their presentation of approaches for children with cerebral palsy. The first treatment they discuss is NDT and cite the "extensive report" (p. S82) by Butler and Darrah (2001) to conclude that there is "no strong evidence supporting the effectiveness of neurodevelopmental treatment for children with cerebral palsy" (p. S82). This is accurate except that they subsequently note that conductive education has not demonstrated any differences between samples either. BUT they go on to assert in quite positive terms that the underlying theory of conductive education makes it worthwhile. Constraint induced treatment (CIT) is discussed next, and again findings demonstrate no difference between groups. BUT the positive results found in adults treated with CIT is praised. These are two examples of interpretive bias.

Confirmatory bias is also evident in the article by Hielkema and colleagues (2011), who studied graduates of an NICU. One group of infants was treated with traditional PT that the authors state is NDT. The other group was treated with Coping with Caring (COPCA) which is a program with a motor component based on neuronal group selection theory (NGST). It becomes obvious that the authors had previously written extensively about NGST. Outcome scores for the two groups did not differ significantly although the outcome measurement, the Infant Motor Profile (IMP), was based on NGST. However, the authors conclude that the study "suggests" (p. e14) that motor development is improved using COPCA.

EBP-Research Versus the Clinic

Schlosser and Raghavendra (2004) note that good clinical practice may not be the same as good research. Research is funded for intensive treatment under well-controlled conditions. Clinicians do not have the freedom to apply a treatment in a predefined way to their clients and then withhold treatment from another group of children (Howle, 2002). In fact, it would be unethical for therapists to apply a treatment IF they did not believe the treatment to be optimal for the client.

Ideally, studies aim to be well designed with a high level of evidence. However, the clinical significance of a study may be elusive. Children with cerebral palsy have many difficulties that the SLP must address. This may be one reason why it is typical to use multiple intervention approaches with these children. However, multiple approaches are rarely researched and are often criticized for not being standardized (Butler & Darrah, 2001). However, that is exactly what good clinicians do—and should do. For example, the use of LSVT for children with cerebral palsy may be appropriate for a specific subgroup of these children, but there are few children with cerebral palsy who have vocal loudness as their primary speech-language goal. This protocol may, however, be a worthwhile supplement to other treatments. This is an example of the beneficial use of multiple approaches to address the specific needs of children.

The disparity between the clinic and academic world is often demonstrated by the lack of respect for clinicians in developing approaches based on the immediate needs of children. For example, many feeding techniques for infants and children were developed by clinicians because they recognized a need in their young clients although it was not being addressed in research. This occurred prior to ASHA's recognition of swallowing. However, this pragmatic approach has been considered a mistake (Ruark, 2004). In addition, although the sequence of developmental milestones are important, the need for "precise" developmental stages, as has been stated as a need by researchers, is viewed as unnecessary by clinicians because the range of "normal" is so great. Precise norms may, in fact, lead to unwarranted diagnoses and poor intervention decisions.

Example of Disparity Between Clinic and Research

I read a truly wonderful study on respiratory development. It was the study I wished I had done! I had conducted similar research using the same instrumentation and I understood the results. Yet, I vehemently disagreed with the authors' conclusions. Then I realized that we came to the study from completely different places: I from a strong clinical background and the researchers from the laboratory. That made all the difference. Both interpretations were right or both were wrong, but each had been influenced by our biases.

The "One-Size-Fits-All" Mistake

Many techniques and approaches for various clinical conditions have been researched, but the determination of what is best for which child has not been elucidated. We base our EBP decisions on the statistics that find the strategy to be effective on most of the individuals in a group. But there are always participants who do not benefit, and some who benefit only slightly. Studies and meta-analyses pool results despite any differences among individuals (Pennington et al., 2009; Ratner, 2006). It is important to realize that although a study did not demonstrate statistical evidence to support a technique, it may have been worthwhile for a percentage of the participants. Clinicians need to determine whether their specific client will benefit from a well-supported technique. Also, when evidence is lacking to support a technique, it may still be worthwhile for a specific client. It is imperative that decisions be made on the basis of each client's needs. This can be done through available research evidence in combination with "knowledge and reasoning" as well as intuition (Schlosser & Raghavendra, 2004, p. 3).

There is acknowledgment of this problem in many of the medical sciences. The Mayo Clinic notes that there was a time quite recently when hormone replacement therapy was considered to be a fountain of youth for menopausal women. Then new evidence suggested health risks and the treatment was discontinued (Ratner, 2006). Nonetheless, a new review suggests that this treatment may be a good choice for certain women after all (Mayo Clinic Staff, 2013).

In our field, Fox and Boliek's (2012) study using LSVT on children with cerebral palsy reports individual findings for its four participants and notes that two of their young participants benefited. Research needs to focus on the characteristics that made the intervention successful for these children. Clinicians need to determine if protocols might be worthwhile for their clients rather than assume they are not, solely because there is no Level I support. The former is practicing good EBP whereas the latter is considered "evidence-obsessed" (Larner, 2004, p. 28). Kent (2006) notes the importance of clinical experience as it relates to EBP. The important question is—who benefits from what intervention? Remember, these are the types of decisions that clinicians need to make daily.

Most good therapy involves combining approaches and techniques to best serve clients. In fact, Arvedson et al. (2010) note that approaches for infants in the NICU have evolved to become more individualized and include multiple interventions. This, however, makes it difficult for researchers to determine what is working. It is DIFFICULT. Could you imagine providing an intervention just to satisfy a researcher's need for consistency?! The purpose of professional publications is to give the clinician many, many, many options to choose from. An article or review should not give the impression that one study is THE answer. Just because an RCT may suggest that an intervention is worthwhile does not mean that it will work for every client.

Therapy or Therapist?

In the last several years, this question has arisen often (Kent, 2006; Ratner, 2006). Kent (2006) notes that the same technique used by two different therapists may have very different outcomes. This phenomenon has been referred to as nonspecific treatment effect. Ratner (2006) warns against the use of interventions without considering who is offering them. Providing a clinical service requires a combination of science and art (Larner, 2004). This is echoed by Howle (2002) when discussing NDT outcomes. She acknowledges that there is an art to good NDT intervention.

Do we really know what makes a good clinician? Most of us "know it when we see it" but cannot easily define it. To make this determination we typically gauge the progress achieved in therapy by our clients. However, the clinician's skill may also be apparent from the exercise of clinical judgment to determine the choice of interventions as part of EBP (Montgomery & Turkstra, 2006). Hopefully, this type of skill is learned in graduate education. It is definitely stressed in postgraduate training such as NDT with its emphasis on clinical problem solving.

As with ASHA, the quality of NDT therapists is maintained through certification. This indicates at least a minimum level of competency. Training for other continuing education (CE) certifications in our field such as LSVT or PROMPT can often be attained within a weekend. However, the basic NDT course requires the commitment of 40 hours a week for 8 weeks, during which time children are treated and constant feedback from instructors is provided. This is a far different model and considerably more extensive than most other CE certification courses.

Conclusions

NDT is a worthwhile intervention for children with cerebral palsy and is extremely valuable training for SLPs working with children with cerebral palsy. There is either very little or largely equivocal evidence for most SLP interventions, in general, and for interventions for children with cerebral palsy, in particular. Nonetheless, NDT has all the qualities that Sugden (2007) considers important for approaches that have equivocal evidence. An intervention should have good theoretical underpinnings, and it should target function, incorporate family, and encourage active participation of the child. NDT has all of these attributes. Moreover, NDT has as much evidence as any other approach for children with cerebral palsy or, for that matter, for SLP interventions in general.

The fact is, the use of multiple interventions is the best answer for children with cerebral palsy. The study by Pennington et al. (2006) found that the traditional interventions for breath control may be effective for *some* children with cerebral palsy. I suggest that these authors would have been more successful by incorporating NDT techniques to supplement the traditional respiratory interventions. Ratner (2006) notes that it is rare for a clinician to stick to a strict set of treatment techniques. There are similar findings in the area of physical therapy (Uyanik, Bumin, & Kayihan, 2003). NDT is but one approach in the therapeutic arsenal of the SLP working with children with cerebral palsy. It should be used along with other interventions (DeGangi & Royeen, 1994) which may or may not have strong evidence to support them, but are well founded and are based on reason, clinical judgment, and experience.

There are many interventions available in our field. We need to determine what works and for whom. What approach, technique, or combination of techniques is best for a specific client? Reviews, meta-analyses, and RCTs give us direction only. There is no one answer. Right now, it appears that too many educators and professionals in our field are trying to make it seem as if there is an answer. But no two clients, or clinicians, are the same. Therefore, no single procedure will work for every child, and a recipe approach is not suitable for our discipline. That is why NDT should be used along with the other interventions that SLPs learn in schools, in continuing education courses, and read about in journals. In addition, it is critical to evaluate one's work continually and make changes when necessary.

It is admirable that Sackett (1997), the father of EBM, states that "the practice of evidence-based medicine is a process of life-long, self-directed learning in which caring for our own patients creates the need for clinically important information" (p. 4). Law (as cited in Ratner, 2006) describes EBP as a "journey" (p. 262). We need to remember that although there is little well-documented support for NDT, this is equally true for many other treatment approaches and clinical disciplines. The NDT approach is, however, supported by several studies addressing motor skill development and speech–language techniques, as well as the prevailing theories of motor control and development.

Until we have the possibility of controlled studies, using approaches that are more clinically realistic with large numbers of homogenous participants, a treatment approach such as NDT is important. It is particularly significant for SLPs who rarely get the opportunity to learn about the influence of gross motor skills on speech control and language development.

Nine Items to Remember

1. EBP incorporates *clinical expertise*, the best research available, and client values.
2. Because insufficient evidence has been found to support a technique does not mean it is not worthwhile.

3. NDT is worthwhile because it has a good theoretical base; its techniques for SLPs have been studied although many are part of accepted practice; and it has as much evidence as other approaches or techniques.

4. If the best Level I evidence does not apply to your client, it is not worthwhile for that client. You need to evaluate this based on specific data from your client.

5. It is important to use good clinical judgment to evaluate techniques presented in courses or articles. Do not automatically accept any input, even from the most prestigious sources.

6. Individualization of any approach for every client is necessary.

7. There are inherent problems gaining valuable clinical information from Level I studies in our discipline. This includes a lack of information regarding individual participants and an inability to structure clinical sessions as described in studies.

8. There are few RCTs in our field due to the problems of running rigorous studies. There are many biases that influence studies, leading to questionable interpretations.

9. Cerebral palsy is a motor disorder. NDT is one approach for SLPs to address this disorder.

Think Critically for Self-Study or Classroom Discussion

1. Why is NDT an appropriate approach for children with cerebral palsy?

2. Why does it not have a good evidence base?

3. Describe how NDT might be used with other SLP interventions.

4. Why does our discipline have difficulty providing evidence for many techniques?

5. What are some sources of bias in research?

References

Adams, M. A., Chandler, L. S., & Shuhmann, K. (2000). Gait changes in children with cerebral palsy following a neurodevelopmental treatment course. *Pediatric Physical Therapy, 12,* 114–120.

Alexander, R. (1987). Oral-motor treatment for infants and young children with cerebral palsy. *Seminars in Speech and Language, 8,* 87–100.

American Speech, Language, and Hearing Association. (2004). *Evidence-based practice in communication disorders: An introduction* (Technical report). Retrieved March 11, 2013, from http://www.asha.org/policy/TR2004-00001.htm

American Speech, Language, and Hearing Association. (2005). *Evidence-based practice in communication disorders* (Position statement). Retrieved on March 11, 2013, from http://www.asha.org/docs/html/PS2005-00221.html

American Speech, Language, and Hearing Association. (2013). *Introduction to evidence-based practice: What it is (and what it isn't).* Retrieved on March 11, 2013, from http://www.asha.org/members/ebp/intro/

Ansel, B. M., & Kent, R. D. (1992). Acoustic-phonetic contrasts and intelligibility in the dysarthria associated with mixed cerebral palsy. *Journal of Speech and Hearing Research, 35,* 296–308.

Arndt, S. W., Chandler, L. S., Sweeney, J. K., Sharkey, M. A., & McElroy, J. J. (2008). Effects of a neurodevelopmental treatment-based trunk protocol for infants with posture and movement dysfunction. *Pediatric Physical Therapy, 20,* 11–22.

Arvedson, J. (n.d.). *Treatment efficacy summary.* Retrieved March 11, 2013, from http://www.asha.org/uploadedFiles/public/TESPediatricFeedingandSwallowing.pdf

Arvedson, J. C., & Brodsky, I. (2002). *Pediatric swallowing and feeding: Assessment and management* (2nd ed.). San Diego, CA: Singular.

Arvedson, J., Clark, H., Lazarus, C., Schooling, T., & Frymark, T. (2010). Evidence-based systematic review: Effects of oral motor interventions on feeding and swallowing in preterm infants. *American Journal of Speech-Language Pathology, 19,* 321–340.

Autti-Ramo, I. (2011). Physiotherapy in high-risk infants—a motor learning facilitator or not? *Developmental Medicine & Child Neurology, 53,* 200–202.

Bahr, D. (2008). A topical bibliography on oral motor assessment and treatment. *Oral Motor Institute, 2*(1). Retrieved February 28, 2013, from http://www.oralmotorinstitute.org/mons/v2n1_bahr.html

Baker, E., & Mcleod, S. (2004). Evidence-based management of phonological impairment in children. *Child Language Teaching & Therapy, 20*, 261–286.

Ballard, K. J. (2001). Principles of motor learning and treatment of AOS. *Neurophysiology and Neurogenic Speech and Language Disorders Newsletter, 11*, 13–18.

Barry, M. (2001). Evidence-based practice in pediatric physical therapy. *PT Magazine, 9*, 38–52.

Bartlett, D. J., & Palisano, R. J. (2000). A multivariate model of determinants of motor change for children with cerebral palsy. *Physical Therapy, 80*, 598–614.

Blauw-Hospers, C. H., & Hadders-Algra, M. (2005). A systematic review of the effects of early intervention on motor development. *Developmental Medicine & Child Neurology, 47*, 421–432.

Boehme, R. (1988). *Improving upper body control: An approach to assessment and treatment of tonal dysfunction.* Tucson, AZ: Therapy Skill Builders.

Boiron, M., Da Nobrega, L., Roux, S., Henrot, A., & Saliba, E. (2007). Effects of oral stimulation and oral support on non-nutritive sucking and feeding performance in preterm infants. *Developmental Medicine & Child Neurology, 49*, 439–444.

Butler, C., & Darrah, J. (2001). Effects of neurodevelopmental treatment (NDT) for cerebral palsy: An AACPDM evidence report. *Developmental Medicine & Child Neurology, 43*, 778–790.

Cirrin, F. M., Schooling, T. L., Nelson, N. W., Diehl, S. F., Flynn, P. F., Staskowski, M., . . . Adamczyk, D. F. (2010). Evidence-based systematic review: Effects of different service delivery models on communication outcomes for elementary school-aged children. *Language, Speech, and Hearing Services in Schools, 41*, 233–264.

Clark, E. G., & Clark, E. A. (2002). Using evidence-based practice to guide decision making in AAC. *Perspectives on Augmentative and Alternative Communication, 11*, 6–9.

Costigan, F., & Light, J. (2011). Functional seating for school-age children with cerebral palsy: An evidence-based tutorial. *Language, Speech, and Hearing Services in Schools, 42*, 223–236.

Darrah, J., Watkins, B., Chen, L., & Bonin, C. (2004). Conductive education intervention for children with cerebral palsy: An AACPDM evidence report. *Developmental Medicine & Child Neurology, 46*, 187–203.

DeAmicis, F., Giordano, F., Vivacqua, A., Pellegrino, M., Panno., M. L., Tramontano, D., . . . Andò, S. (2011). Resveratrol, through NF-Y/p53/sin#/HDAC1 complex phosphorylation, inhibits estrogen receptor a gene expression via p38^{MAPK}/CK2 signaling in human breast cancer cells. *Journal of the Federation of American Societies for Experimental Biology, 25,* 3695–3707.

DeGangi, G. A., & Royeen, C. B. (1994). Current practice among Neurodevelopmental Treatment Association members. *The American Journal of Occupational Therapy, 48,* 803–809.

Duffy, J. R. (2005). Pearls of wisdom—Darley, Aaronson, and Brown and the classification of the dysarthrias. *Perspectives in Neurophysiology and Neurogenic Speech and Language Disorders, 15,* 22–27.

Duffy, J. R., & Josephs, K. A. (2012). The diagnosis and understanding of apraxia of speech: Why including degenerative etiologies may be important. *Journal of Speech, Language, and Hearing Research, 55,* S1518–S1522.

Einarsson-Backes, L. M., Deitz, J., Price, R., Glass, R., & Hays, R. (1994). The effect of oral support on sucking efficiency in preterm infants. *The American Journal of Occupational Therapy, 48,* 490–498.

Elman, R. J. (2007). Sources of possible bias in evidence-based reviews. *Perspectives in Neurophysiology and Neurogenic Speech and Language Disorders, 17,* 3–6.

Emby, D., Yates, L., & Mott, D. (1990). Effects of neurodevelopmental treatment and orthoses on knee flexion during gait: A single-subject design. *Physical Therapy, 70,* 626–637.

Feeney, P. (2006, May 2). Primer on research: An introduction. *ASHA Leader.*

Fetters, L., & Kluzik, J. (1996). The effects of neurodevelopmental treatment versus practice on the reaching of children with spastic cerebral palsy. *Physical Therapy, 76,* 346–358.

Finn, P. (2006, June 13). Bias and blinding: Self-fulfilling prophecies and intentional ignorance. Primer on research. Part 2. *ASHA Leader.*

Folkman, F. R. (1992). *The effects of seating position on the respiratory patterns of four- to five-year-old normal and cerebral palsy children during rest and speech.* (Unpublished doctoral dissertation). University of Colorado.

Fox, C. M., & Boliek, C. A. (2012). Intensive voice treatment (LSVT LOUD) for children with spastic cerebral palsy and dysarthria. *Journal of Speech, Language, and Hearing Research, 55,* 930–945.

Girolami, G., & Campbell, S. K. (1994). Efficacy of a neuro-developmental treatment program to improve motor control in infants born prematurely. *Pediatric Physical Therapy, 6,* 175–184.

Glogowska, M., Roulstone, S., Enderby, P., & Peters, T. J. (2000). Randomized controlled trial of community based speech and language therapy in preschool children. *British Medical Journal, 321,* 1–5.

Hielkema, T., Blauw-Hospers, C. H., Dirks, T., Drijver-Messelink, M., Bos, A. F., & Hadders-Algra, M. (2011). Does physiotherapy intervention affect motor outcome in high risk infants? An approach combining a randomized controlled trial and process evaluation. *Developmental Medicine & Child Neurology, 53*, e8–e15.

Hill, A. J., Kurkowshi, T. B., & Garcia, J. (2000). Oral support measures used in feeding the preterm infant. *Nursing Research, 49*, 2–10.

Howle, J. M. (2002). *Neurodevelopmental treatment approach: Theoretical foundations and principles of clinical practice.* Laguna Beach, CA: NDTA.

Hulme, J. B., Bain, B., Hardin, M., McKinnon, A., & Waldron, D. (1989). The influence of adaptive seating devices on vocalization. *Journal of Communication Disorders, 22*, 137–145.

Hulme, J. B., Shaver, J., Acher, S., Mullette, L., & Eggert, C. (1987). Effects of adaptive seating devices on the eating and drinking of children with multiple handicaps. *The American Journal of Occupational Therapy, 41*, 81–89.

Hustad, K. C., Gorton, K., & Lee, J. (2010). Classification of speech and language profiles in 4-year-old children with cerebral palsy: A prospective preliminary study. *Journal of Speech, Language, and Hearing Research, 53*, 1496–1513.

Hustad, K. C., Schueler, B., Schultz, L., & DuHadway, C. (2012). Intelligibility of 4-year-old children with and without cerebral palsy. *Journal of Speech, Language, and Hearing Research, 55*, 1177–1189.

Hwang, Y. S., Lin, C. H., Coster, W. J., Bigsby, R., & Vergara, E. (2010). Effectiveness of cheek and jaw support to improve feeding performance of preterm infants. *The American Journal of Occupational Therapy, 64*, 886–894.

Jenicek, M. (2006). Evidence based medicine: Fifteen years later. Golem the good, the bad, and the ugly in need of a review? *Medical Science Monitor, 12*, RA 241–251.

Justice, L. (2008). Treatment research. *American Journal of Speech-Language Pathology, 17*, 210–211.

Kamhi, A. G. (2006). Treatment decisions for children with speech-sound disorders. *Language, Speech, and Hearing Services in Schools, 37*, 271–279.

Kent, R. D. (2006). Evidence-based practice in communication disorders: Progress not perfection. *Language, Speech, and Hearing Services in Schools, 37*, 268–270.

Kluzik, A., Fetters, L., & Coryell, J. (1990). Quantification of control: A preliminary study of effects of neurodevelopmental treatment on reaching in children with cerebral palsy. *Physical Therapy, 70*, 65–78.

Knox, V., & Evans, A. L. (2002). Evaluation of the functional effects of a course of Bobath therapy in children with cerebral palsy: A preliminary study. *Developmental Medicine and Child Neurology, 44*, 447–460.

Kuehn, D. P. (1997). The development of a new technique for treating hypernasality: CPAP. *American Journal of Speech-Language Pathology, 6*, 5–8.

Larner, G. (2004). Family therapy and the politics of evidence. *Journal of Family Therapy, 26*, 17–39.

Lass, N. J., & Pannbacker, M. (2008). The application of evidence-based practice to oral motor nonspeech treatments. *Language, Speech, and Hearing Services in Schools, 39*, 408–421.

Law, J., Garrett, Z., & Nye, C. (2004). The efficacy of treatment for children with developmental speech and language delay/disorder: A meta-analysis. *Journal of Speech, Language, and Hearing Research, 47*, 924–943.

Majnemer, A. (1998). Benefits of early intervention for children with developmental disabilities. *Seminars in Pediatric Neurology, 5*, 62–69.

Mayo Clinic Staff. (2013). *Hormone therapy: Is it right for you?* Retrieved February 15, 2013, from http://www.mayoclinic.com/health/hormone-therapy

McCauley, R. J., Strand, E., Lof, G. L., Schooling, T., & Frymark, T. (2009). Evidence-based systematic review: Effects of nonspeech oral motor exercises on speech. *American Journal of Speech-Language Pathology, 18*, 343–360.

McCullough, G. H. (2006). Zen and the art of swallowing maintenance: Best evidence, best practice. *Perspectives in Swallowing and Swallowing Disorders, 15*, 7–10.

McDonald, E. T., & Schultz, A. R. (1973). Communication boards for cerebral palsied children. *Journal of Speech and Hearing Disorders, 38*, 73–88.

McEwen, I. R., & Lloyd, L. L. (1990). Positioning students with cerebral palsy to use augmentative and alternative communication. *Language, Speech, and Hearing Services in Schools, 21*, 15–21.

Montgomery, E. B. Jr., & Turkstra, L. S. (2006). Judgment in evidence-based practice. *Perspectives in Swallowing and Swallowing Disorders, 15*, 11–15.

Nwaobi, O., Brubaker, C., Cusick, B., & Sussman, M. (1983). Electromyographic investigation of extensor activity in cerebral-palsied children in different seating positions. *Developmental Medicine & Child Neurology, 25*, 175–183.

Olswang, L. B., & Pinder, G. L. (1995). Preverbal functional communication and the role of object play in children with cerebral palsy. *Infant-Toddler Intervention: The Transdisciplinary Journal, 5*, 277–300.

Ottenbacher, K. J., Biocca, Z., DeCremer, G., Gevelinger, M., Jedlovec, K. B., & Johnson, M. B. (1986). Quantitative analysis of the effectiveness of pediatric therapy: Emphasis on the Neurodevelopment Treatment approach. *Physical Therapy, 66,* 1085–1101.

Pennington, L., Marshall, J., & Goldbart, J. (2003). Speech and language therapy to improve communication skills of children with cerebral palsy (Review). *Cochrane Review, 3,* Art. No. CD 003466466. doi:10.1002/14651858.CD003466.pub2

Pennington, L., Marshall, J., & Goldbart, J. (2005). Direct speech and language therapy for children with cerebral palsy: Findings from a systematic review. *Developmental Medicine & Child Neurology, 47,* 57–63.

Pennington, L., Miller, N., Robson, S., & Steen, N. (2010). Intensive speech and language therapy for older children with cerebral palsy: A systems approach. *Developmental Medicine & Child Neurology, 52,* 337–344.

Pennington, L., Smallman, C., & Farrier, F. (2006). Intensive speech and language therapy for older children with cerebral palsy: Findings from six cases. *Child Language Teaching and Therapy, 22,* 255–273.

Pennington, L., Thomson, K., James, P., Martin, L., & McNally, R. (2009). Effects of It Takes Two To Talk—The Hanen program for parents of preschool children with cerebral palsy: Findings from an exploratory study. *Journal of Speech, Language, and Hearing Research, 52,* 1121–1138.

Pinder, G. L., & Olswang, L. B. (1995). The development of communicative intent in young children with cerebral palsy: A treatment efficacy study. *Infant-Toddler Intervention: The Transdisciplinary Journal, 5,* 51–70.

Pinder, G. L., Olswang, L. B., & Coggins, K. (1993). The development of communicative intent in a physically disabled child. *Infant-Toddler Intervention: The Transdisciplinary Journal, 3,* 1–17.

Ratner, N. B. (2006). Evidence-based practice: An examination of its ramifications for the practice of speech-language pathology. *Language, Speech, and Hearing Services in Schools, 37,* 257–267.

Redstone, F. (1991). Respiratory components of communication. In M. B. Langley & L. J. Lombardino (Eds.), *Neurodevelopmental strategies for managing communication disorders in children with severe motor dysfunction.* Austin, TX: Pro-Ed.

Redstone, F. (2005). Seating position and length of utterance of preschoolers with cerebral palsy. *Perceptual and Motor Skills, 101,* 961–962.

Ruark, J. L. (2004). Little research on the development of oral skills for swallowing: Is ignorance bliss? *Perspectives on Swallowing and Swallowing Disorders, 13,* 20–22.

Sackett, D. L. (1997). Evidence-based medicine. *Seminars in Perinatology, 21,* 3–5.

Salario, C., Brandys, E., Morozova, O., Pidlock, F. S., Trovato, M. K., Sadowsky, C., et al. (2008). Neurorehabilitation. In P. J. Accardo (Ed.), *Caputo & Accardo's neurodevelopmental disabilities in infancy and childhood* (pp. 651–672). Baltimore, MD: Paul H. Brookes.

Schertz, M., & Gordon, A. M. (2009). Changing the model: A call for a re-examination of intervention approaches and translational research in children with developmental disabilities. *Developmental Medicine & Child Neurology, 51,* 6–7.

Schlosser, R. W., & Raghavendra, P. (2004). Evidence-based practice in augmentative and alternative communication. *Augmentative and Alternative Communication, 20,* 1–21.

Scott, K. S., Bahr, D., & Reardon-Reeves, N. (2009). *Creating effective and efficient research teams.* Handout of paper presented at convention of American Speech, Language, and Hearing Association, New Orleans, LA. Retrieved February 28, 2013, from http://www.asha.org/events/convention/handouts/2009/1926

Sheppard, J. J. (2005). The role of oral sensorimotor therapy in the treatment of pediatric dysphagia. *Perspectives on Swallowing and Swallowing Disorders, 14,* 6–10.

Solomon, N. P., & Charron, S. (1998). Speech breathing in able-bodied children and children with cerebral palsy: A review of the literature and implications for clinical intervention. *American Journal of Speech-Language Pathology, 7,* 61–78.

Stanger, M., & Oresic, S. (2003). Rehabilitation approaches for children with cerebral palsy: Overview. *Journal of Child Neurology, 18,* S79–S88.

Steele, C. M. (2004). Food for thought: Reflections on evidence-based practice. *Perspectives on Swallowing and Swallowing Disorders, 13,* 1–5.

Sugden, D. (2007). Current approaches to intervention in children with developmental coordination disorder. *Developmental Medicine & Child Neurology, 49,* 467–471.

Tomlin, G., & Borgetto, B. (2011). Research pyramid: A new evidence-based practice model for occupational therapy. *American Journal of Occupational Therapy, 65,* 189–196.

Trahan, J., & Malauin, F. (1999). Changes in the gross motor function measure in children with different types of cerebral palsy: An eight-month follow-up study. *Pediatric Physical Therapy, 11,* 12–17.

Uyanik, M., Bumin, G., & Kayihan, H. (2003). Comparison of different therapy approaches in children with Down syndrome. *Pediatrics International, 45,* 63–78.

Wolf, L. S., & Glass, R. P. (1992). *Feeding and swallowing disorders in infancy: Assessment and management.* Tucson, AZ: Therapy Skill Builders.

Workinger, M. S., & Kent, R. D. (1991). Perceptual analysis of the dysarthrias in children with athetoid and spastic cerebral palsy. In. C. A. Moore, K. M. Yorkston, & D. R. Beukelman (Eds.), *Dysarthria and apraxia of speech: Perspectives on management* (pp. 109–126). Baltimore, MD: Paul H. Brookes.

Yorkston, K. M. (1996). Treatment efficacy: Dysarthria. *Journal of Speech and Hearing Research, 39,* S46–S57.

Index

368 Effective SLP Interventions for Children with Cerebral Palsy

Assessment *(continued)*
  of respiratory function, 174,
    175, 176–178
  of speech. *See* Speech
    assessment
Assistive technology (AT), 274,
    276
  See also Augmentative and
    alternative communication
Asymmetrical tonic neck reflex
    (ATNR), 94, 100, 106, 255
Ataxia, 72
Ataxic cerebral palsy, 63
Athetoid cerebral palsy, 7, 77,
    100, 171, 191
Athetosis, 72, 76
ATNR. *See* Asymmetrical tonic
    neck reflex
Auditory scanning, 283
Augmentative and alternative
    communication (AAC), 8,
    273–297, 307
  access, 279–283
  aided systems, 277, **278**,
    279–283
  ASHA and, 348
  assessment, 284
  augmented input, 292–293,
    294
  case studies, **283**, **294**,
    295–296
  cerebral palsy and, 275–277
  defined, 274, 276–277
  direct selection, 279–280
  displays, 291–292, **292**
  early intervention and, 287–289
  feature matching, 284–285
  for interaction, 294–295
  interface adjustments, 280
  mobile technology and,
    296–297
  modeling, 293
  myths about, 274, 288–289

new directions for, 296–297
positioning for, 285–286, 343
scanning, 280–283
unaided strategies, 276–277
vocabulary, 289–291
Augmentative communication,
    276
Augmented input, 292–293, **294**
Augmented input interventions,
    293
Austin, L., 255, 259
Autism spectrum disorders,
    cerebral palsy and, 69
Azrin, N.H., 234

B

Babbling, 16, 17, 191, 198, 207
"Big Mack," 281
Bahr, D., 347
Bahr, D.C., 18
Baker, E., 346
Balaghi, M., 66
Ballard, K.J., 33
Barry, M., 345
Basal ganglia, 6
Beecher, R., 101
Behavioral issues, cerebral palsy
    and, 68–69
Behavioral programs, for saliva
    control, 233–235
Behaviorist theory of language
    development, 246
Bell, R., 246
Belly breathing, 195
Benigna, J.P., 286
Berninger, V., 306
Bernstein, N.A., 33–34, 35, 37
Bias
  blind review, 349
  disparity between clinic and
    research, 351–352, **352**
  editorial bias, 349–350